Clinical topics in cultural psychiatry

Clinical topics in cultural psychiatry

Edited by Rahul Bhattacharya, Sean Cross
and Dinesh Bhugra

RCPsych Publications

RCPsych Publications is an imprint of the Royal College of Psychiatrists,
17 Belgrave Square, London SW1X 8PG
http://www.rcpsych.ac.uk

British Library Cataloguing-in-Publication Data.
A catalogue record for this book is available from the British Library.
ISBN 978-1-904671-82-4

Distributed in North America by Publishers Storage and Shipping Company.

Printed by Bell & Bain Limited, Glasgow, UK.

To Sir David Goldberg

A great teacher, clinician and researcher

Contents

Tables

Boxes

Figures

Contributors

Gwen Adshead Consultant Forensic Psychotherapist, Broadmoor Hospital, Berkshire, UK

Sheraz Ahmad Specialist Registrar in General Adult Psychiatry, Charing Cross Higher Training Scheme, London, and Psychosexual Therapist

Peter J. Aspinall Reader in Population Health, Centre for Health Services Studies, University of Kent, and Honorary Special Advisor to the London Health Observatory, UK

Oyedeji Ayonrinde Consultant Psychiatrist, South London and Maudsley NHS Trust, London, UK

Rahul Bhattacharya Consultant Psychiatrist, East London NHS Foundation Trust, London, UK

Dinesh Bhugra Professor of Mental Health and Cultural Diversity and Head of the Section of Cultural Psychiatry, Health Services Research Department, Institute of Psychiatry, King's College London, UK

Kamaldeep Bhui Professor of Cultural Psychiatry and Epidemiology, Bart's and The Royal London School of Medicine and Dentistry, Queen Mary and Westfied College, London, UK

Carole J. Bramley Freelance researcher, Nottingham, UK

Zarrar A. Chowdary Consultant in General Adult Psychiatry, Park House, North Manchester General Hospital, Manchester, UK

Frances Connan Consultant Psychiatrist, Vincent Square Eating Disorders Service, London, UK

Sean Cross Specialist Registrar in Liaison Psychiatry, St Thomas' Hospital, London, UK

Simon Dein Senior Lecturer in Anthropology and Medicine and Visiting Professor in Psychology of Religion, Glyndwr University, Wales, UK

Manisha Desai Consultant Psychiatrist, West London NHS Trust, London, UK

Nisha Dogra Senior Lecturer and Honorary Consultant in Child and Adolescent Psychiatry, Greenwood Institute of Child Health, University of Leicester, UK

Saeed Farooq Professor and Head of Department of Psychiatry, Post-Graduate Medical Institute, Lady Reading Hospital, Peshawar, Pakistan

Chris Fear Consultant General Psychiatrist, Gether Foundation NHS Trust, Gloucester, UK

Gideon Felton Year 6 (ST6) Specialist Training in Psychiatry, Ealing Hospital, London, UK

Scott Ferris Locum Consultant Psychotherapist, Broadmoor Hospital, Berkshire, UK

Peter Jones Professor of Psychiatry, University of Cambridge, Cambridge, UK

Khalid Karim Senior Lecturer and Honorary Consultant in Child and Adolescent Psychiatry, Greenwood Institute for Child Health, University of Leicester, Leicester, UK

Brendan D. Kelly Senior Lecturer in Psychiatry, University College Dublin and Mater Misericordiae University Hospital, Dublin, Ireland

Gill Livingston Professor of Psychiatry of Old Age, Department of Mental Health Sciences, University College London, and Honorary Consultant in Mental Health Care of Older People, Camden and Islington NHS Foundation Trust, London, UK

Kwame McKenzie Senior Scientist, Social Equity and Health Research, Centre for Addiction and Mental Health, Toronto, and Professor of Psychiatry, Social Equity and Health Research, University of Toronto, Canada

Neil Morgan Consultant Psychiatrist in Psychotherapy, Psychotherapy Department, Mile End Hospital, East London & City Mental Health Trust, London, UK

Vijaya Murali Consultant Psychiatrist, Birmingham and Solihull Mental Health Foundation Trust, UK

David Ndegwa Consultant Forensic Psychiatrist, South London and Maudsley NHS Foundation Trust, London, UK

Jean O'Hara Consultant in the Psychiatry of Intellectual Disability, and Clinical Director, South London and Maudsley NHS Foundation Trust and the Estia Centre, Institute of Psychiatry, King's College London, UK

Femi Oyebode Professor of Psychiatry, Queen Elizabeth Psychiatric Hospital, Birmingham, UK

Bhaskar Punukollu Consultant in Addiction Psychiatry, South West London and St George's NHS Trust, London, UK

Gopinath Ranjith Consultant Liaison Psychiatrist, St Thomas' Hospital, London, and Honorary Lecturer, Institute of Psychiatry, King's College London, UK

Justine Schneider Professor of Mental Health and Social Care, Nottinghamshire Healthcare NHS Trust and the University of Nottingham, UK

Sati Sembhi Consultant Psychiatrist, Suffolk Mental Health Partnership Trust, St Clement's Hospital, Ipswich, Suffolk, UK

Rachel Tribe Professor of Psychology, School of Psychology, University of East London, London, UK

Anish Unadkat Specialist Registrar in Psychiatry, Charing Cross Psychiatric Training Scheme, London, UK

Preface

Culture is what makes us who we are. We are born into a culture and gradually absorb its cultural values and mores, often without realising it. Culture influences our cognitive schema, the way we deal with stress and respond to others. More importantly, culture influences the way individuals perceive and express distress and how they seek help. Cultures also dictate how healthcare systems develop and deliver care. In this era of globalisation, cultures are directly and indirectly influenced by each other. Under these circumstances, it is imperative that clinicians are aware of cultural factors in the genesis and management of psychiatric disorders. Every individual has a culture and cultural roots do go deep. It behoves clinicians to understand their patients in their social and cultural contexts so that the therapeutic alliance can be strengthened.

Advances in Psychiatric Treatment as a journal set a precedent in 1997 when it started a series of articles on culture and psychiatric disorders. Over the past decade or so it has published several contributions in this field and is continuing to do so. With the new curriculum developed by the Royal College of Psychiatrists in 2005 and since, cultural psychiatry has become a significant part of training of psychiatrists. It was decided to put articles from *Advances* together in a single volume not only so that practising clinicians can benefit from the cumulative knowledge, but also that other mental health practitioners may have access, thereby helping to ensure that clinical teams can work together effectively and provide optimal care to their patients, irrespective of their ethnicity, culture or religion. We chose a number of existing articles and asked their authors to revise them. However, in the process we discovered that many subjects had not been previously covered so we commissioned several new chapters We are most grateful to all our authors, old and new, for providing updated reviews in a field that is changing fairly rapidly. Thanks are also due to Professor Peter Tyrer, Dr Joe Bouch and Dr Jonathan Green for their vision and encouragement.

Rahul Bhattacharya, East London NHS Foundation Trust, London
Sean Cross, St Thomas' Hospital, London
Dinesh Bhugra, Institute of Psychiatry, King's College London

Part 1
Theoretical and general issues

CHAPTER 1

Globalisation, psychiatry and human rights: new challenges for the 21st century

Brendan D. Kelly

Summary Globalisation is a complex, large-scale social phenomenon that presents mental health services with both challenges and opportunities. These relate to the increased cultural diversity of service users and service providers; the effects of migration on mental health; and the implementation of international protocols in relation to: training, policy and education. In the aftermath of the terrorist attacks of 11 September 2001 in the USA, the relationship between large-scale social change and mental health has also focused attention on the concepts of anomie and social capital. An explicit return to the principles of biopsychosocial psychiatry and a positive engagement with globalisation will advance the development of effective, evidence-based models of care appropriate to the changing needs of patients.

Globalisation means crossing borders. All of the social and economic forces driving globalisation relate to the opening or dismantling of borders: instant communication, easy travel, deregulation of commerce and widened access to information and technology. The internet is often hailed as a good example of globalisation, as it allows people in far-flung corners of the planet to communicate rapidly with each other regardless of their geographical location. Other examples include the establishment of supranational political bodies, enhanced cross-border cultural interaction and globalised approaches to environmental issues (Box 1.1).

From the start, globalisation has attracted robust criticism, chiefly related to the social inequities it appears to accentuate. Critics point out that the internet, for example, remains the realm of a privileged minority as most of the world's population have never made a telephone call, let alone sent an email. The free flow of capital into and out of unstable economies also presents problems, often compounded by the waves of migration that tend to follow financial downturns (Stiglitz, 2002). Perhaps the greatest criticism of globalisation, however, relates to the management of cultural diversity, a phenomenon that presents very great challenges, as well as

---

Box 1.1   Key features of globalisation

Instant communication (e.g. by the internet)

Fast, efficient means of travel

Deregulation of commerce

Widened access to technology

Supranational political bodies

Cross-border cultural interaction

Globalised approaches to environmental issues

---

opportunities, in many societies around the world. These criticisms, along with the terrorist attacks of 11 September 2001 in the USA, have stimulated a worldwide re-evaluation of globalisation and a reconsideration of the strategies that societies and individuals use to manage global change.

In this chapter, I examine the effects of globalisation on the practice of psychiatry and suggest strategies for their optimal management in relation to mental health, with a view to exploiting the opportunities that globalisation presents for the development of psychiatric services.

Socioeconomic effects and their impact on mental health

There is considerable disagreement among economists about the likely long-term economic effects of globalisation. On the one hand, it is argued that the process of globalisation offers individuals more freedom to choose how they live, where they work and what they buy (Economist, 2001). Opening borders, deregulating trade and using government chiefly to maintain social justice should, it is argued, lead to a more integrated, more equitable and more sustainable global society. This view actively informs the current policies of international organisations such as the World Bank, the International Monetary Fund and the World Trade Organization.

Critics of globalisation argue the opposite case, maintaining that current globalisation policies serve to widen the gap between rich and poor (Stiglitz, 2002). Market deregulation favours the dominant, strong economies of the West and fails to offer low- and middle-income countries an opportunity to strengthen their infrastructure sufficiently to compete in a global economy. Globalisation, by this logic, will lead to further poverty, inequality and social injustice.

The majority of commentators from both sides, however, are united on one point: that globalisation presents opportunities that could, at least in theory, be used for the greater good. The chief point of disagreement is the sequencing of change, with certain critics arguing that it is wrong to deregulate markets without first preparing an economy and a society for change. They point to evidence from the World Bank that shows little decrease in world poverty and a possible increase in inequality between countries (World Bank, 2001).

Socioeconomic and other inequalities are significantly related to mental health. Psychiatric disorders are more common in people from lower socioeconomic groups (Goldberg & Morrison, 1963; Wiersma *et al*, 1983). This relationship is likely to be bi-directional, with health affecting socio-economic status and socioeconomic status affecting health (Lewis & Araya, 2002). Thus, if globalisation truly increases poverty, it is likely to have a proportionately negative effect on mental health. This effect would be compounded by the decreasing ability of an increasingly poor country to provide adequate healthcare to its citizens. An effect on social capital would also be evident, with reduced community cohesion, resulting in weakened social support and increased psychosocial morbidity (Putnam, 2000).

It is likely that a disproportionate part of this burden would be borne by women, who, in addition to performing the majority of domestic and child care tasks, may find themselves satisfying a growing need for relatively low-paid labour (Lewis & Araya, 2002). In light of the particular importance of psychosocial stressors in relation to depression in women (Avotri & Walters, 1999), such a change would be expected to increase the incidence of depression and anxiety among them.

This is the worst-case scenario: increased poverty, increased illness burden and decreased ability to provide mental healthcare. The socioeconomic effects of globalisation, however, need not be entirely negative. Indeed, several important features of this process suggest that globalisation, if properly managed, can serve as a force for the promotion of economic growth and the enhancement of social capital both in low- and middle-income and in high-income countries. Communication technology is a good example.

At present, advances in communication technology are not equitably distributed around the world. However, this technology is spreading rapidly from high-income countries to low- and middle-income ones and it has a strong enabling power when it arrives. The internet, for example, can be used to inform farming and fishing practice by providing information relating to prices, markets and weather forecasts (Economist, 2001). In countries such as Bangladesh, mobile telephone networks are proving far more efficient than traditional terrestrial telephones, as each person in a village might make only one or two calls per week and terrestrial telephone systems are either unavailable or administered by inefficient, bureaucratic government bodies. Advances in communication technology have much to offer high-income nations too: even critics of globalisation use the internet extensively to organise protests and coordinate campaigns.

5

There is no compelling reason to believe that globalisation must necessarily increase the gap between rich and poor. Globalisation on this scale and at this speed is a new phenomenon. Our economic and social policies in response to it are probably responsible, at least in part, for any perceived negative effects. Just as Stiglitz (2002) argues for an urgent reconsideration of economic policies in response to globalisation, there is a similar need to re-evaluate social policy. There is a strong relationship between socioeconomic change and mental health, and this relationship should form an important part of social, economic and health planning. This point is well illustrated by the significant challenges that increased migration currently presents to mental health services.

Migration and mental illness

Globalisation has led to a significant increase in migration. People are now moving further, faster and in greater numbers than ever before: in the 1980s, 2.3 million asylum applications were lodged in 37 industrialised countries, and in the 1990s, the number of applications submitted in the same countries almost tripled, to 6.1 million (Ryan *et al*, 2009). Migration is known to have significant effects on health, with migrants showing higher rates of both physical (Gleize *et al*, 2000) and mental illness (Gavin *et al*, 2001).

In the UK, Irish, Caribbean and Pakistani immigrants have significantly higher rates of suicidal thoughts and deliberate self-harm (Nazroo, 1997). Egyptian and Asian immigrants have increased rates of bulimia and anorexia nervosa (Chapter 2, this volume). Asylum seekers present particular challenges to mental health services as they come from a wide variety of cultural backgrounds and have sharply diminished social support. Many have experienced human rights abuse, torture or displacement in their homeland (Box 1.2). On arrival in a new country, they might face confinement in detention centres, enforced dispersal and ongoing discrimination (Silove *et al*, 2000). Rates of post-traumatic stress disorder among asylum-seeking migrants vary between countries, but can be as high as 48% (Ryan *et al*, 2009).

Schizophrenia is six times more common in African–Caribbeans living in the UK than in the native population (Harrison, 1990) and four times more common among migrants to The Netherlands (Selten *et al*, 1997). This is difficult to explain: incidence of schizophrenia is not increased in migrants' countries of origin (Hickling & Rodgers-Johnson, 1995), nor do migrants have increased exposure to environmental risk factors such as obstetric complications (Hutchinson *et al*, 1997). It is notable, however, that the increase in risk of schizophrenia among migrants shows a powerful inverse relation with the size of the migrant group, a finding that, at the present state of biological psychiatry, lends itself more readily to psychosocial explanations than to biological ones (Boydell *et al*, 2001).

Box 1.2 Mental health of asylum seekers: particular challenges

In their home country
- Human rights abuse
- Torture
- Displacement
- Poor mental healthcare

In their new country
- Diminished social support
- Confinement in detention centres
- Enforced dispersal
- Ongoing discrimination
- Adjustment disorder
- Post-traumatic stress disorder
- Depression
- Increased rates of other illnesses

Globalisation, then, affects the pattern of occurrence of mental illness and, through migration, has had a significant effect on the epidemiology of schizophrenia. The increased diversity of mental health service users presents an urgent challenge to service providers in high-income countries. People from different ethnic backgrounds often have different views about mental health and are accustomed to substantially different models of care. This can result in a damaging mismatch between the needs of patients and the services provided. In London, for example, the pathway to care for migrants is characterised by a high rate of involuntary admission and increased involvement of police, as opposed to general practitioners (Davies *et al*, 1996).

In response to these problems, it is necessary to address issues in psychiatric training, service provision and social policy. In the first instance, it is important to increase the emphasis placed on transcultural psychiatry in mental health curriculums. The World Psychiatric Association (2002) has developed its Institutional Program on the Core Training Curriculum for Psychiatry, which places significant emphasis on transcultural issues. Similarly, the Royal College of Psychiatrists (2009) has developed a Competency Based Curriculum for Specialist Training in Psychiatry, which places similar emphasis on sociocultural competencies for postgraduate trainees in psychiatry. An enhanced appreciation of cultural factors as they affect mental health will serve both to deepen the understanding of cultural diversity and to enhance the quality and acceptability of the mental healthcare provided to all.

The development of ethnically segregated services, however, would tend to maintain racism and compound psychological stressors, and thus represents an inappropriate model for service development (Bhui *et al*, 2000). It is generally more helpful to increase knowledge of mental illness among migrants themselves and to provide appropriate training for mental health team workers to provide effective, needs-based interventions for specific migrant communities. There is also a strong need to reconsider the effects of social policies on the psychological well-being of migrants, as current policies of dispersal of large groups of refugees to smaller communities in disparate locations within host countries may serve to increase the psychological stresses and social disadvantages experienced by certain migrant groups.

Globalisation and human rights in psychiatry

Opponents of current models of globalisation often claim that it has negative effects on human rights, particularly in relation to financial well-being and economic stability. This is an issue of special concern in relation to people with mental illness – particularly those with long-term illness who have reduced ability to advocate for themselves. In 1991, the rights of those with mental illnesses were 'globalised' in the United Nations' Principles for the Protection of Persons with Mental Illness (United Nations, 1991) (Box 1.3). These principles, however, do not have the status of a formal international treaty and there is no obligation on UN member states to use the principles to define a minimum standard of care (Harding, 2000).

In 2001, the World Health Organization renewed its emphasis on human rights and mental health by devoting World Health Day 2001 to global advocacy on mental health issues. There were compelling social, political and legislative reasons for this choice, many of which relate to the effects of globalisation. Migration, for example, presents particular challenges in terms of both healthcare and human rights. In the first instance, there is a basic human right to adequate healthcare and it is likely that migrants are being denied this in many countries around the world. Indeed, the quality and availability of mental healthcare for both migrants and native populations present a real problem in many countries. As recently as 2009, for example, Zambia had only one psychiatric hospital, seven smaller psychiatric units with a few beds each, and virtually no access to psychological therapies (Ngungu & Beezhold, 2009).

Alleged abuses of psychiatry around the world also provide cause for increasing concern. Certain countries, such as China, are of particular interest in this regard, owing, for example, to alleged abuse of the language and practice of psychiatry to assist with the persecution of individuals who practice Falun Gong in China (Munro, 2000). Various other issues relating to training, access to service and quality of care are also important considerations in this context, both in China and in many other countries (Morrall & Hazelton, 2004).

Box 1.3   Key rights of people with mental illnesses and principles regarding their mental healthcare

All people are entitled to receive the best mental healthcare available and to be treated with humanity and respect

There shall be no discrimination on the grounds of mental illness. All people with mental illnesses have the same rights to medical and social care as other ill people

All people with mental illnesses have the right to live, work and receive treatment in the community, as far as possible

Mental healthcare shall be based on internationally accepted ethical standards, and not on political, religious or cultural factors

The treatment plan shall be reviewed regularly with the patient

Mental health skills and knowledge shall not be misused

Medication shall meet the health needs of the patient and shall not be administered for the convenience of others or as a punishment

In the case of voluntary patients, no treatment shall be administered without their informed consent, subject to some exceptions (e.g. patients with personal representatives empowered by law to provide consent). In the case of involuntary patients, every effort shall be made to inform the patient about treatment

Physical restraint or involuntary seclusion shall be used only in accordance with official guidelines. Records shall be kept of all treatments

Mental health facilities shall be appropriately structured and resourced

An impartial review body shall, in consultation with mental health practitioners, review the cases of involuntary patients

(United Nations, 1991)

The evolution of a globalised approach to these issues, as demonstrated by the World Psychiatric Association, has many advantages. Most importantly, it provides a unified, authoritative voice with which to advocate for change. However, it is important to recognise that definitions of 'mental health' and 'psychiatry' can vary considerably between cultures. A solution that meets the needs of one country may not be appropriate for others. Furthermore, most legislatures have their own mental health laws, which often have substantially different approaches to issues such as involuntary admission and quality assurance. This is also a time of considerable legislative change in Europe, with many countries introducing amendments to existing laws (e.g. the 2007 amendments to the Mental Health Act 1983 in England and Wales) or entirely new mental health legislation (e.g. the Mental Health Act 2001 in Ireland).

The best way to ensure that human rights are respected on a global scale is to increase awareness and implementation of the United Nations' principles regarding people with mental illnesses (United Nations, 1991). These principles provide a framework that can usefully inform legislative change in individual countries. They should also form an important part of psychiatric education and can be used to help shape service developments and planning. The implementation of these principles is a challenging task, best accomplished when mental health professionals and policy makers work in partnership with advocacy groups and service-user representatives.

One of the central contributions that psychiatrists can make to this process is the continued provision of high-quality, evidence-based mental healthcare. Healthcare, however, is delivered in a specific social and political context, which is often largely determined by policy makers and politicians. Nevertheless, psychiatrists are well placed to educate colleagues, policy makers and the public about mental health and human rights. International psychiatric organisations such as the World Psychiatric Association have a particular role to play as powerful advocates for improved psychiatric care and for better working conditions for mental health workers around the globe.

Psychological effects of large-scale social change

On 11 September 2001 the city of New York experienced the largest act of terrorism in the history of the USA, which took the lives of about 3000 people in New York alone ('Dead and missing', New York Times, 26 December 2001, B2). While certain commentators stated that these events heralded the 'end of globalisation', many others took the opposite view and concluded that there was now an even more urgent need for globalisation to proceed in a timely and equitable fashion (Economist, 2001).

In the months following the attacks, Galea et al (2001) studied the prevalence of PTSD and depression in residents of Manhattan, the area most affected by the events. They interviewed over 1000 adults and found that 7.5% reported symptoms consistent with PTSD related to the attacks and 9.7% reported symptoms consistent with current depression. These prevalences were double those described in similar populations in the previous year. The authors then examined predictors of psychopathology and found that Hispanic ethnicity was associated with both PTSD and depression and that this association was independent of other covariates. Post-traumatic stress disorder and depression were also related to low social support. The authors emphasise that social ties have a positive and protective role in mental health.

Social ties, however, are rapidly decreasing in the USA, as evidenced by reduced participation in community organisations, local representation and national politics (Putnam, 2000). The events of 11 September were devastating not only because of their nature, magnitude and unpredictability, but also because they occurred in the context of a society with rapidly depleting social capital.

The combination of poor social ties and large, unpredictable events evokes the concept of 'anomie'. This term was famously used by Emile Durkheim, a French sociologist, to describe a state in which norms are confused, unclear or absent, and where there are large-scale social changes that the individual cannot understand, let alone control (Durkheim, 1947). Anomie is traditionally related to suicide, but the concept has also been suggested as one of a range of factors that might help to explain the increased incidence of schizophrenia in progressively smaller migrant groups (Boydell *et al*, 2001).

The concept of anomie has renewed importance in an era of globalisation. Changes in society are increasingly occurring on a global level and the magnitude of such change is greater than ever before. International political bodies are introducing directives and legislation over which many individuals feel they have little or no control. The threat of international terrorism is greater than ever and many individuals feel that they cannot effectively defend themselves or their families. Increasingly, the world of the individual is shaped by global events that appear to lie beyond the individual's control.

Rebuilding social capital is a key stage in reducing feelings of anomie. This is important for society in general, but has added urgency in relation to mental illness. The reduction of the stigma of mental illness is a particularly important step and is best accomplished through a multidisciplinary approach over a sustained period. Community treatment programmes and social skills courses have critical roles to play in reducing stigma, increasing community reintegration and rebuilding social capital. This process would be advanced by a strong return to the principles of biopsychosocial psychiatry, which takes a systematic, multidimensional approach to treating mental illness (Gabbard & Kay, 2001).

Conclusion

Globalisation is a complex, large-scale social phenomenon which is intrinsically neither good nor bad. The effects of globalisation depend largely on our engagement with it. There is a strong need to re-evaluate our economic and social policies in response to globalisation, particularly with regard to the effects of socioeconomic change on mental health. There are overwhelming humanitarian reasons why the relationship between socioeconomic change and mental illness should form an important part of social, economic and health planning. There are also financial reasons: schizophrenia, for example, already costs the US economy some $40 billion per year – three times as much as the entire US space programme (Torrey, 2001).

The likely effects of globalisation on clinical practice in psychiatry are summarised in Box 1.4. Globalisation presents significant opportunities for the development of psychiatric services. Whether or not we take advantage of these opportunities depends largely on our responses to phenomena such

---

Box 1.4 Summary of the likely effects of globalisation on clinical practice

Increased ethnic and cultural diversity of service users, with a wider range of attitudes and beliefs in relation to mental illness

Increased ethnic and cultural diversity of service providers, with a wider range of approaches and beliefs in relation to mental healthcare

In high-income countries, increased rates of inward migration and increased rates of migration-associated mental illnesses

In rapidly developing low- and middle-income countries, increased rates of mental illnesses associated with social change, economic change and life events

In all countries, increased access to a range of healthcare information through global media such as the internet

Increased emphasis on the implementation of international protocols in psychiatric training, mental health policy and the protection of human rights

Increased examination of the concept of social capital and its influence on the mental health of populations

---

as increased migration and the increasingly diverse needs of mental health service users. The World Psychiatric Association's introduction of a 'core curriculum' for psychiatric training should assist in placing new emphasis on transcultural issues in psychiatry. In terms of service provision, there is a strong need to train mental health team workers to provide effective, needs-based interventions for specific migrant communities. Social policies in relation to migration (e.g. enforced dispersal) also require reconsideration as they can increase the psychological stresses and social disadvantages experienced by migrant groups.

The best way to protect the rights of mentally ill people on a global scale is to work with advocacy groups and service-user representatives to implement the United Nations' principles for their protection (United Nations, 1991). Psychiatrists can make a major contribution to this process by providing high-quality, evidence-based mental healthcare. International psychiatric organisations have a crucial role as powerful advocates for improved psychiatric care and working conditions for all mental health workers. There, developments are usefully underpinned by the growing literature examining relationships between globalisation, mental healthcare and the incidence of specific disorders (Bhugra & Mastrogianni, 2004; Okasha, 2005; Eddy et al, 2007; Walker, 2007; McColl et al, 2008), as well as related issues in training and professional development (Kirmayer et al, 2008).

Finally, research performed in the aftermath of 11 September 2001 in the USA emphasises the importance of social ties and social capital in protecting mental health. Emile Durkheim's concept of anomie has new relevance in light of the dramatic decrease in social capital recently described in the USA and elsewhere. Rebuilding social capital is important for society in general, but is particularly urgent in relation to mental illness. Integrated treatment programmes have a critical role to play in reducing the stigma of mental illness, enhancing community reintegration and increasing social capital.

Rebuilding social capital is a challenging task that depends on a careful interplay of local, national and international strategies. Globalisation can contribute positively to this process, provided that social and economic policies in response to globalisation are planned with care. As mental health professionals, we are well positioned to advocate that such planning takes adequate account of the needs of people with psychiatric illness and facilitates the delivery of mental healthcare that is effective, acceptable, evidence-based and appropriate to the needs of patients.

References

Avotri, J. Y. & Walters, V. (1999) 'You just look at our work and see if you have any freedom on earth': Ghanaian women's accounts of their work and their health. *Social Science and Medicine*, **48**, 1123–1133.

Bhugra, D., Mastrogianni, A. (2004) Globalisation and mental disorders: overview with relation to depression. *British Journal of Psychiatry*, **184**, 10–20.

Bhui, K., Bhugra, D. & McKenzie, K. (2000) *Specialist Services for Minority Ethnic Groups? (Maudsley Discussion Paper no. 8)*. Institute of Psychiatry.

Boydell, J., van Os, J., McKenzie, K., *et al* (2001) Incidence of schizophrenia in ethnic minorities in ecological study into interactions with environment. *BMJ*, **323**, 1336–1338.

Davies, S., Thornicroft, G., Leese, M., *et al* (1996) Ethnic differences in risk of compulsory psychiatric admission among representative cases of psychosis in London. *BMJ*, **312**, 533–537.

Durkheim, E. (1947) *The Division of Labour in Society* (trans. George Simpson). Free Press.

Economist (2001) *Globalisation*. Economist/Profile.

Eddy, K. T., Hennessey, M. & Thompson-Brenner, H. (2007) Eating pathology in east African women: the role of media exposure and globalisation. *Journal of Nervous and Mental Diseases*, **195**, 196–202.

Gabbard, G. O. & Kay, J. (2001) The fate of integrated treatment: whatever happened to the biopsychosocial psychiatrist? *American Journal of Psychiatry*, **158**, 1956–1963.

Galea, S., Ahern, J., Resnick, H., *et al* (2001) Psychological sequelae of the September 11th terrorist attacks in New York City. *New England Journal of Medicine*, **346**, 982–987.

Gavin, B. E., Kelly, B. D., Lane, A., *et al* (2001) The mental health of migrants. *Irish Medical Journal*, **94**, 229–230.

Gleize, L., Laudon, F., Sun, L. Y., *et al* (2000) Cancer registry of French Polynesia: results for the 1900–1995 period among native and immigrant population. *European Journal of Epidemiology*, **16**, 661–667.

Goldberg, E. M. & Morrison, S. L. (1963) Schizophrenia and social class. *British Journal of Psychiatry*, **109**, 785–802.

Harding, T. W. (2000) Human rights law in the field of mental health: a critical review. *Acta Psychiatrica Scandinavica Supplementum*, **399**, 24–30.

Harrison, G. (1990) Searching for the causes of schizophrenia: the role of migrant studies. *Schizophrenia Bulletin*, **16**, 663–671.

Hickling, F. W. & Rodgers-Johnson, P. (1995) The incidence of first contact schizophrenia in Jamaica. *British Journal of Psychiatry*, **167**, 193–196.

Hutchinson, G., Takei, N., Bhugra, D., *et al* (1997) Increased rate of psychosis among African–Caribbeans in Britain is not due to an excess of pregnancy and birth complications. *British Journal of Psychiatry*, **171**, 145–147.

Kirmayer, L. J., Rousseau, C., Corin, E., *et al* (2008) Training researchers in cultural psychiatry: the McGill–CIHR Strategic Training Program. *Academic Psychiatry*, **32**, 320–326.

Lewis, G. & Araya, R. (2002) Globalization and mental health. In *Psychiatry in Society* (eds N. Sartorius, W. Gaebel, J. J. Lopez-Ibor, *et al*), pp. 57–78. John Wiley & Sons.

McColl, H., McKenzie, K. & Bhui, K. (2008) Mental healthcare of asylum-seekers and refugees. *Advances in Psychiatric Treatment*, **14**, 452–459.

Morrall, P. & Hazelton, M (eds) (2004) *Mental Health: Global Policies and Human Rights.* Whurr Publishers.

Munro, R. (2000) Judicial psychiatry in China and its political abuses. *Columbia Journal of Asian Law*, **14**, 1–128.

Nazroo, J. (1997) *Ethnicity and Mental Health.* PSI.

Ngungu, J. & Beezhold, J. (2009) Mental health in Zambia – challenges and way forward. *International Psychiatry*, **6**, 39–40.

Okasha, A. (2005) Globalization and mental health: a WPA perspective. *World Psychiatry*, **4**, 1–2.

Putnam, R. D. (2000) *Bowling Alone: The Collapse and Revival of American Community.* Touchstone.

Royal College of Psychiatrists (2009) *A Competency Based Curriculum for Specialist Training in Psychiatry.* Royal College of Psychiatrists (http://www.rcpsych.ac.uk/PDF/Core_Feb09.pdf).

Ryan, D. A., Kelly, F. E. & Kelly, B. D. (2009) Mental health among persons awaiting an asylum outcome in western countries: a literature review. *International Journal of Mental Health*, **38**, 88–111.

Selten, J. P., Slaets, J. P. & Kahn, R. S. (1997) Schizophrenia in Surinamese and Dutch Antillean immigrants to The Netherlands: evidence of an increased incidence. *Psychological Medicine*, **27**, 807–811.

Silove, D., Steel, Z. & Watters, C. (2000) Policies of deterrence and the mental health of asylum seekers. *JAMA*, **284**, 604–611.

Stiglitz, J. (2002) *Globalization and its Discontents.* Penguin.

Torrey, E. F. (2001) *Surviving Schizophrenia.* HarperCollins.

United Nations (1991) *Principles for the Protection of Persons with Mental Illnesses and the Improvement of Mental Health Care.* United Nations.

Walker, C. (2007) *Depression and Globalization: The Politics of Mental Health in the Twenty-First Century.* Springer-Verlag.

Wiersma, D., Giel, R., De Jong, A., *et al* (1983) Social class and schizophrenia in a Dutch cohort. *Psychological Medicine*, **13**, 141–150.

World Bank (2001) *World Development Report 2000/2001.* Oxford University Press.

World Psychiatric Association (2002) *Institutional Program on the Core Training Curriculum for Psychiatry.* WPA (http://www.wpanet.org/education/core-curric-psych-stu.shtml).

CHAPTER 2

Migration and mental illness

Dinesh Bhugra and Peter Jones

Summary   Human beings have moved from place to place since time immemorial. The reasons for and the duration of these migrations put extraordinary stress on individuals and their families. Such stress may not give rise to comparable increases in all types of mental illness across all migrant groups. In this chapter, we provide an overview of some observations in the field of migration and mental health, hypothesise why some individuals and groups are more vulnerable to psychiatric conditions, and consider the impact of migration experiences on provision of services and care.

Migration is the process of social change whereby an individual moves from one cultural setting to another for the purposes of settling down either permanently or for a prolonged period. Such a shift can be for any number of reasons, commonly economic, political or educational betterment. The process is usually stressful and stress can lead to mental illness.

The preparation that migrants undertake, their acceptance by the new host community and the process of migration itself are some of the macro-factors in the origin of subsequent mental disorders. The micro-factors include personality traits, psychological robustness, cultural identity, and the social support and acceptance of others in their own ethnic group.

Migration to the UK has had many peaks. In the 20th century there were several: the first was the refugee influx during and around the Second World War; the second occurred in the 1960s, when able-bodied young men and women were recruited from the former colonies to fill jobs created by the belated expansion of the post-war economy. A decade later, following the political upheaval in East Africa, a large number of individuals migrated with their families, en masse.

Migrants can be classified using several different criteria, one of which is the legal definition. There needs to be a distinction between actual settlers and temporary migrant workers. The reasons for migration as defined by Rack (1982) include both 'push' and 'pull' factors. Settlers, as well as political exiles, asylum seekers and refugees, may well have to deal with very stringent legal procedures, which will test their psychological stamina. Refugees fleeing war and other conflict may face even rougher

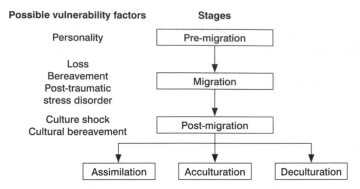

Fig. 2.1 Stages of migration.

times. Factors such as language, communication and the existence of social networks will play a role in the processes of dealing with initial adversity, settling down and assimilation.

The migratory process can be seen as having three stages. The first, pre-migration, is when the individual decides to migrate and plans the move. The second involves the process of migration itself and the physical transition from one place to another, involving all the concomitant psychological and social steps. The third stage, post-migration, is when the individual has to deal with the social and cultural frameworks of the new society, learn new roles and become interested in transforming their own functioning (Fig. 2.1). Primary migrants may be followed by others. Once they have settled down and had children, the second generation is not a generation of migrants, but it will have some similar experiences in terms of cultural identity and stress.

A more complex model has been developed to explain the diverse range of acculturation patterns, taking into account the dynamics between the ethnic identities of the immigrant and the host communities (Fig. 2.2). An international study of immigrant youth revealed four consistent patterns (Berry et al, 2006). Integration with a multicultural society was observed when both the immigrant and host communities had strong ethnic identities. In face of a strong ethnic identity of the host, immigrants tended to assimilate in the 'melting pot'. With a weak host identity but strong immigrant identity the immigrant population was separated and segregated. When neither the host nor the immigrant populations had strong ethnic identity, the immigrant minority community was marginalised and excluded from the mainstream.

We shall now review some of the key studies related to specific psychiatric conditions and highlight some key assessment and treatment strategies. Readers should note that our discussion cannot reflect the heterogeneity inherent in each migratory setting. Not all migrants have the same experiences or even the same reasons for migration and certainly the new societies' responses are not likely to be similar either.

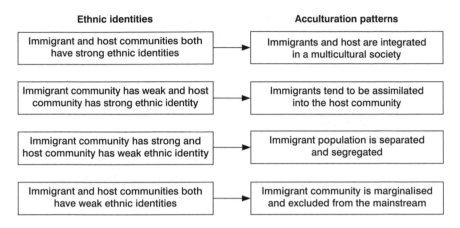

Fig. 2.2 Acculturation patterns (after Berry *et al*, 2006).

Psychiatric conditions and migration

Schizophrenia

Ödegaard (1932) reported that Norwegians who had migrated to the USA had higher rates of schizophrenia (with a peak prevalence occurring 10–12 years post-migration). This study has been cited frequently as indicating that all migrant groups will have high rates of schizophrenia. However, Sashidharan (1993) argues cogently that this model should not be applied without critical evaluation to minority ethnic groups in the UK as their migratory experiences differ.

Several studies of second-generation immigrants in the 1980s and 1990s showed that rates of schizophrenia were higher among immigrant groups than among native White people in the UK (for a review see Bhugra, 2000). Cochrane & Bal (1987) observed that immigrants in the UK had higher rates of psychiatric admissions than the native population. Similar high rates of schizophrenia have been reported in the migrant populations in The Netherlands (Selten & Sijben, 1994) and Sweden (Zolkowska *et al*, 2001). Regardless of whether rates reported were for in-patient or community samples, some common themes emerge. First, incidence of schizophrenia in the African–Caribbean immigrant population was 2.5–14.6 times higher than in the White population (Harrison *et al*, 1988, 1997). Second, the rates among Asians were not as elevated and were not consistently high (Bhugra *et al*, 1997).

The key difference between two studies from London was that King *et al* (1994) collected their data from an area of London in which the population density of Asians was lower, whereas Bhugra *et al* (1997) collected data from a London catchment area in which Asians formed 50% of the population.

A number of hypotheses may be put forward to explain these high rates, some of which are listed in Box 2.1 and examined below. Hypotheses 1–4

> **Box 2.1** Six hypotheses for the higher incidence of schizophrenia in immigrant groups
>
> 1   The immigrants' countries of origin have high rates of schizophrenia
> 2   People with schizophrenia are predisposed to migrate
> 3   Migration produces stress, which can initiate schizophrenia
> 4   Immigrants are misdiagnosed with schizophrenia
> 5   Immigrants present different patterns of symptoms
> 6   Increased population density of migrant ethnic groups can show elevated rates of schizophrenia

were postulated by Cochrane & Bal (1987); hypothesis 6 is discussed in the section Ethnic density *v.* social isolation.

Hypothesis 1: Factors in countries of origin

It was long believed that the countries from which people had migrated had high rates of schizophrenia, thereby suggesting a biological vulnerability to the illness among their populations. Before the 1990s, very few studies had considered the rates in 'sending countries', especially the Caribbean. With the Determinants of Outcome in Severe Mental Disorders (DOSMD) study (Jablensky *et al*, 1992) and studies in Jamaica (Hickling & Rodgers-Johnson, 1995), Trinidad (Bhugra *et al*, 1996) and Barbados (Mahy *et al*, 1999), it was observed that rates of narrow-definition schizophrenia were not elevated compared with those in populations who had emigrated. This suggests that biological causation is less likely, although biological vulnerability to environmental exposures cannot entirely be ruled out. Biological factors such as neurodevelopmental abnormalities, pregnancy and birth complications, and genetic vulnerability have not been reported consistently as having different prevalence in minority ethnic groups.

Hypothesis 2: Predisposition to migrate

'Selective migration' has been put forward as a plausible hypothesis to explain the high rates of schizophrenia among immigrants, on the basis of the suggestion that more vulnerable people are more restless and rootless. This superficially attractive hypothesis cannot be supported, on several accounts. First, high rates of schizophrenia are found in second-generation rather than original immigrants (Harrison *et al*, 1998, 1997). Significantly different rates have been found among older Asian women who were not primary immigrants, thereby making it less likely that illness had predisposed them to move (Bhugra *et al*, 1997). Second, the physical process of migration and dealing with official immigration procedures is so a difficult and stressful that individuals with schizophrenia are unlikely to complete it. Third, if such selective migration were the case, rates would be high among all immigrant groups, which they are clearly not.

Hypothesis 3: Migratory stress

The key question here is whether migration itself is a stressor that produces elevated rates of schizophrenia, or whether the stressors occur later. If it were a straightforward association then rates of common mental disorders would be elevated among all immigrant groups, which is clearly not the case (see below). Furthermore, as mentioned above, Ödegaard (1932) had demonstrated that rates of schizophrenia were at their highest more than 10–12 years after immigration, thus making it less likely that the actual process of migration is contributing directly. The finding of raised rates in the second generation but not in the first also argues against this.

However, the stress and chronic difficulties of living in societies in which racism is present both at individual and institutional levels may well contribute to ongoing distress. These factors may also interact with social class, poverty, poor social capital, unemployment and poor housing. For example, 80% of the African–Caribbeans in one sample of people with first-onset schizophrenia were unemployed, compared with 40% of Whites and Asians (Bhugra *et al*, 1997). However, such differential rates of unemployment and high rates of schizophrenia among African–Caribbeans may not be causally related and the high rates of unemployment cannot be explained away by general unemployment only.

Hypothesis 4: Misdiagnosis

The notion that misdiagnosis alone can explain the high rates of schizophrenia among African–Caribbeans has caught the public and professional imaginations. However, this belief cannot be true. If misdiagnosis is the sole explanation, why is it that Asians are not misdiagnosed as readily, bearing in mind language differences? By using standardised definitions and assessments, as well as operational criteria, researchers should be able to reduce any discrepancy in diagnosis. As the same criteria are used in the sending countries, it would be likely that patients in those countries are being misdiagnosed too, and if they are not, why not?

Hypothesis 5: Symptom patterns

A key hypothesis that has been excluded from Cochrane & Bal's (1987) list is that of symptom patterns in schizophrenia. There is considerable evidence from the DOSMD study that there are cultural differences between inception rates of narrow- and broad-definition schizophrenia (Jablensky *et al*, 1992). Rates of narrow-definition schizophrenia vary across cultures within a narrow band, whereas the band for broad-definition schizophrenia is much wider. It is possible that different migrant groups show different increases in specific symptoms, particularly in broad-definition schizophrenia.

Mood disorders

Migration as a risk factor for schizophrenia has been researched extensively, but there are only a few studies looking into migration and mood disorders.

A recent meta-analysis (Swinnen & Selten, 2007) found an increase in mood disorders with migration, although the mean relative risk was relatively low. The relative risk of bipolar affective disorder in migrants was 2.47. Interestingly, for studies conducted in the UK, this risk was no longer significant after people of African–Caribbean origin were excluded. The relative risk of 'any mood disorder' was 1.38. However, it is always important to differentiate between poorly planned migration and 'uprooting' with planned migration. In a survey of Irish-born people in London, poorly planned migration was associated with an increase in the relative risk of subsequent depression, although adequate social support was found to be protective (Ryan et al, 2006).

Common mental disorders

The findings on prevalence of common mental disorders across different ethnic and migrant populations are equivocal. In the UK, Murray & Williams (1986) found that Asian men were more likely to consult a general practitioner (GP) than White British men, although they reported fewer long-standing illnesses and less emotional distress. In contrast, no differences were found between Asian and White women. Cochrane & Stopes-Roe (1981) found lower rates of emotional disorders among patients of Indian and Pakistani origins compared with Whites. Maveras & Bebbington (1988) reported that Greek Cypriots in London had higher rates of anxiety than White UK-born Londoners (but similar rates to Greeks in Athens), whereas White Londoners had higher rates of depression. Gillam et al (1989) reported that White British people consulted a GP more frequently for GP-defined psychological problems, and that consultation rates for psychiatric problems were lowest among Caribbean and Asian women. Another UK study found that Black African patients had lower rates of 'common mental illness' (compared with Black Caribbean or White English). However, GPs were less likely to detect common mental illness in Black Africans and this was associated with patients' decisions not to talk about psychological problems rather than any other reason (Maginn et al, 2004).

In a UK community survey, Nazroo (1997) found lower rates of anxiety in Indian, Pakistani, Bangladeshi, Chinese and Caribbean women than among White British or White Irish women. Rates of depressive neurosis did not differ significantly across the different ethnic groups. Irrespective of clinical scores, Indian, Pakistani and Caribbean women and men were more likely to have visited a GP in the previous month. Jacob et al (1998) reported from their GP surgery sample that 30% of Asian women had common mental disorders that were not dissimilar to those reported by White British women. On balance it would appear that rates of common mental disorders are no higher among minority ethnic populations across all groups and both genders than among White populations. This would suggest that either these populations are psychologically robust or their expressions of distress are different.

Suicidal thoughts and self-harm

In the same community survey, Nazroo (1997) also reported that Irish, Caribbean and Pakistani men were more likely to consider that life was not worth living. Among women, however, there were no differences between ethnic groups. On comparing these groups by age and migration status, Nazroo found that UK-born individuals (or immigrants below the age of 11) of Caribbean, Indian or Pakistani origin were more likely to suffer from anxiety, depression and suicidal thoughts, although in some groups these differences were marginal.

Merrill & Owens (1986) reported much higher rates of attempted suicide among Asian women than their White counterparts. Bhugra *et al* (1999a,b) too found that Asian women aged 18–24 were 2.5 times more likely to attempt suicide. The authors of both studies attributed these findings to increased culture conflict arising from a disparity between individuals' traditional and modern attitudes within themselves as well as to the social and gender role expectations of significant others.

Eating disorders

Although some UK studies, for example Mumford & Whitehouse (1988), have demonstrated that rates of bulimia nervosa are higher among Asian schoolgirls than among their White counterparts, as has Nasser (1986) for anorexia among Egyptian girls in London, these findings are not universal. Very little work has been done in the UK on eating disorders in minority ethnic groups and both the studies cited above highlight the role of culture conflict in the causation of abnormal eating patterns. It is also possible that such conflict will be raised in geographical areas where ethnic density of the population is greater. Bhugra & Bhui (2003) found that African–Caribbean teenagers in London were more likely to eat 'sensibly' in front of others and to make up for this in private and that Asians were more likely to indulge in compulsive eating.

Post-traumatic stress disorder

Eisenbruch (1991) suggests that the cultural bereavement experienced by refugees is interlinked with symptoms and experiences of post-traumatic stress disorder (PTSD). Depending upon the type and urgency of migration and reasons for such an drastic step, PTSD can prove to be a significant finding across different ethnic groups and migrants. Further research is urgently required among refugees and migrants to understand their culture-specific experiences and explanations so that appropriate services can be delivered.

Personality disorder

There is very little literature on migration and personality disorder. A recent study looking into a tertiary-referral emergency service in Spain found that all subgroups of immigrants had a lower likelihood of being diagnosed with borderline personality disorder, and the rates were considerably lower in Asian and sub-Saharan populations (Pascual *et al*, 2008).

Ethnic density *v.* social isolation

In common with Murphy (1977), Mintz & Schwartz (1964) and Faris & Denham (1960), we believe that ethnic density, that is, the number of people of the same ethnic group around an individual, plays a significant role in the genesis and maintenance of some types of psychological distress. For example, rates of schizophrenia among Asians may be high in geographical areas where they are scattered and not so high where the Asian population is significant. Social support and low expressed emotion in an ethnically dense environment may act as protective factors against onset and relapse (as the relapse rates are lower as well). Among African–Caribbeans, both the scattering of the population, altered cultural and social identity, and low self-esteem may contribute to high rates, low and delayed recognition, and poor outcome. It would appear that African–Caribbean males in London are more likely to have been separated from their fathers for longer than 4 years and thus patterns of secure attachment and lower self-satisfaction and achievement may also play a role (Bhugra *et al*, 1997).

It is also likely that in ethnically dense populations, especially where the emphasis is on sociocentrism and collective responsibility, underlying culture conflict is more likely to take centre stage and produce high rates of attempted suicide and suicidal thoughts but not anxiety or depression. In such a setting, cultural identity, self-concept – including self-esteem – and social support are likely to play important roles.

Krupinski (1975) failed to find any impact of ethnic density on rates of psychiatric disorders among immigrant groups in Australia. Rates of schizophrenia were lower among Dutch and British groups, whereas alcoholism was higher among the British but rare among Italians and Greeks. Murphy (1968) posited that rates of psychiatric disorders are lower among immigrants in countries in which they constitute a larger proportion of the total population. This may well explain lower rates of schizophrenia in Asian samples from Southall in west London, where the Asian population forms nearly 50% of the total (Bhugra *et al*, 1997), and the high rates reported by King *et al* (1994) in north London, where Asians are in the minority. Kraus (1969) too demonstrated a highly significant negative correlation between the rate of schizophrenia and the size of the particular immigrant group. Social change, assimilation and protection in cultural identity may prove to be significant factors.

Analysis of data from the ÆSOP schizophrenia study in south-east London found that ethnic density and social capital (measured by proxy through voter turn-out) were both independently associated with a 5% reduced risk of non-affective psychosis (Kirkbride *et al*, 2008).

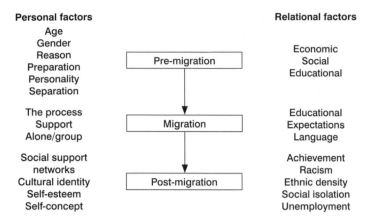

Fig. 2.3 Factors in migration and psychological distress

We propose that phases of migration, interlinked with significant life events and chronic ongoing difficulties, as well as personal factors (e.g. self-concept, self-esteem) and relational factors (e.g. social support, cultural identity), must be considered separately and continually (Fig. 2.3). In the first phase of migration the psychological distress will be different from that experienced at a later date.

Implications for care

Psychiatric assessment of immigrants requires consideration of many factors specific to their situation (see Chapter 19, this volume). Duration since the migration, preparation prior to migration and post-migration assimilation, acceptance and deculturation can be the most destructive for the individual. Insidious ongoing racism, with both chronic and acute difficulties related to racial life events, can be particularly pathogenic in producing various psychiatric conditions (Chapter 9, this volume). We hypothesise that this operates within a social context: if ethnic density is sparse, with a related paucity of support and other protective factors, the risk of illness will increase. It is very likely that such interactions can contribute not only to symptom formation, but also to persistence of symptoms (Box 2.2).

In assessing and planning treatments the clinician must take into account the individual's experiences and explanatory models of illness and their expectations of treatment. The patient's assessment of, and adaptation to, illness, and the attitudes of the patient and their carers to prevention of future illness are key aspects of treatment adherence. Differing attitudes towards symptoms have been demonstrated in different immigrant communities: for example, there is evidence that African–Caribbean people are less likely to view unusual thought content as a symptom and Bangladeshi people are less likely to view suspiciousness or hallucinatory behaviour as symptoms (Pote & Orrell, 2002).

Box 2.2 Factors to consider in assessing the mental health of immigrants

The patient's explanatory models of illness

Patient and carer attitudes to illness

Migration status

Experiences of migration

Phase of migration

Adjustment

The host society's attitudes

Cultural identity

Cultural conflict

Ethnic density

Achievements and expectations

The cultural acceptability of certain interventions varies between ethnic groups, and strategies might need modification to be effective. This might explain why a randomised controlled trial showed cognitive–behavioural therapy for insight to be generally efficacious, whereas subgroup analysis revealed a statistically significant drop-out rate among the African–Caribbean and Black African participants (Rathod *et al*, 2005).

The clinician should explore how migration came about. The distinction between voluntary migration (and uprooting) and forced resettlement is important, as is whether the patient migrated alone or as part of a group. These factors are likely to have a major effect on the individual and their social functioning and support (Kuo & Tsai, 1986). The effect of racial stratification combined with ethnic density will also influence an individual's functioning. As social support is related to social networks, the clinician should be aware of the latter and encourage the patient to link with them.

Liu (1986) suggests that the attributes, as well as the structure, of network support systems should be seen in the context of the cultural blueprint of a society. We believe that clinicians must also take into account the heterogeneity of networks in conjunction with the individual's personality, self-concept, self-esteem and self-sufficiency. The role of culture and the impact of migration on social structures is crucial in understanding social support and social networks. With increased ethnic density, social support may well be more easily available and may work to an individual's advantage in some sociocentric societies and yet may prove to be disadvantageous in others, especially if there is an underlying cultural conflict. The clinician must assess the quality of networks and social support, as well as the type of society and culture that the individuals come from.

Conclusion

Migration remains an enigma for the clinician because not all migrants go through the same experiences and or settle in similar social contexts. They do not all prepare in the same way and reasons for migration vary. The process of migration and subsequent cultural and social adjustment also play a key role in the mental health of the individual. Clinicians must take a range of these factors into account when assessing and planning intervention strategies aimed at the individual and their social context.

References

Berry, J. W., Phinney, J. S., Sam, D. L., et al (2006) Immigrant Youth in Cultural Transition: Acculturation, Identity and Adaptation across National Context. Lawrence Erlbaum.

Bhugra, D. (2000) Migration and schizophrenia. Acta Psychiatrica Scandinavica Supplementum, 102, 68–73.

Bhugra, D. & Bhui, K. (2003) Eating disorders in teenagers in east London: a survey. European Eating Disorders Review, 11, 46–57.

Bhugra, D., Hilwig, M., Hossein, B., et al (1996) First-contact incidence rates of schizophrenia in Trinidad and one-year follow-up. British Journal of Psychiatry, 169, 587–592.

Bhugra, D., Leff, J., Mallett, R., et al (1997) Incidence and outcome of schizophrenia in whites, African–Caribbeans and Asians in London. Psychological Medicine, 27, 791–798.

Bhugra, D., Baldwin, D., Desai, M., et al (1999a) Attempted suicide in West London. I: Rates across ethnic communities. Psychological Medicine, 29, 1125–1130.

Bhugra, D., Baldwin, D., Desai, M., et al (1999b) Attempted suicide in West London. II: Inter group comparisons. Psychological Medicine, 29, 1131–1139.

Cochrane, R. & Bal, S. S. (1987) Migration and schizophrenia: an examination of five hypotheses. Social Psychiatry, 22, 181–191.

Cochrane, R. & Stopes-Roe, M. (1981) Psychological symptom levels in Indian immigrants in England. Psychological Medicine, 11, 319–327.

Eisenbruch, M. (1991) From post-traumatic stress disorder to cultural bereavement. Social Science and Medicine, 33, 673–680.

Faris, R. & Denham, W. (1960) Mental Disorders in Urban Areas. Hafner Publishing.

Gillam, S., Jarman, B., White, P., et al (1989) Ethnic differences in consultation rates in urban general practice. BMJ, 299, 953–958.

Harrison, G., Owens, D., Holton, A., et al (1988) A prospective study of severe mental disorder in Afro-Caribbean patients. Psychological Medicine, 18, 643–657.

Harrison, G., Glazebrook, C., Brewin, J., et al (1997) Increased incidence of psychotic disorders in migrants from the Caribbean in the UK. Psychological Medicine, 27, 799–807.

Hickling, F. W. & Rodgers-Johnson, P. (1995) The incidence of first contact schizophrenia in Jamaica. British Journal of Psychiatry, 167, 193–196.

Jablensky, A., Sartorius, N., Ernberg, G., et al (1992) Schizophrenia: manifestations, incidence and course in different cultures. A World Health Organization ten-country study. Psychological Medicine Monograph Supplement, 20, 1–97.

Jacob, K. S., Bhugra, D., Lloyd, K., et al (1998) Common mental disorder, explanatory models and consultation behaviour among Indian women living in the UK. Journal of the Royal Society of Medicine, 91, 66–71.

King, M. B., Coker, E., Leavey, G., et al (1994) Incidence of psychotic illness in London. BMJ, 309, 1115–1119.

Kirkbride, J. B., Boydell, J., Ploubidis, G. B., et al (2008) Testing the association between the incidence of schizophrenia and social capital in an urban area. Psychological Medicine, 38, 1083–1094.

Kraus, J. (1969) Some social factors and the rates of psychiatric hospital admissions of immigrants in New South Wales. *Medical Journal of Australia*, **2**, 17.

Krupinski, J. (1975) Psychological maladaptations in ethnic concentrations in Victoria. In *Cultures in Collision* (ed. I. Pilowsky), pp. 49–58. Australian National Association for Mental Health.

Kuo, W.-H. & Tsai, Y.-M. (1986) Social networking, hardiness and immigrant's mental health. *Journal of Health and Social Behaviour*, **2**, 133–149.

Liu, W. T. (1986) Culture and social support. *Research on Aging*, **3**, 57–83.

Maginn, S., Boardman, A. P., Craig, T., *et al* (2004) The detection of psychological problems by general practitioners. *Social Psychiatry and Psychiatric Epidemiology*, **39**, 464–471.

Mahy, G. E., Mallett, R., Leff, J., *et al* (1999) First-contact incidence rate of schizophrenia on Barbados. *British Journal of Psychiatry*, **175**, 28–33.

Maveras, V. & Bebbington, P. (1988) Greeks, British Greek Cypriots and Londoners. *Psychological Medicine*, **18**, 433–442.

Merrill, J. & Owens, J. (1986) Ethnic differences in self-poisoning: a comparison of Asian and White groups. *British Journal of Psychiatry*, **148**, 708–712.

Mintz, N. & Schwartz, D. (1964) Urban ecology and psychosis. *International Journal of Social Psychiatry*, **10**, 101–118.

Mumford, D. & Whitehouse, A. (1988) Increased prevalence of bulimia nervosa among Asian school girls. *BMJ*, **297**, 718.

Murphy, H. B. M. (1968) Socio-cultural factors in schizophrenia. In *Social Psychiatry* (eds A. Zubin & V. Freyhan), pp. 74–92. Grune & Stratton.

Murphy, H. B. M. (1977) Migration, culture and mental illness. *Psychological Medicine*, **7**, 677–684.

Murray, J. & Williams, P. (1986) Self reported illness and general practice consultations in Asian born and British born residents of west London. *Social Psychiatry*, **21**, 136–145.

Nasser, M. (1986) Comparative study of prevalence of abnormal eating attitudes among Arab female students at both London and Cairo universities. *Psychological Medicine*, **16**, 621–625.

Nazroo, J. (1997) *Ethnicity and Mental Health*. PSI.

Ödegaard, O. (1932) Emigration and insanity: a study of mental disease among the Norwegian-born population of Minnesota. *Acta Psychiatrica et Neurologica Scandinavica Supplementum*, **4**, 1–206.

Pascual, J. C., Malagón, A., Córcoles, D., *et al* (2008) Immigrants and borderline personality disorder at a psychiatric emergency service. *British Journal of Psychiatry*, **193**, 471–476.

Pote, H. L. & Orrell, M. W. (2002) Perceptions of schizophrenia in multi-cultural Britain. *Ethnicity and Health*, **7**, 7–20.

Rack, P. (1982) *Race, Culture and Mental Disorder*. Tavistock.

Rathod, S., Kingdon, D., Smith, P., *et al* (2005) Insight into schizophrenia: the effects of cognitive behavioural therapy on the components of insight and association with socio-demographics: data on a previously published randomised controlled trial. *Schizophrenia Research*, **74**, 211–219.

Ryan, L., Leavey, G., Golden, A., *et al* (2006) Depression in Irish migrants living in London: case–control study. *British Journal of Psychiatry*, **188**, 560–566.

Sashidharan, S. (1993) Afro-Caribbeans and schizophrenia. *International Review of Psychiatry*, **5**, 129–144.

Selten, J.-P. & Sijben, N. (1994) First admission rates for schizophrenia in immigrants to the Netherlands. *Social Psychiatry and Psychiatric Epidemiology*, **29**, 71–77.

Swinnen, S. G. H. A. & Selten, J.-P. (2007) Mood disorders and migration. Meta-analysis. *British Journal of Psychiatry*, **190**, 6–10.

Zolkowska, K., Cantor-Graae, E. & McNeil, T. F., (2001) Increased rate of psychosis among immigrants to Sweden. Is migration a risk factor for psychosis? *Psychological Medicine*, **31**, 669–678.

CHAPTER 3

Mental health of refugees and asylum seekers

Rachel Tribe

Summary This chapter reviews contextual factors relating to people seeking asylum in host countries and becoming internally displaced within their country of origin. These are major life events for individuals, their families and communities and are likely to involve substantial changes and losses at a number of levels. Related terminology is defined and some of the more common exile-related stressors are considered, as is the resourcefulness of many refugees who overcome substantial obstacles and build productive lives in their new environments. Some of the issues that may require particular attention by psychiatrists when working with refugees and asylum seekers are examined. Finally, some implications for practice are reviewed, with consideration of issues relating to working across languages and cultures and to cultural constructions of mental health.

Refugees are not a recent phenomenon. Since the time of the Roman Empire people have fled their homes and sought refuge and protection in other countries. Refugees flee war, internal unrest and persecution because of their ethnic origin or their political, religious or social activities. Estimates of the number of refugees worldwide stand at 15.2 million; there are 827 000 asylum-seekers (pending cases) and 26 million internally displaced people (United Nations High Commission on Refugees, 2009). This number is larger than the entire population of Australia and it is perhaps pertinent to the debate to realise that it is almost the same as the number of refugees resulting from the Second World War. Refugees represent a variety of cultures, races and nations from all over the world. Summerfield (2000) reported that nearly 1% of the world's population were refugees or displaced persons as a result of about 40 violent conflicts.

The terms 'asylum seeker' and 'refugee' (see Box 3.1 for definitions) are frequently used in a negative and derogatory way, often associated with words such as bogus and scrounger. This type of language obscures the reality of who can be called refugees and why they seek sanctuary abroad. The status of those fleeing persecution is enshrined in international law, the United Nations Convention on Refugees, which resulted from a need to deal with the massive movements of people displaced by or fleeing the

Second World War. Countries that have signed the Convention are obliged to consider the application of anyone who claims refugee status and grant that person refuge on the basis of the evidence. This is never an easy process for either party. Although not a subject for this chapter, it is inevitable that the quality of decision-making in different countries is variable and that some people, although genuinely fearing persecution in their own country, are refused asylum.

Normally, the receiving or host country decides whether or not to grant an individual the right to refugee status, although in some countries the UNHCR may be asked to make this decision. In general, each case is decided on its merits. An asylum seeker is someone who is requesting asylum or refuge and has asked to be given formal legal refugee status (Box 3.1).

Box 3.1 Definitions

Refugees

The 1951 United Nations Convention relating to the Status of Refugees states that a refugee is a person who, owing to a well-founded fear of being persecuted for reasons of race, religion, nationality, membership in a particular social group, or political opinion, is outside the country of his nationality, and is unable to or, owing to such fear, is unwilling to avail himself of the protection of that country (United Nations High Commission on Refugees, 1951: Article 1A(2)).

Once recognised under the Convention, refugees have different rights to health, welfare and social services depending on the policies and resources of the host country concerned.

Asylum seekers

Asylum seekers may describe themselves as refugees, as this is what they hope to achieve, but they remain asylum seekers while they are awaiting a decision on their application for refugee status.

Internally displaced persons (IDPs)

An internally displaced person is usually someone who has been forced to flee his or her home and community owing to civil war or persecution, often on political or religious grounds, but has been displaced within his or her country of origin, rather than to a different country.

Exceptional leave to remain (ELR): granted before April 2003

An individual has been granted permission to remain in the host country for a specific period of time. Someone granted ELR status was generally ascribed fewer rights than someone with full refugee status.

Humanitarian protection (HP): granted from 1 April 2003

Humanitarian protection may be granted if an individual does not qualify for refugee status but their application is allowed on human rights grounds. Permission is granted to remain in the host country for a specific period of time.

Without formal refugee status, asylum seekers may find their access to services and legal rights curtailed. Asylum seekers experience fear and uncertainty relating to whether their asylum applications will be rejected and they will be deported.

Internally displaced people residing in collapsing states are extremely vulnerable, usually possessing even fewer rights than refugees, particularly when human rights violations have occurred. For example, in the 1990s, the conflicts in Kosovo and the genocide in Rwanda demonstrated the difficulties faced by international organisations in trying to protect civilians. The UNHCR tries to tackle such situations 'by encouraging states and other institutions to create conditions which are conducive to the protection of human rights and the peaceful resolution of disputes' (United Nations High Commission on Refugees, 2002: p. 1). In pursuit of the same objective, the UNHCR actively 'seeks to consolidate the reintegration of returning refugees in their country of origin, thereby averting the recurrence of refugee-producing situations' (United Nations High Commission on Refugees, 2002: p. 1). In 2008, the UNHCR identified some 6.6 million stateless persons in 58 countries (United Nations High Commission on Refugees, 2009).

The UNHCR is probably the most useful agency for further information, in particular its Refworld. In addition, the International Committee of the Red Cross/Crescent runs a tracing service for people who have lost contact with family members through a war or disaster (contact: itms2@redcross.org.uk or call 0845 053 2004). Both the UNHCR and the Red Cross/Crescent play an important role in providing services to refugees around the world and act as humanitarian intermediaries.

Where do refugees go?

Most refugees flee across borders from one low- or middle-income country to another. At the close of 2008, 20% of the world's refugees were hosted by high-income countries, whereas low- or middle-income countries hosted the remaining 80% (United Nations High Commission on Refugees, 2009: p. 7). Many find themselves in refugee camps, which can be extremely hostile and frightening places, with shifting populations and little, if any, personal space. As a patient in an Asian country told the author, 'We are the innocent victims in the big people's war, we all want it to stop… What life is there for me and my children? We do not live in the refugee camp, we exist.'

A number of national and non-governmental health agencies around the world provide an impressive service, frequently with very limited resources, in an attempt to meet some of the physical and psychological health needs of people forced to live in refugee camps. The work of many of these organisations is coordinated by the Inter-Agency Standing Committee (IASC; www.humanitarianinfo.org/iasc).

At certain times in history various countries have sought out refugees in the same way that countries are currently actively seeking immigrants with particular skills, for example, people in India with computer skills are being sought by the USA and the UK. Countries that have sought refugees have included the USA, Canada and Australia. At the launch of Refugee Week in the UK in 2006, the then Prime Minister Tony Blair is quoted as saying 'Like those from all continents to whom Britain has been a safe haven before and since, they have repaid our hospitality by enriching our culture, our society and country. Refugee Week celebrates this contribution. It also reminds us of the courage and resilience of those who must continue to leave family, friends and home to escape prosecution' (Refugee Action 2006). Thus, although refugees are often viewed as a burden, they may also prove to be a considerable asset. Refugees have contributed significantly to knowledge around the world. Refugees in Britain have included the inventor of the contraceptive pill and the first governor of the Bank of England. These individuals are among many with prestigious achievements in the fields of medicine, law, music, art and architecture, to name but a few.

Into exile

Refugees differ from immigrants in that the latter have usually made a positive choice to change their country of residence and have been able to plan the move practically, psychologically and systematically over time. Refugees, on the other hand, usually have to flee in fear of their lives, at short notice and often to unknown destinations. It is not a decision that is taken lightly, to risk losing everything your life has been built upon. The UNHCR uses the words of Euripides (431 BC) to describe the state of being a refugee or asylum seeker: 'There is no greater sorrow on earth than the loss of one's native land'. To flee to a destination where an unknown future awaits can never be an easy decision and individuals will face many very stressful issues (Box 3.2). Nevertheless, refugees may also feel immense relief if they feel that they have reached a safe haven and know that their lives are no longer under threat.

The period between applying for refugee status and a decision being made varies between countries from hours to years. This is an extremely stressful and uncertain time, when asylum seekers are unable to make plans for the future and may be terrified of being returned to their country of origin. It is a time when psychological well-being may be extremely fragile.

In the resettlement environment, family loss is a predictor of psychological distress (Rumbaut, 1991). Michelson & Sclare (2009) undertook a small-scale comparative study of two groups of asylum seekers and refugees, one of which comprised unaccompanied minors and the other children accompanied to the UK by a parent or one or more primary caregivers. They noted that the unaccompanied minors had experienced significantly more traumatic events prior to resettlement, and were more likely to exhibit symptoms of post-traumatic stress disorder (PTSD) than their accompanied

---

Box 3.2   Possible issues faced by refugees

Causes

- War
- Human rights abuses
- Persecution on grounds of politics, religion, gender or ethnicity

Resultant losses

- Country
- Culture
- Family
- Profession
- Language
- Friends
- Plans for future

Issues in country of asylum

- Multiple change
- Psychological and practical adjustment
- Uncertain future
- Traumatic life events
- Hardship
- Racism
- Stereotyping by host community
- Unknown cultural traditions

---

peers. Families may suffer acute disruption and close families may be split. A frequent pattern is that one of the adults flees, with the possibility that their partner and children may follow later. Sometimes families send unaccompanied children to seek asylum in the West, but this is usually done only when parents fear that their child's life may be at risk in their country of origin. In 2008, about 16 300 asylum applications were lodged by unaccompanied and separated children in 68 countries; 44% of refugees and asylum-seekers are children below 18 years of age (United Nations High Commission on Refugees, 2009). The immense loss of attachment figures and anyone or anything that is familiar may place unaccompanied refugee children in need of special provision (Ressler *et al*, 1988).

Exile-related stressors

Several studies suggest that exile-related stressors may be as powerful as events prior to flight (Pernice & Brook, 1996; Gorst-Unsworth & Goldenberg, 1998). Among potential predisposing factors for psychological health problems in immigrants and refugees, the Canadian Task Force on Mental Health Issues (1998) lists: separation from family and community; an unwelcoming host community; prolonged or severe suffering prior to exile; being elderly or adolescent; lacking knowledge of the host language; and loss of socioeconomic status.

The media often focus on issues of economic migration rather than on refugee issues. This has had the effect of further marginalising genuine asylum seekers and refugees. Responding clinically to the needs of individuals who become refugees may have implications and challenges for existing models of psychological intervention (Tribe, 1999a). The idea of talking to a psychiatrist, who is a stranger, about feelings may be an extremely alien and culturally incongruous concept, particularly given the associations with 'madness' and the way different cultural groups may position or construct these issues. Somatisation among refugee clients (patients) is frequently high: physical pain may be deemed more acceptable than psychological pain (Tribe, 1999b).

Case vignette 1   The stigma of mental health problems

Pedro, a refugee from Latin America, once rushed back into my office several minutes after our session had finished, in a highly anxious and aroused state. He told me he had bumped into a friend, Enriques, in the corridor. He begged me to tell Enriques that his appointment with me was in connection with an arm injury and to say nothing of any emotional dilemmas. It appears that it was fine to have physical health problems, but to have psychological ones was not acceptable as they were viewed as too stigmatising.

Implications for practice

It is now recognised that refugees and asylum seekers have a complex set of interwoven physical and mental healthcare needs (Burnett & Peel, 2001). If an asylum seeker or refugee approaches you for psychiatric help, one of the least helpful things you can do is contact the local embassy of their country of origin. Most refugees have fled their country of origin because of perse- cution or atrocities and in fear of their lives; they are usually terrified that their embassy, which is part of their government structure, may find them and take action against them or their families. It is impossible to assess the likelihood or not of this happening. It is also a high-risk strategy to assume that patients from the same country will have a lot in common and might, for example, be put in the same therapy group. There will be refugees in the UK who share a nationality but are drawn from totally opposing political or religious groups. Given that refugees may have been forced to flee because somebody had spoken about their political, religious or ethnic views or background means that issues of trust may be problematic and require careful consideration. Refugees may also be extremely anxious about personal information getting into the wrong hands and being used against them or their family members in their country of origin (Box 3.3).

Psychiatrists may be asked to write and present legal reports for patients as evidence supporting their claim of asylum/refugee status. This task does not always sit comfortably with the traditional role and may require careful consideration. It may mean a change of role for the psychiatrist or that the patient is asked to disclose experiences and give information at a pace that

---

Box 3.3   Points to consider when treating asylum seekers or refugees

The patient may be extremely anxious about the security of personal information

The patient may find it difficult to trust anyone, including the psychiatrist and fellow refugees

Never contact the local embassy of the patient's country of origin for information; instead, use refugee-specific organisations such as Human Rights Watch and the UNHCR

It is usually unwise to put patients from the same country in the same therapeutic group

---

is seriously out of alignment with the psychiatric treatment. Refugees may also assume that you are familiar with the politics and human rights record of their country. This may mean that they do not immediately disclose episodes of human rights abuse or even of torture. They may assume that you will know from the place where they were imprisoned or their personal history what has happened to them.

Individuals may present for help many years after becoming refugees, in the same way as those who have been through any traumatic experience. Miller (1999) cites McSharry & Kinney's unpublished findings that 43% of a randomised community sample of Cambodian refugees living in the USA were suffering from PTSD 12–14 years after resettling there.

The people that a refugee associates with a healing role may be community elders or family members, rather than psychiatrists, and these people may not be available to the refugee in exile. Refugee community organisations often play a vital role and frequently operate with very little funding. Miller (1999) suggests that the mental health needs of refugees might be better served by complementing clinic-based treatments with a range of community-based initiatives, which may be viewed as more culturally acceptable. These may have the added benefit of providing opportunities for culturally familiar social and community support, and may be able to help refugees to deal with the many exile-related stressors that exist, but are generally viewed as outside the remit of the psychiatrist. Visiting a refugee community organisation may not carry the same connotations as visiting a mental health centre; furthermore, for many refugees the latter may not even be within their repertoire of help-seeking behaviour.

Refugees have experienced many losses, including perhaps a view of the world as a safe and benevolent place on which they could have an impact. In various countries around the world psychiatrists have worked alongside community leaders, helping them to develop community-based interventions and to recognise when referral may be appropriate (Tribe & de Silva, 1999). Culture may also be an extremely important variable in assisting people to maintain their equilibrium. A refugee's sense of familiarity and identity may be severely threatened when they flee to a country so different from their own. In addition, many refugees have learned that talking about their beliefs and experiences can lead to their capture and perhaps organised violence and torture. Consequently, the idea of a talking cure may seem initially not only unlikely but frightening (Tribe, 1999a). This may mean that the process will have to take a rather different pace.

Working with unfamiliar languages and cultures

Resources in the West vary, particularly in the area of mental health, which is frequently not viewed as a priority in a resource-limited healthcare environment. However, the World Health Organization has recently accorded greater priority to the mental health of refugees and internally displaced people (Brundtland, 2010). Cultural interpretations of psychological distress, trauma and mental health differ around the world, and this appears to require careful consideration by mental healthcare practitioners.

Evidence-based clinical practice may be relatively easy to implement in the West, but it is not so easy with the very limited resources typically found in poorer countries. This issue may be further compounded by the fact that refugees are often resented by the host nation, which may feel less than inclined to put resources into refugee health and may attribute to refugees marginal or 'out-group' status.

A recently arrived asylum seeker may not be fluent in the spoken language of the receiving country and a psychiatrist may need to work with an interpreter or bicultural worker (Box 3.4). The time at the beginning and end of the consultation can be used to develop a working alliance with the interpreter as well as to discuss cultural factors and technical terminology. It may also be used to clarify procedural, organisational or ethical matters and to agree on the way in which the interpreter will work. The most common models for interpreting (Tribe, 1999b; Tribe & Raval, 2002) are:

- the linguistic or literal interpretation
- the psychotherapeutic model, which is more concerned with ensuring that the expressed emotions are conveyed by the interpreter to the psychiatrist
- the advocacy model, where the advocate interprets and advocates for the patient
- a combination of the three.

Explanatory health beliefs and constructions of psychological health or well-being for a refugee may bear little resemblance to those held by psychiatrists trained and practising in the West. Blackwell (1989: p. 2) writes:

> It is all too easy to repeat the colonising process by imposing a therapeutic ideology rooted in the culture of the host community, giving meaning to the survivor's experience in the language and symbols of that host community and its professionals, and failing to recognise the rich sources of meaning and symbolism available to the survivor from his or her own culture.

Box 3.4 Some issues to consider when a language and culture are not shared

Spend a few minutes with the interpreter before the session to clarify objectives, and review the meeting afterwards

Try to use the same interpreter for all the meetings with an individual or family; it is important to consider matching on age, gender and religious issues

Using an interpreter may mean that more time should be allocated for the meeting

Avoid specialist terminology

Use trained and experienced interpreters whenever possible; remember that they are part of the consultation and respect their contribution and different training

Always remain aware that you are interviewing someone from a different culture and who may therefore put different interpretations on events or feelings

Health beliefs about many aspects of psychiatry may be different across cultures

Remember that words may not translate exactly across languages

---

The role and healing powers of different cultural practices and those of psychological interventions appear to be well-established. Rather than rejecting either, it would therefore appear most useful to try to isolate the positive factors within both frameworks. This may be necessary if the consultation is to be optimal for the patient (see Kleinman, 1980; Heigel, 1983; Fernando, 1995; de Silva, 1999).

Refugees, trauma and the language of mental health

The debate about whether most refugees require a psychiatrist and whether the language of mental health/illness is the most appropriate for their situation is a complicated issue and one that raises strong opinions. It appears that few refugees present themselves to mental health services (Miller, 1999; Summerfield, 2003). Three major hypotheses dominate the literature on refugees, trauma and mental health:

- anyone who has been through the experiences of an asylum seeker and has lost so much must be 'damaged' or traumatised;
- people are very resilient and any reaction they have must be a normal one to abnormal events;
- many refugees go through immensely trying times that can be extremely distressing; some will benefit from psychological help but not necessarily that of the Western psychiatric model.

In reality, refugees are as diverse a group as any other and any of the above discourses may be true.

Case vignette   The importance of individual meaning-making

Mr A had been a young medical student in Africa and had suffered horribly at the hands of the authorities, who had tortured him for his political beliefs. He had a vision of what he thought would be a better world if his ideals for a more democratic system became established in his home country. Those in power did not agree. At this time Mr A had viewed himself as a brave martyr or hero, standing up for his political views and what he saw as a better political system. His major coping strategy during this period appeared to relate to his membership of a tight-knit political group that provided a strong and rigid support network. The group believed absolutely in its own identity and purpose. Subsequently, Mr A fled to Britain, as he feared for his life in his country of origin. Several years after his flight, he was referred to me by his general practitioner, who was concerned about his mental state.

My initial hypothesis was that Mr A's current distress was related to what I saw as his traumatic experiences in Africa and subsequent exile in Britain, but I was wrong. It was not related to the trauma of being tortured, to his flight from a repressive regime or to the difficulties of living in exile. What was causing him immense distress (he had active suicidal ideation) was that he had recently lost his political beliefs. He now thought of them merely as an adolescent rebellion and was devastated to think that his suffering and the subsequent loss of his country, family, profession and culture had all been for what he now viewed a developmental phase. His past political activities meant that he could not return to his country of origin as he was likely to be imprisoned and tortured. His torture and exile had felt bearable when he constructed them in terms of a political struggle and set of values. Without those political beliefs they felt unbearable and meaningless.

It is vital that individual diversity is considered when establishing resources or offering treatment or help to refugees. This is just as important as considering cultural differences and meanings. As asylum continues to present a major political challenge for the West, it also provides a focus for strong debate on the importance of psychiatric categorisations and trauma presentations. Vociferous debate occurs between those who believe that such constructs as PTSD are useful and those who believe that they are an unhelpful and culturally inappropriate response (McNally, 2003; Roberts *et al*, 2009). It is important to remember that becoming an asylum seeker is always a major event in an individual's life. However, it is not the defining characteristic but rather a part of the whole. Some services for refugees have established themselves to deal almost exclusively with this part of refugees' lives. This may mean that the service they offer is skewed and may be over-reductionist. That is not to say that becoming a refugee is not a major life event and may not require specialist care, but when treating refugees we should recognise the immense power of survival that people possess and use these in our clinical work (Tribe, 1999*a*).

Research into the mental health needs of refugees

Refugees are a vulnerable group and a strict ethical code should govern research in this population. Leaning (2001) has suggested guidelines on conducting such research.

The first widely published studies into the mental health of refugees were conducted after the Second World War and appeared to show a relationship between the severity of war experiences and psychiatric breakdown (e.g. Krupinski *et al*, 1973). The next major group of studies was undertaken soon after the Vietnam war, when numbers of South-East Asian refugees fled to the West. These studies widened the focus of research from the earlier work and started to incorporate cultural variables and their role in the presentation of distress, as well as psychosocial factors relating to displacement. Much of the earlier work attempted to find a link between numbers and severity of traumatic events without due consideration of the meaning of these events to the individual. More recent studies have considered this important factor (e.g. Norris, 1992; Steil & Ehler, 2000; Gisoni *et al*, 2009).

Summary

This chapter has attempted to define how and why individuals are forced to become asylum seekers, refugees or displaced people and to flee, often at very short notice, to a foreign country, to a refugee camp or to a designated 'safe place in their country of origin. Arrival in another country or region may not, in itself, give refugees peace of mind, as the intricacies of the asylum system and basic welfare and safety needs require immediate attention, as does living in a foreign country with a different culture, language and structure. In addition, individuals must come to terms with the immense losses frequently associated with flight and, perhaps most important, with loss of a belief in an imagined future.

References

Blackwell, R. D. (1989) *The Disruption and Reconstitution of Family, Network and Community Systems following Torture, Organised Violence and Exile*. Medical Foundation.

Brundtland, G. H. (2010) Mental health of refugees, internally displaced persons and other populations affected by conflict. WHO (http://www.who.int/hac/techguidance/pht/mental_health_refugees/en).

Burnett, A. & Peel, M. (2001) Health needs of asylum seekers and refugees. *BMJ*, **322**, 544–7.

Canadian Task Force on Mental Health Issues (1998) *After the Door Has Been Opened: Mental Health Issues Affecting Immigrants and Refugees in Canada*. Health and Welfare, Canada.

de Silva, P. (1999) Cultural aspects of post-traumatic stress disorder. In *Post-Traumatic Stress Disorders, Concepts and Therapy* (ed. W. Yule), pp. 116–138. John Wiley & Sons.

Fernando, S. (ed.) (1995) *Mental Health in a Multi-Ethnic Society*. Routledge.

Gisoni, C., Malta, L., Jayasinghe, N., *et al* (2009) Relationships between memory inconsistency for traumatic events following 9/11 and PTSD in disaster restoration workers. *Journal of Anxiety Disorder*, **23**, 557.

Gorst-Unsworth, C. & Goldenberg, E. (1998) Psychological sequelae of torture and organised violence suffered by refugees from Iraq. Trauma-related factors compared with social factors in exile. *British Journal of Psychiatry*, **172**, 90–94.

Heigel, J. P. (1983) Collaboration with traditional healers: experience in refugee's mental care. *International Journal of Mental Health*, **12**, 30–43.

Kleinman, A. (1980) *Patients and Healers in the Context of Culture*. University of California Press.

Krupinski, J., Stoller, A. & Wallace, L. (1973) Psychiatric disorders in East European refugees now in Australia. *Social Science and Medicine*, **7**, 31–49.

Leaning, J. (2001) Ethics of research in refugee populations. *Lancet*, **357**, 1432.

McNally, R. (2003) Progress and controversy in the study of post traumatic stress disorder. *Annual Review of Psychology*, **54**, 229–252.

Michelson, D. & Sclare, I. (2009) Psychological needs, service utilization and provision of care in a specialist mental health clinic for young refugees: a comparative study. *Clinical Child Psychology and Psychiatry*, **14**, 273–296.

Miller, K. (1999) Rethinking a familiar model: psychotherapy and the mental health of refugees. *Journal of Contemporary Psychotherapy*, **29**, 283–306.

Norris, F. H. (1992) Epidemiology of trauma: frequency and impact of different potentially traumatic events on different demographic groups. *Journal of Consulting and Clinical Psychology*, **60**, 409–418.

Pernice, R. & Brook, J. (1996) Refugees' and immigrants' mental health: association of demographic and post-migration factors. *Journal of Social Psychology*, **136**, 511–519.

Refugee Action (2006) 'Different pasts, shared future' – unique collaboration as party leaders praise the contribution of refugees. Refugee Action (http://www.refugee-action.org.uk/news/2006/RefugeeWeeklaunch.aspx).

Ressler, E. M., Boothby, N. & Steinbock, D. J. (1988) *Unaccompanied Children*. Oxford University Press.

Roberts, N. P., Kitchener, N. J., Kenardy, J., *et al* (2009) Multiple session early psychological interventions for the prevention of post-traumatic stress disorder. *Cochrane Database of Systematic Reviews*, issue 3, CD006869 (doi: 10.1002/14651858.CD006869.pub2).

Rumbaut, R. G. (1991) The agony of exile: a study of the migration and adaptation of Indochinese refugee adults and children. In *Refugee Children: Theory, Research, and Services* (eds F. L. Ahearn & J. L. Athey), pp. 59–91. Johns Hopkins University Press.

Steil, R. & Ehler, A. (2000) Dysfunctional meaning of post traumatic intrusions in chronic PTSD. *Behaviour Research and Therapy*, **38**, 537–558.

Summerfield, D. (2000) War and mental health: a brief overview. *BMJ*, **321**, 3323–3325.

Summerfield, D. (2003) Mental health of refugees. *British Journal of Psychiatry*, **183**, 459–460.

Tribe, R. (1999a) Therapeutic work with refugees living in exile: observations on clinical practice. *Counselling Psychology Quarterly*, **12**, 233–242.

Tribe, R. (1999b) Bridging the gap or damming the flow? Using interpreters/bicultural workers when working with refugee clients, many of whom have been tortured. *British Journal of Medical Psychology*, **72**, 567–576.

Tribe, R. & de Silva, P. (1999) Psychological intervention with displaced widows in Sri Lanka. *International Review of Psychiatry*, **11**, 186–192.

Tribe, R. & Raval, H. (2002) *Working with Interpreters in Mental Health*. Routledge.

United Nations High Commission on Refugees (1951) *Convention and Protocol Relating to the Status of Refugees: The 1951 Refugee Convention*. UNHCR.

United Nations High Commission on Refugees (2002) *UNHCR Mission Statement*. UNHCR.

United Nations High Commission on Refugees (2009) *2008 Global Trends: Refugees, Asylum-Seekers, Returnees, Internally Displaced and Stateless Persons*. UNHCR (http://www.unhcr.org/4a375c426.html).

CHAPTER 4

Racism, racial life events and mental ill health

Dinesh Bhugra and Oyedeji Ayonrinde

Summary Life events are a universal experience that everyone undergoes, However, the individual response to life events, whether they are negative (loss, bereavement, etc.) or positive (new house, new job) must be seen in a cultural context. Different cultures place differing emphasis on the significance of these events. Coping strategies are also influenced by cultures. Life events which are attributed to racism can affect vulnerable individuals. In this chapter, we review the literature, focusing on work related to racism, racial life events and mental illness. Race is a biological aspect and race is behaviour related to control of power and resources away from races deemed to be inferior.

The association of life events with the onset of various psychiatric disorders is well known. The body of evidence has highlighted the impact of negative or positive life events on the genesis of common mental disorders, especially depression. These findings have been replicated across different cultures, although the effect of different life events varies between cultures. In addition, the role of chronic difficulties (see p. 43) and resulting ongoing chronic stress have been shown to contribute to vulnerability to certain mental illnesses. However, data on the impact of life events, especially those perceived as racial, on members of minority ethnic groups are rather sparse. The questions that need to be addressed concern the perception of life events as racial, the role of pervasive and perceived institutional and individual racism, and chronic difficulties. In this review, we aim to draw the clinician's attention to some of these key factors, which may precipitate or perpetuate ongoing psychiatric problems.

Race, ethnicity and racism

Race and ethnicity

Until the middle of the 20th century race was used as a Darwinian tool to emphasise that Black people were inferior and savage compared with White people. This was accepted as a biological fact by the scientific community, thereby giving it a scientific legitimacy. Racism takes several forms and occurs both at individual and institutional levels.

The term 'race' has three usages: biological, common and political (Fuller & Toon, 1988). In biological usage, 'race' refers to the genetic separateness of different groups: each 'racial' group has an average genetic make-up that differs in some forms from the genetic make-up of other groups. However, genetic differences within each race are so wide that two individuals within the same racial group may have differences greater than the average differences between two different groups. Races are not separate, and the boundaries between them are arbitrary. In medicine, race is often used as a category that allows clinicians to link specific illnesses with particular races, for example cystic fibrosis and some White groups. Such distinctions can legitimise racist thinking. In common usage, race has become synonymous with physical appearance, and skin colour is given undue importance.

The political use of the term allows the majority of society to consolidate power and minority groups to politicise their identity.

'Ethnicity' is often used both to remove the pejorative implications of 'race' and in recognition that different races may share a similar culture. Essentially, ethnicity refers to a psychological sense of belonging, which will often be cemented by similarities in physical appearance or social behaviour (MacLachlan, 1997).

Racism

In its *Lexicon of Cross-Cultural Terms in Mental Health*, the World Health Organization (1997) defines racism, prejudice and ethnocentrism as follows. Racism is the belief that there is an inherent connection between perceived hereditary and cultural traits, and that some groups are biologically superior to others. Prejudice is the negative attitudinal and emotional set against an individual or group based on selected social or cultural characteristics. Ethnocentrism is the overvaluing of one's own culture in relation to other cultures, so that biased judgements are made regarding what is good, correct, beautiful, moral, normal, sane or rational. Individual racism differs from institutional racism, which is a collective view within an organisation that is deeply embedded in the way in which it functions. Although most professionals would not favour the theory of (genetic) inherited psychological inferiority, it remains a standard way of thinking among the lay public, where individual traits are described away as being 'in the blood' (Thomas & Sillen, 1991).

The Macpherson Report (Macpherson, 1999: para. 6.34) defines institutional racism as:

> The collective failure of an organisation to provide an appropriate and professional service to people because of their colour, culture, or ethnic origin. It can be seen or detected in processes, attitudes and behaviour which amount to discrimination through unwitting prejudice, ignorance, thoughtlessness and racist stereotyping which disadvantage minority ethnic people.

A key difficulty with such a definition is that it argues for detecting flaws in the processes by which an organisation (as a living organism) works, and it is not always clear what these processes are, who identifies the flaws and who should deal with them. Subjective experiences or interpretations of racism are even more difficult to define, as some are directly linked with an individual's personality traits, previous experiences and support systems (social and economic).

Subjugation of ethnic minorities by the majority using historical, social, biological and economic factors is common throughout history (Bhugra & Bhui, 1999). There is no doubt that racism and ideas pertaining to it date back to the pre-Christian era. In 100 BC, Cicero advised Atticus not to buy slaves from Britain as they were stupid, lazy and incapable of learning. However, the ideology behind racism is based on the wish to maintain the status quo and on the belief in the superiority of one group or another on purely racial or biological grounds. Race is a taxonomic concept of limited usefulness, and over the past 30 years it has started to give way to ethnicity or cultural groupings, which are very much more amorphous. Racism can be seen as ideology, as practice and as social structure.

Racism must be distinguished from racial discrimination. The former is restricted to discourses about grouping human populations into racial stocks (which may lead to ethnocentrism). The latter, however, is to do with actual behaviours. Racism takes many forms, some of which are described in Box 4.1.

It must be emphasised that racism is not a static phenomenon. Furthermore, it should be distinguished from racialism, which is the acting out of racial prejudice by one individual towards another. Racism includes

---

Box 4.1 Types of racism

Dominative   Hatred turns into actions

Aversive   The individual feels superior but is unable to act

Regressive   The individual's views on racism result in regressive behaviour

Pre-reflecting gut racism   Fear of strangers

Post-reflecting gut racism   Rationalisation, justification of fear of strangers

Cultural   Rejection and denigration of leisure and social customs

Institutional   An organisation's views on perceived inferiority

Paternalistic   The majority 'know' what is good for the minority

Colour-blind   The acceptance of differences is seen as culturally divisive

New racism   Hidden in 'individualism': positive action is objected to and existing racism criticised on the grounds of the present achievements of the group

> **Box 4.2** The therapists' self-assessment
>
> Therapists must always be aware of:
> - their own likes and dislikes
> - their own identity, e.g. race, gender, ethnicity, culture, power
> - mutual learning from the patient
> - the possibility of idealising a particular culture
> - the strengths and weaknesses of the patient's culture and of their own culture

the use of beliefs or practices to justify and maintain inequity, exclusion or domination. An interesting development is the use of 'colour-blindness' as a form of racism. When the 'colour-blind' look at subordinate groups of people of different skin colour they do not see them as people with their own history, culture, spiritual and socioeconomic realities. Racism can also exacerbate the health effects of poverty. Moore (2000) suggests that the psychology of colonialism and the control of information, communications and liberty are important factors in the development of racism. A dominative racist is one who acts on bigotry, whereas the aversive racist exhibits dislike and avoidance. There are those who do not reveal their racist tendencies except as unconscious aspects of mass behaviour (Kovel, 1984). The hatred of the 'out-group' (see p. 45) and authoritarianism also contribute to the maintenance of the status quo. It is also important to acknowledge that the sudden arrival of a large number of people who are perceived as competing for limited resources (benefits, housing, education, healthcare) can be worrying to the host population and it might be unfair to attribute all such anxieties to racism (Ghodse, 2003).

Psychiatry reflects dominant social values and can both be oppressive and be seen to be oppressive, particularly when individuals are detained against their will. This leads to a sense of alienation, and with time and experience individuals from minority groups may feel further let down. The relationship of racism with research and clinical conditions is extremely complex. It is essential that clinicians assessing an individual from a different ethnic and cultural background recognise their own views on race (Box 4.2).

The stress diathesis model in mental illness

The stress diathesis model in the aetiology of mental illness proposes that individuals vulnerable to stress may develop psychiatric disorders under certain circumstances and if adequate social networks or protective factors are not available. It is clear that adverse life events can influence the adaptive potential and mental health of human beings (Rutter, 1985), thereby contributing significantly to psychiatric morbidity. The strongest and most consistent associations have been reported in the aetiology of depression (Brown & Harris, 1978; Paykel, 1994), although associations have also been found with the onset of psychotic illness (Brown & Harris, 1978). The association between life events and common mental disorders has likewise been reported in non-Western cultures (Vadher & Ndetei, 1981; Guereje, 1986; Bebbington et al, 1998). Studies of genetic factors and shared familial life events have suggested that those who are more prone to depression are more likely to perceive events as threatening. Loss events may be particularly important in the onset of depression and dangerous events in the onset of anxiety disorders (Finlay-Jones & Brown, 1981).

Brown & Harris (1978) define a 'chronic difficulty' as a problem that has gone on for at least 4 weeks and a 'life event' as a traumatic or stressful event that occurred within a specific period of time. They observed that in a sample of attenders at a general practice surgery, 38% of patients with depression had experienced severe life events. Those who had experienced chronic major difficulties (during the previous 2 years) and severe life events comprised 62% of the depression sample. Chronic major difficulties are likely to be associated with depression, as they are most likely to interfere with cognition and may produce negative cognitions. Social class, economic factors and the help of a close confidant (i.e. social support) provide a degree of buffer for individuals.

The significance of experiences of hopelessness, entrapment, humiliation and defeat in the aetiology of depression has been discussed by Brown (1998). Other depressogenic events include attacks on self-esteem, which force the individual into a subordinate position, undermining their sense of rank, attractiveness and value and seemingly blocking escape routes (Gilbert & Allan, 1998). These relationships, however, are far from linear. A recent survey found that, although 'older gay black men' in the USA reported significantly higher levels of perceived stigma and greater use of 'less effective coping strategies', they did not experience more negative mental health outcomes as a result (Steven & Knight, 2008).

It is very likely that similar aetiological models will operate in individuals from ethnic minorities, and clinicians must assess their patients' feelings of self-esteem, sense of entrapment and lack of social support.

Racial life events

Racial life events are problems that can be directly attributed to racial behaviour, and they occur in many different domains (Box 4.3). Racial difficulties may be defined as ongoing difficulties in an individual's life that can be attributed to racial components and last for more than 1 month. They include problems with housing, employment, social functioning and education.

Box 4.3 Domains of racial life events

- Accommodation
- Education
- Employment
- Finance
- Health
- Incidents of harassment
- Damage to property
- Law and welfare

The impact of racial life events on ethnic minorities is varied and wide-ranging (Bhugra & Ayonrinde, 2001), from migration itself to racially motivated attacks after migration. Migration may have significant effects on the individual and the group (see Bhugra & Cochrane, 2001). Accurate data on the prevalence of racial attacks, violence and racially motivated crime (victimisation, attacks and harassment) are difficult to obtain. There are several reasons for this: the individual may not perceive these attacks as racial and therefore not report them as such; the ethnicity of the perpetrator may not be known; victims may wrongly attribute a racial motive to an incident; further victimisation may prevent reporting; and insufficient evidence may lead to under-reporting.

Another reason for the difficulty in obtaining representative data in the UK is that the British Crime Survey (BCS) and police records have different methods of data collection. The BCS records reported both actual offences (such as vandalism, burglary, theft, wounding of persons, assault or robbery) and threatened offences; the police, however, record only reported crimes, although they do also note any alleged racial motive or if the investigating officer suspects a racial motive. Fitzgerald & Hale (1996) cite BCS findings that only 2% of all crimes were considered by victims to be motivated by racism, and nearly a quarter of these occurred in inner-city areas. However, perceptions of the crime need to be studied in detail.

There are ethnic differences too in reporting of crimes (Commission for Racial Equality, 1999). Bearing in mind the type of crime, method of reporting and delay in reporting, it is important to emphasise that this area remains under-researched.

Chahal & Julienne (1999) observed that between 43% and 62% of racial incidents in the UK went unreported. Among those that were reported were injuries to the person, harassment, assault and criminal damage to property; incidents related to failure to get a job, a mortgage, or support in schools, hospitals and so on are not even likely to be recorded. In a qualitative study of subjective experiences of racism, they found that participants described the routine nature of racial incidents in their lives. They also used different pathways for disclosing these events – most of which were in personal or social sectors. Failure to disclose was often due to feelings of shame, inadequacy, hopelessness or mistrust. Only a significant increase in incidents led individuals to disclose to statutory agencies. General practitioners (GPs) were most frequently approached, but the resulting action was often limited (e.g. a GP might write a letter to the housing authority in support of re-housing, but do nothing else). Thus, even if events are identified, their impact can easily be ignored. Commonly recurring emotional themes in the group were those of anger, stress, depression, heightened arousal and poor sleep.

In a survey of employed 'White UK', Bangladeshi and African–Caribbean people, the African–Caribbean respondents reported greater stress than the other two groups in the workplace. The racial discrimination reported by the African–Caribbean women was associated with increased work stress and higher levels of psychological distress (Wadsworth et al, 2007). Data collected from the ÆSOP study showed that 'perceived disadvantage' was associated with higher incidence of psychosis (after controlling for other factors). Interestingly, Black respondents in the 'non-psychotic' group attributed their disadvantage to racism, whereas Black people with psychosis attributed disadvantage to their own situation (Cooper et al, 2008).

Racial discrimination is associated not only with mental ill health: it is also associated with physical health problems. An association between perceived racism and blood pressure levels in African Americans has been revealed (Brondolo et al, 2003). Specific associations have been found between perceived racism and night-time ambulatory blood pressure in Black Americans and Latinos even after controlling for socioeconomic status and personality factors (Brondolo et al, 2008) and between perceived racial discrimination with respiratory illness and ill health across different ethnic groups (Karlsen & Nazroo, 2002).

In addition to stressors that are common to all, minority groups may experience stress resulting from their minority status. These include stressor stimuli (e.g. prejudice, hostility and discrimination); external mediating forces (social support); and internal mediating forces (cognitive factors) that influence the individual's perception of life events. Smith (1985) has suggested the terms 'out-group' and 'in-group' to describe the situation of minority groups (the out-group) in a majority culture (the in-group). Out-group status results in social isolation, social marginalisation and status inconsistency, which increase the individual's state of arousal. The incomplete or partial assimilation by minority individuals of the new (host) majority culture and the complete or partial rejection of their own culture may lead to additional stresses.

Racism and mental disorders

Racism at either the individual or the institutional level may lead to problems such as those illustrated in Box 4.4. A sense of status inconsistency may occur, in which the individual has two or more distinct and incompatible

Box 4.4 Problems related to racism

Institutional racism

- Stereotyping
- Rejection
- Prejudice
- Devaluation of culture

Individual racism

- Stereotyping
- Rejection
- Prejudice
- Devaluation of culture
- Threats
- Attacks

social statuses (e.g. the individual's social status is contaminated by the status associated with their ethnicity). This contradiction in role and status is likely to lead to adjustment difficulties or psychopathology (Smith, 1985). As individuals from ethnic minorities are more 'visible' among the majority population, their actions take on a symbolic meaning and stereotypes tend to take over. Smith (1985) argues that high visibility, over-observation, lack of anonymity, polarisation and role entrapment are some of the factors that contribute to the stress and chronic difficulties.

A systematic review has revealed that, in the UK, Black patients are 3.83 times more likely than White patients to be compulsorily detained under the Mental Health Act 1983 (Singh *et al*, 2007). Compulsory detention is 3.35 times more likely for all Black and ethnic minorities (BME) patients overall, and 2.06 times more likely for Asian patients. In exploring the potential causes of these increased levels of detention, Singh and his colleagues felt that there is no clear evidence base that racism within mental health services is among them. There is a debate to be had regarding whether the failure to provide equitable care to minority ethnic groups represents institutional racism and if so to what extent. In a commentary on the Macpherson Report, Singh (2007) proposed that the lack of diagnostic clarity, coherent treatment plans and appropriate treatment for patients from ethnic minorities revealed at a national level are a direct result of individual clinical encounters. However, this explanation has been challenged as too simplistic and not in line with the concept that institutional racism is complex and covert (Patel & Heginbotham, 2007).

Racism is a multidimensional phenomenon, and a number of instruments have been developed to measure racial life events in domains such as those shown in Box 4.3. Many of these scales have been developed for specific ethnic groups, sometimes for specific ethnic contexts and studies.

Box 4.5 Factors mitigating or exacerbating the effect of individual and institutional racism

Mitigating factors

- Social support: ethnic group, cultural identity

Exacerbating factors

- Stress
- Mental illness
- Powerlessness

Potentially mitigating or exacerbating factors

- Age
- Gender
- Socioeconomic status

Box 4.5 lists key factors that influence the effects that racism has on individuals. In summary, racism has:

- the ability to create differential social status that results in differential health consequences
- a role in determining differential exposure to risk factors and available resources
- an effect on the individual's psychological well-being and functioning (Herman, 1996; Jackson *et al*, 1996; William-Morris, 1996; Williams, 1996). Cumulative perceptions of racism and racial discrimination have a greater adverse effect on mental than on physical health (Jackson *et al*, 1996). The role of 'locus of control' as an intervening variable for psychological well-being has to be explored further in the context of minority ethnic groups.

Racial events and psychiatric disorders

Depression

The limited data available show that adverse social life events are, like adverse life events in general, significantly associated with depression. Several community studies have shown higher rates of depression in minority ethnic groups (Nazroo, 1997; Shaw *et al*, 1999), with possible explanations including exposure to differential environmental losses, unemployment, poverty and racism. A study of self-harm by Asian women revealed that nearly a quarter of the sample had experienced racial life events, although a causal association cannot be ascertained from the data (Bhugra *et al*, 1999). There is always the argument that it is the biological component of 'race' rather than racial discrimination that makes a particular ethnic group more vulnerable to depression. A recent study from multi-ethnic urban Brazil found adolescents who reported (possibly perceived) racial discrimination were more likely to suffer from major depression, but their actual skin colour was not independently associated with depression (Santana et al, 2007).

Looking at specific groups, a study of the maternity experiences of asylum seekers in England found that half the women interviewed reported encountering explicit hostility and racism in maternity services, and the majority described feelings and behaviour consistent with post-natal depression (McLeish, 2005). Perceived racial discrimination during pregnancy is associated with low birth weight of offspring (Collins et al, 2004).

Anxiety

Stress models suggest an increase in anxiety in the face of threatening life events. Anxiety symptoms are known to develop following racial threats (Jones et al, 1996; Thompson, 1996). In a study from New Zealand, Pernice & Brook (1996) reported that racial discrimination was significantly associated with high levels of anxiety among immigrants in Black and minority ethnic groups. They found surprisingly high anxiety levels among those who spent a lot of leisure time with their own ethnic group. It is possible that individuals made anxious by racial discrimination sought solace in the company of their own ethnic group.

Post-traumatic stress disorder

Increased levels of stress with symptoms akin to post-traumatic stress disorder following experiences of racial discrimination have been reported (Ritsner et al, 1997). Symptoms of hypervigilance, increased arousal, poor concentration, increased levels of frustration, denial, social withdrawal, anxiety and repeated flashbacks occur following a significant racial life event in the same way as post-traumatic stress disorder does.

Psychosis

Anecdotal evidence suggests links between racial events and psychosis, and institutional racism is said to play a key role in adherence to treatment and follow-up. The empirical data, however, are inconclusive. However, one study in England found experience of perceived interpersonal racism to be independently associated with psychosis and common mental disorders after controlling for socioeconomic status, gender and age (Karlsen et al, 2005).

The relationship between racial life events and onset of psychiatric disorders is complex and it is only relatively recently that researchers have started working on disentangling it.

Racism and mental distress

Racism, be it individual or institutional, is likely to act as a constant stressor and to result in chronic difficulties preventing individuals from progressing. They may feel that, although they are capable of achieving more, other people or the system are hindering their progress. Such obstacles may give individuals a sense of entrapment and bewilderment, knocking their self-esteem and self-concept. This may further alienate them from their own ethnic group, especially if their methods of dealing with chronic difficulties are at variance with those of their peers, thereby adding further to their stress.

Conclusion

Individuals, whatever their ethnic background, interact with their social and cultural milieux and respond to ongoing difficulties or sudden stress in different ways. Actual racial life events, a perception of such events and chronic racism are all likely to precipitate psychiatric disorders. However, the research data remain sparse, and in the studies that have been carried out data-collection methods have sometimes been unclear, making any interpretations and generalisations very difficult.

References

Bebbington, P., Hamdi, E. & Ghubash, R. (1998) The Dubai Community Psychiatry Survey IV. *Social Psychiatry and Psychiatric Epidemiology*, **33**, 501–509.

Bhugra, D. & Ayonrinde, O. (2001) Racial life events and psychiatric morbidity. In *Psychiatry in Multicultural Britain* (eds D. Bhugra & R. Cochrane), pp. 91–111. Gaskell.

Bhugra, D. & Bhui, K. S. (1999) Racism in psychiatry: paradigm lost, paradigm regained. *International Review of Psychiatry*, **11**, 236–243.

Bhugra, D. & Cochrane, R. (eds) (2001) *Psychiatry in Multicultural Britain*. Gaskell.

Bhugra, D., Baldwin, D., Desai, M., *et al* (1999) Attempted suicide in West. II. *Psychological Medicine*, **29**, 1130–1139.

Brondolo, E., Reippi, R., Kelly, K., *et al* (2003) Perceived racism and blood pressure. A review of the literature and conceptual and methodological critique. *Annals of Behavioral Medicine*, **25**, 55–65.

Brondolo, E., Libby, D. J., Denton, E.-G., *et al* (2008) Racism and ambulatory blood pressure in a community sample. *Psychosomatic Medicine*, **70**, 49–56.

Brown, G. (1998) Genetic and population perspective on life events and depression. *Social Psychiatry and Psychiatric Epidemiology*, **33**, 363–372.

Brown, G. & Harris, T. (1978) *Social Origins of Depression*. Tavistock Press.

Chahal, K. & Julienne, L. (1999) *We Can't All Be White*. York Publishing Services.

Collins, J., David, R., Handler, A., *et al* (2004) Very low birth weight in African American infants: the role of maternal exposure to interpersonal racial discrimination. *American Journal of Public Health*, **94**, 2132–2138.

Commission for Racial Equality (1999) *Ethnic Minorities in Britain*. CRE.

Cooper, C., Morgan, C., Byrne, M., *et al* (2008) Perceptions of disadvantage, ethnicity and psychosis. *British Journal of Psychiatry*, **192**, 185–190.

49

Finlay-Jones, R. & Brown, G. (1981) Types of stressful life events and onset of anxiety and depression disorders. *Psychological Medicine*, **11**, 813–815.

Fitzgerald, M. & Hale, C. (1996) *Ethnic Minorities, Victimisation and Racial Harassment* (Home Office Research Findings no. 39). Home Office.

Fuller, J. H. S. & Toon, P. D. (1988) *Medical Practice in a Multicultural Society*. Heinemann.

Ghodse, A. H. (2003) Invited commentary on: Globalisation and psychiatry. *Advances in Psychiatric Treatment*, **9**, 470–473.

Gilbert, P. & Allan, S. (1998) The role of defeat and entrapment (arrested flight) in depression: an exploration of an evolutionary view. *Psychological Medicine*, **28**, 585–598.

Guereje, O. (1986) Social factors and depressions in Nigerian women. *Acta Psychiatrica Scandinavica*, **74**, 392–395.

Herman, A. (1996) Toward a conceptualisation of ease in epidemiologic research. *Ethnicity and Disease*, **6**, 7–20.

Jackson, J. S., Brown, T., Williams, D., *et al* (1996) Racism and the physical and mental health of African Americans. *Ethnicity and Disease*, **6**, 132–147.

Jones, D. R., Harrell, J. P., Morriss-Prather, C., *et al* (1996) Affective and physiological responses to racism. *Ethnicity and Disease*, **6**, 109–122.

Karlsen, S. & Nazroo, J. Y. (2002) Relation between racial discrimination, social class, and health among ethnic minority groups. *American Journal of Public Health*, **92**, 624–631.

Karlsen, S., Nazroo, J. Y., McKenzie, K., *et al* (2005) Racism, psychosis and common mental disorder among ethnic minority groups in England. *Psychological Medicine*, **13**, 1795–1803.

Kovel, J. (1984) *White Racism: A Psychohistory*. Columbia University Press.

MacLachlan, M. (1997) *Culture and Health*. John Wiley & Sons.

Macpherson, W. (1999) *The Stephen Lawrence Inquiry. Report of an Inquiry by Sir William Macpherson of Cluny*. TSO (The Stationery Office).

McLeish, J. (2005) Maternity experiences of asylum seekers in England. *British Journal of Midwifery*, **13**, 782–785.

Moore. L. (2000) Psychiatric contributions to understanding racism. *Transcultural Psychiatry*, **37**, 147–182.

Nazroo, J. (1997) *Ethnicity and Mental Health*. PSI.

Patel, K. & Heginbotham, C. (2007) Institutional racism in mental health services does not imply racism in individual psychiatrists. Commentary on: Institutional racism in psychiatry. *Psychiatric Bulletin*, **31**, 367–368.

Paykel, E. S. (1994) Life events, social support and depression. *Acta Psychiatrica Scandinavica Supplementum*, **377**, 50–58.

Pernice, R. & Brook, J. (1996) Refugees' and immigrants' mental health. *Journal of Social Psychology*, **136**, 511–519.

Ritsner, M., Ponizoysky, A. & Ginath, Y. (1997) Changing patterns of distress during the adjustment of recent immigrants. *Acta Psychiatrica Scandinavica*, **95**, 494–499.

Rutter, M. (1985) Resilience in the face of adversity. Protective factors and resistance to psychiatric disorder. *British Journal of Psychiatry*, **147**, 598–611.

Santana, V., Almeida-Filho, N., Roberts, R., *et al* (2007) Skin colour, perception of racism and depression among adolescents in urban Brazil. *Child and Adolescent Mental Health*, **12**, 125–131.

Shaw, C. M., Creed, F., Tomenson, B., *et al* (1999) Prevalence of anxiety and depressive illness and help seeking behaviour in African Caribbeans and white Europeans. *BMJ*, **318**, 302–305.

Singh, S. P., (2007) Institutional racism in psychiatry: lessons from inquiries. *Psychiatric Bulletin*, **31**, 363–365.

Singh, S. P., Greenwood, N., White, S., *et al* (2007) Ethnicity and the Mental Health Act 1983. *British Journal of Psychiatry*, **191**, 99–105.

Smith, E. (1985) Ethnic minorities: life stress, social support and mental health issues. *Counseling Psychologist*, **4**, 537–579.

Steven, D. & Knight, B. (2008) Stress and coping among gay men: age and ethnic differences. *Psychology and Aging*, **23**, 62–69.

Thomas, A. & Sillen, S. (1991) *Racism and Psychiatry*. Citadel Press.

Thompson, V. L. (1996) Perceived experiences of racism as stressful life events. *Community Mental Health Journal*, **32**, 223–233.

Vadher, A. & Ndetei, D. M. (1981) Life events and depression in a Kenyan setting. *British Journal of Psychiatry*, **139**, 134–137.

Wadsworth, E., Dhillon, K., Shaw, C., *et al* (2007) Racial discrimination, ethnicity and work stress. *Occupational Medicine*, **57**, 18–24.

Williams, D. (1996) Racism and health: a research agenda. *Ethnicity and Disease*, **6**, 1–6.

William-Morris, R. S. (1996) Racism and children's health. *Ethnicity and Disease*, **6**, 69–82.

World Health Organization (1997) *Lexicon of Cross-Cultural Terms in Mental Health*. WHO.

CHAPTER 5

Expressed emotion across cultures

Dinesh Bhugra and Kwame McKenzie

Summary   Expressed emotion (EE) has been used as a construct in understanding the interaction between patients and their carers and families. A considerable amount of data from Western cultures suggests that living in high-EE families can lead to relapse of schizophrenia in vulnerable individuals, even when they are on medication. However, the data from other cultures are less solid. This chapter reviews some of the existing findings and recommends that various components of EE must be seen in the cultural context and embedded in the normative data of the population before the concept can be considered in association with the pathogenesis of relapse.

Some 40 years ago, the hypothesis was put forward that ordinary aspects of family life are crucial to an understanding of how families interact with those among them who have mental illnesses (Brown, 1985). The concept and measurement of the 'expressed emotion' (EE) within families were developed in the 1960s, initially for use in schizophrenia. They were subsequently used for a number of physical and psychiatric conditions, ranging from dementia to diabetes and Parkinson's disease. They have been a major impetus for the development and evaluation of social treatments of schizophrenia (Kuipers & Bebbington, 1990). The family's EE has been shown to be predictive of outcome in mental and physical illnesses in a variety of cultural settings.

Family environment is crucial both in the development of the individual and in creating and sustaining psychopathology in vulnerable individuals. There are studies which look at a socialisation paradigm, explaining how parental negativity can undermine children's learning about emotions and their management (Hoffman, 1983). Thus, the child may grow up without really understanding the implicit and explicit messages carried in the way the emotions are expressed. Externalising behaviours may be strongly influenced by family interactions that reinforce escalating negative affect and aggression (Beauchaine et al, 2007). One example of this has been in the field of self-harm, where the quality of communication and social problem-solving in the families has been studied (Tulloch *et al*, 1997; Speckens & Hawton, 2005; Nock & Mendes, 2008). There is also plenty of evidence and ongoing research regarding the role of attachment patterns in the later development of psychopathology, which will influence the way adult interpersonal relationships work, especially during times of stress (Bowlby, 1969). Insecure attachment models may inhibit the development of adaptive emotion-regulation skills, which may be of direct importance in self-harm (Yates, 2004). The process of 'scapegoating' by individuals who self-harm reflects their parents' anxiety and perceptions of their own well-being (Sabbath, 1969).

Measuring EE

The Camberwell Family Interview

The first research instrument to record the range of feelings and emotions found in ordinary families was the Camberwell Family Interview (CFI), developed by G. W. Brown and colleagues. This is conducted with the patient's key carers, and from it the interviewer tries to create a picture of how things have been in the household in the months leading to the onset of illness. In the first phase of development of the interview (Brown, 1959; Brown *et al*, 1958, 1962, 1972), Brown and colleagues reported that its theoretical constructs were being worked out at the same time as the interviews were being conducted. In a historical account of the process, Brown (1985) suggested that the term 'expressed emotion' emerged only after several studies had been carried out. After the instrument had been in use for a while, the researchers developed a semi-standardised interview distinguishing between critical comments and dissatisfaction (although they clearly go together).

The original interview was very long and a shortened version was produced (Vaughn & Leff, 1976*a*) that can be completed in 1–2 hours. The interview is in a 'mental conversational style ... rather than a clinical one' (Leff & Vaughn, 1985). All judgements on relatives' EE are based on this interview.

The components of EE

The original version of the CFI describes five components of EE: critical comments, hostility, emotional over-involvement, warmth and positive comments (Brown 1985). Critical comments are simply counted over the period of the interview. Hostility is rated as being absent or present and in terms of generalisation and rejection. Emotional over-involvement is an extremely complex construct and it often causes difficulties for both researchers and clinicians. It is also the most likely of the five components to vary across cultures. Many attitudes and behaviours relevant to this rating may be evident during the interview, for example exaggerated emotional response, excessive self-sacrifice or devoted behaviour, and marked over-protectiveness. Warmth is rated on a 6-point scale and positive comments are rated as present or absent and counted.

It was decided to exclude both warmth and positive remarks from the final index of EE, because of complex associations identified during the development of the assessment interview (Brown *et al*, 1962, 1972). Warmth measured in the parents of people with schizophrenia correlated positively with emotional over-involvement and moderately negatively with critical comments. Warmth in the absence of emotional over-involvement or criticism was associated with better outcome. Relatively little is known about the influence of the positive-comments dimension and this aspect of the scale has been typically overlooked (Wearden *et al*, 2000).

The short-form CFI

The shortened version of the CFI (Vaughn & Leff, 1976*a*) has become the standard tool for assessing EE. Two types of information are elicited: objective information about events and circumstances in the home in the months before the admission/current episode of illness and subjective information concerning the relative's feelings and attitudes towards the patient when talking about the illness. The interview is usually audio-taped and its transcript is rated on three primary subscales:

- critical comments, indicating dislike or disapproval of the patient's behaviour or personality
- hostility, expressed as a generalised critical attitude towards or rejection of the patient
- emotional over-involvement, related to expressions of over-protectiveness, over-concern, self-sacrificing behaviour and exaggerated emotional responses.

Ratings on these primary subscales are combined to provide an overall dichotomous categorisation of 'high' or 'low' EE, with cut-off points that vary according to individual studies and cultures. The index of EE can be seen as an indicator of the 'emotional temperature' in the home – it is a marker of intensity, although it is not necessarily a constant.

The shortened CFI can also be used to derive two subscales reflecting the positive attributes of warmth (based on evidence of sympathy, affection and empathy) and positive comments, although, as mentioned above, these scales are not involved in the overall classification of EE.

The FMSS

As the CFI requires an interview of 1–2 hours' duration, with an equivalent or greater amount of time needed for rating, a number of more economical methods have been developed for measuring EE (Hooley & Parker, 2006). Among the most widely used alternatives is the Five-Minute Speech Sample (FMSS; Magaña *et al*, 1986), in which a key relative is asked to speak about the patient for 5 minutes, describing them as a person and their mutual relationship. High criticism is scored when the respondent makes a negative initial statement, provides evidence of a negative relationship with the patient, or makes one or more critical comments during the speech sample. A 'borderline' critical rating is given when evidence of dissatisfaction is expressed in the speech sample. The emotional over-involvement component is derived from criteria similar to those used in the CFI:

- emotional display during the speech sample
- evidence of self-sacrifice or over-protectiveness
- 'statement of attitude' reflecting very strong feelings of love or willingness to do anything for the patient
- excessive detail about the patient's birth or infancy, reflecting a preoccupation with the past
- exaggerated praise, based on five or more positive remarks (Magaña-Amato, 1993).

Unlike in the CFI, hostility is not rated separately, in recognition of the facts that hostility is rarely present in the absence of criticism and that it has relatively little value as an independent predictor of psychiatric outcome (Kuipers & Bebbington, 1988). Respondents are classified as high EE if they are rated as being high in criticism and/or emotional over-involvement. The family EE is rated on the basis of the highest score from both parents. On overall EE ratings, the FMSS has shown significant agreement with the CFI in adult samples (Magaña et al, 1986; Halford, 1991; Leeb et al, 1991; Moore & Kuipers, 1999), as well as in studies with children (Calam & Peters, 2006) and adolescents (Rein et al, 2006).

EE and patient outcome

Since the original investigations in patients with schizophrenia (Brown et al, 1962, 1972), high EE (Box 5.1) has been consistently implicated as a predictor of poor clinical outcomes for a number of psychiatric as well as physical conditions (Butzlaff & Hooley, 1998; Wearden et al, 2000; Hooley, 2007). In a systematic review and meta-analysis of this literature, Butzlaff & Hooley (1998) examined the predictive validity of the construct

---

Box 5.1 Indicators of high expressed emotion

- Critical comments: six or more
- Emotional over-involvement: a score of 3 or higher
- Hostility: present
- Warmth: absent
- Positive regard: absent

in schizophrenia, mood disorders and eating disorders. Surprisingly, even though a majority of the 36 identified outcome studies had involved patients with schizophrenia, the strongest mean effect sizes for EE on relapse rates were found for mood and eating disorders.

The interaction between EE and patient outcome is complex. Research has demonstrated that patients from households with high EE do not differ in their pathology from those in households with low EE. It is the relatives who differ markedly in their response to the patients and their illnesses. Of the five components of EE, critical comments, hostility and emotional over-involvement have been shown to be the most predictive of relapse, i.e. of increased symptoms (Kuipers, 1992).

Cultural variations

In some cultures, for example in parts of India, emotional over-involvement is the norm. If a carer does not show emotional over-involvement it is seen as lack of care. So interviewers must try to understand and follow cultural norms. Expressed emotion is best measured by a person from the same cultural group: it is difficult for a researcher who is not familiar with the nuances of the language and cultural expression of an interviewee to rate any of the components of EE. If measures of EE are being applied in cultures where they have not been used before, they must be accompanied by fieldwork to establish the norms and the context. The most important factor for the researcher is to embed emotional over-involvement, hostility and warmth in the specific cultural context. Measurement is also dependent on an assessment of the interviewee's general style of emotional expression.

Findings from Western countries

Meta-analyses

There have been more than 30 studies of outcome in schizophrenia for a total of over 1500 patients. A meta-analysis of the relationship between EE and outcome examined the predictive validity of the construct in relapse of schizophrenia, mood disorders and eating disorders (Butzlaff & Hooley, 1998). Using 27 of the studies that focused on outcome in schizophrenia, the authors concluded that EE is a significant and robust predictor of relapse in the disorder. Additional analyses demonstrated that the relationship between EE and relapse was strongest for patients with more chronic schizophrenic illness. Interestingly, although the EE construct is most closely associated with research in schizophrenia, the mean effect sizes for EE for both mood disorders and eating disorders were significantly higher than the mean effect size for schizophrenia.

Butzlaff & Hooley's study agrees with Bebbington & Kuipers' (1994) aggregate analysis of 25 studies involving 1346 patients. This found that for patients living in situations rated as showing high EE (the 'high-EE group'; $n = 705$) the relapse rate was 50%, whereas in the 'low-EE group' ($n = 641$) the rate was 21%. In the majority of the studies, high EE was predictive of relapse in symptoms of schizophrenia 9 months later for both genders. A large amount of face-to-face contact (more than 35 hours per week) with a relative with a high EE score increased the risk of relapse, but in households with a low EE score, high levels of contact appeared to be protective. Both warmth and positive comments were predictive of good outcome. Interestingly, medication had an independent effect on relapse rate, suggesting that it is useful for patients irrespective of the EE status in the family. One of the criticisms of the applications of this construct is that it can 'pathologise' the family or specific relatives who might in reality be struggling hard to cope with a difficult home situation.

The UK

Vaughn & Leff (1976b) studied 43 people with schizophrenia and 32 with 'depressive neurosis' who were living with a spouse or family, and were able to follow up 37 and 30 patients respectively in the two groups. Most of the individuals with depression lived with a spouse. The relapse rate for individuals with schizophrenia in homes with high EE was 50%, compared with 12% in homes with low EE. The authors used seven or more critical comments and/or an emotional over-involvement rating of 4 or 5 to rate EE as high. For individuals with schizophrenia living in high-EE homes, the amount of face-to-face contact also predicted relapse. They reported that more than 35 hours of face-to-face contact was the crucial cut-off. Those whose exposure was more than 35 hours had higher relapse rates (89% v. 57%). When they explored the use of medication they found that in the high-EE families, individuals with schizophrenia who were not on medication were more likely to relapse (78%) than those who were on medication (25%). They argue that low EE and regular medication act as additive factors in reducing the risk of relapse. Of the individuals with depression, 67% of those who had a relative with a critical comments score of more than 2 relapsed, compared with 22% if the score was 0 or 1.

The USA

Using similar methods in a study of a group of people with schizophrenia living with their families in California, Vaughn and her colleagues observed that 33% of Californian families had been rated low EE, compared with 52% in the British sample (Leff & Vaughn, 1985). The Californian families were significantly less likely to make no critical comments than the London families, and hostility was more common in the Californian sample, but there were no cultural differences in emotional over-involvement. Once again, patients in high-EE settings were more likely to relapse (56% compared with 17% for low EE). Also, there was a high relapse rate (68%) among those in the non-medicated high-EE group, whereas there were no relapses at all in the medicated low-EE group.

Australia

In Australia, Vaughan *et al* (1992) recruited 91 individuals with schizophrenia and found that 59% from high-EE families relapsed, compared with 36% from low-EE families. Of those with high contact (more than 35 hours per week), 68% from high-EE families relapsed, compared with only 12% from low-EE families. There was no gender difference and those from high-EE households were still more likely to relapse even when on medication (42%), confirming the previous findings from London and California.

Studies in care homes and residential settings

In an interesting development, Moore *et al* (1992) studied EE in group homes and long-term care settings in the UK and found that high-EE settings were characterised by less tolerance, inappropriate expectations of patient progress and frustration in the key worker. Criticisms focused on embarrassing behaviours and negative symptoms. In a follow-up UK study, Ball *et al* (1992) found that higher discharge rates were possible for patients who were ready to return to low-EE hostels.

The study and identification of EE in the relatives of patients with schizophrenia in different settings have led to the development of intervention strategies with families and carers. The aim of such work is to reduce EE by education and also to reduce the patients' face-to-face contact with high-EE individuals to less than 35 hours per week. Most studies have shown that this is possible. Lowering of the EE can be achieved through relatives' groups and individual and family work. Another innovation is the increasing use of the FMSS discussed above to measure levels of EE in relatives (Magaña *et al*, 1986). However, the authors point out that this method may misclassify a proportion of high-EE individuals as low.

Findings from non-Western countries

India

Levels of EE in families in low- and middle-income countries have been assessed in several studies. The levels as well as the prevalence of the various components of the rating scale vary. For example, tone of voice can play a role in the identification of high EE, but in several cultures speaking loudly is the norm. In a Chandigarh-based substudy of the World Health Organization's study of first-onset schizophrenia, 104 relatives were interviewed for the purposes of assessing EE (Wig *et al*, 1987*b*). Of the three centres studied (Chandigarh, Aarhus and London), the Chandigarh sample reported the lowest ratings on all of the following: mean number of critical comments; proportion of relatives showing hostility; positive remarks; mean score on warmth; and level of parental over-involvement. Compared with the 54% of relatives classified as showing high EE in the two European samples, only 23% were classified as showing high EE in the Chandigarh sample. More than a quarter (29%) of the Chandigarh sample showed hostility but low criticism. The authors concluded that the Chandigarh relatives commonly express both high criticism and high warmth simultaneously. One-year follow-up suggested that the better outcome in people with schizophrenia in Chandigarh may be related to the high proportion of relatives with low EE. In a further report, the authors suggest that expression of anger in the form of hostility is relatively unmodified by cultural factors (Leff et al, 1987).

Egypt

In a study from Egypt, Kamal (1995) recorded high EE in 55% of the families of patients with schizophrenia. It reported that Egyptian patients tolerated higher levels of criticism (including benign criticism) before relapse than have been reported in Western studies. A similar observation was reported by Okasha et al (1994), who found that criticism is an accepted and acceptable component of interpersonal relations in Egyptian culture and that it might well reflect an element of care. It is also possible that criticism and over-involvement are intertwined and that warmth might act as a key protective factor. Emotional over-involvement is seen in the West as pathological because it crosses individuals' boundaries (i.e. it acts against the individual, egocentric position), whereas in other cultures such an approach may be the norm. In sociocentric societies emotional over-involvement is to be expected because the individual is part of the larger kinship group. (Egocentric or individualistic societies are those in which the individual is seen as predominant, whereas in sociocentric or collectivist societies individuals are an integral part of kinship and it is kinship that takes precedence over individuals: see Hofstede, 1984.)

Israel

Similarly, it has been demonstrated that anger is more openly and more immediately expressed in Israel than in Western countries and a failure to express one's anger is perceived as a weakness (Heresco-Levy et al, 1990). Thus, it is likely that both hostility and critical comments seen in the context of anger may result in false-positive rates of high EE. Heresco-Levy et al also emphasise that EE ratings must be adjusted in relation to the normative levels of overt expression of emotions, which vary across cultures. However, changes in levels may be influenced by processes of acculturation if cultural groups move across national and cultural boundaries.

China

In China, Phillips & Xiang (1995) found that, using conventional assessment criteria, over 42% of Chinese relatives of patients with schizophrenia were rated as showing high EE. They observed a non-significant increase in the relative risk of relapse for Chinese patients from high-EE households when compared with low-EE households. They attribute this to a number of factors. First, the effect on the patient of having a high-EE relative may be less significant in Chinese culture than in other cultures. Second, the fact that the role of families (especially small families) in the context of a political system in which an individual's role is as 'dictated' by the state may well act as a protective factor, as this indicates an external locus of control. It might also reflect the diverging attitudes of the community and the individual regarding the individual's autonomy. Thus, there is a change in role expectations which can then be influenced by family EE.

Japan

From Japan, Mino *et al* (1995) reported that, contrary to their expectations of low EE (as Japanese tend not to display emotions readily), 48% of Japanese households were classified as high EE, with criticism being the most common component (39% of households made six or more critical comments).

Minority ethnic groups

The preceding brief overview of international studies suggests that different components of EE have varying prevalence in different countries. However, it is inevitable that different cultures will place differing emphasis on these components, a particularly important factor for psychiatrists working with minority ethnic groups. For example, in the Indian context, mothers are over-involved with their sons and this over-involvement is not necessarily pathological. Similarly, in Jewish settings, critical comments and over-involvement on part of the mother are culture-related and should not be perceived as necessarily pathological.

Mexican American families

In the study of EE in minority ethnic groups, Jenkins' work, especially that dealing with Mexican American families, has been ground-breaking. Highlighting the anthropological and clinical dimensions of individually variable constructions of family worlds in particular cultural contexts, she argues that emotional over-involvement is clinically rated on the basis of affective and behavioural features (that may include self-sacrificing and extremely overprotective behaviours) but that it should not be (Jenkins, 1992). In her study of Mexican Americans she suggests that Mexican culture encourages relatives to display a high degree of involvement in kin affairs.

Among 70 Mexican American families and 109 key relatives, Karno *et al* (1987) found that only 11% of the relatives were rated as showing high EE. Nearly all of the 11% were female and almost all of the patients were male. The authors had adapted the EE rating scales for the Mexican American cultural context and found that the outcome of schizophrenia in their sample was indeed related to family EE, but they caution that the cross-cultural validity of concepts such as over-involvement must be taken into account.

Asian families in the UK

In Birmingham, UK, Hashemi & Cochrane (1999) reported on EE in 60 families (20 British Pakistani, 20 British Sikh and 20 matched White), all of which included a relative with schizophrenia. They observed that 80% of the British Pakistani, 45% of the White and 30% of the British Sikh families exhibited high levels of EE. Emotional over-involvement was significantly higher among the British Pakistani group (55% v. 10% for the British Sikh group). They observed that the modal score for White and Sikh relatives on emotional over-involvement was 1, whereas for British Pakistanis it was 4. Using the conventional rating criteria, the authors found that White patients with high-EE relatives were significantly more likely to relapse than those with low-EE families, whereas for both Asian groups, high EE did not predict relapse. However, raising the cut-off of emotional over-involvement for Pakistani families led to significantly better prediction of relapse.

Although the numbers are small in this study, these differences indicate that using conventional measures of EE across different ethnic groups is fraught with difficulties. The authors draw our attention to similarities between the UK Asian and North Indian groups. They subsequently carried out a population-based normative study for EE and found that Pakistani families in the UK were more likely than White families to be rated as high EE, indicating that components such as emotional over-involvement may be cultural rather than pathogenic traits (Hashemi & Cochrane, 1999).

Studies of different national and minority ethnic groups show that it is essential that normative data on EE in the population are available before clinicians can assess the prevalence and effects of high EE among the families of patients with psychiatric or physical disorders. Expressed emotion is not a simple unidirectional concept and it should not be seen in isolation of intermediary factors such as the role of kinship, attitudes of the family to mental illness, and family and cultural dynamics.

EE and adolescence

The relationship between child psychopathology and parental EE has been reported in children with depression (Schwartz et al, 1990; Asarnow et al, 1993, 2001), obsessive–compulsive disorder (Hibbs et al, 1991), internalising symptoms (Psychogiou et al, 2007), disorganised attachments (Jacobson et al, 2008), disruptive behavioural disorders (Hibbs et al, 1991), conduct problems (Schwartz et al, 1990; Vostanis et al, 1994; Psychogiou et al, 2007), attention-deficit hyperactivity disorder (ADHD; Psychogiou et al, 2007), overall behavioural problems (Baker et al, 2000) and substance misuse (Schwartz et al, 1990). This indicates that there is a clear association, but this is not always replicated (Asarnow et al, 1993, 2001). Asarnow et al (2001) observed that young people (aged 6–18 years) with depression in a mixed in-patient and out-patient sample were significantly more likely to be living in high-EE families than non-depressed peers with ADHD.

Asarnow *et al* (1994) followed up 26 children admitted to hospital for depression and found that high family EE on the FMSS predicted recovery rates 1 year after discharge. However, this finding has not been replicated with older adolescents. In a Canadian sample of 57 adolescent out-patients and in-patients with depression, McCleary & Sanford (2002) found high EE to be associated with the presence of more depressive symptoms at initial assessment but that EE status did not significantly predict recovery at 1-year follow-up. Different study methods might explain this difference.

It has been suggested that high EE in the parents of adolescents with depression might be a non-specific response to the illness and related to the intergenerational conflict associated with normative development in adolescence (Hill *et al*, 2007).

Maternal and paternal EE have been shown to be correlated (Cook *et al*, 1989), although the determinants of EE may be different for mothers and fathers. Hibbs *et al* (1991) found that history of parental psychopathology is associated with high EE in both mothers and fathers. This factor remained the only significant predictor of high EE in fathers, whereas maternal EE was even more strongly related to the presence of childhood psychiatric illness. Previous episodes of psychiatric illness in parents might be related to an inability to manage their children's difficulties, which may in turn be linked to critical attitudes. Thus, there may be interactive factors between parental psychopathology and child behaviour, with increased levels of maternal anxiety (Hirshfeld *et al*, 1997) which need to be explored further.

These findings of reciprocal effects in the relationship between parental EE and child psychopathology suggest that EE may be a state-dependent product of the interactions between parent and offspring, rather than a stable trait of parental communication: 'EE may reflect disturbances in the organisation, emotional climate, and transactional patterns of the entire family, even if it is only measured in a single caregiver' (Miklowitz, 2004: p. 670).

EE and self-harm

Given the prominence otherwise afforded to EE in the literature, it is perhaps surprising that only three published studies have specifically considered EE and its relationship with self-harm. In the only investigation to have employed the CFI, Tarrier *et al* (2004) measured EE in key relatives recruited from a British clinic sample of adults with recent-onset schizophrenia. Overall, there were no significant differences in any dimensions of EE between the families of patients who had made at least one suicide attempt and the families of patients with no history of suicide. There were also no significant correlations between any EE subscales and patients' current suicidal ideation. Nonetheless, on the basis of a path analysis of putative risk factors, the authors concluded that there might be an indirect role for EE in the suicide process. According to this model, negative psychotic symptoms gave rise to critical comments from relatives. Criticism in turn influenced suicidality by increasing hopelessness, as mediated by increased negative self-evaluation. However, the predictive value and generalisability of this model to other populations remain unclear.

In a study involving adolescents, Wedig & Nock (2007) found that high overall parental EE and high parental criticism were significantly related to self-harm, whereas high emotional over-involvement was not. Further work is required to confirm whether these findings are consistent and whether they can be applied cross-culturally.

Implications for management

There is some evidence that outcome in schizophrenia is better in low- and middle-income countries and this has been attributed to low EE (Wig *et al*, 1987*a,b*). However, although outcome has been shown to be variable for different ethnic groups in the UK, data on EE and its relationship to outcome in minority ethnic groups are sparse. Out of the five constructs of EE (critical comments, emotional over-involvement, hostility, warmth and positive remarks) it is the first three that have been shown to predict outcome for people with schizophrenia. Our conjecture is that these three components are helpful, but that they must be seen in the context of culture and kinship and, more important, they must be considered in the context of warmth and positive regard. Most studies neglect to place warmth and positive regard in the protective light that they should be seen in. In some cultures, positive regard is related not to the individual but to his or her social status and background. These social factors may then interact with hostility and emotional over-involvement, blunting their edge in a more significant way.

For the clinician, several significant factors affect the way prognosis or outcome of schizophrenia can be seen in the context of EE. Most importantly, the role of normative cultural data for the general population (who do not have a relative with a mental illness) needs to be understood. If the normative data show high levels of EE then the significance of these components in mental illness has to be seen in that context. The effects of intermediary factors such as explanation of the illness, attitudes towards the illness, the perceived or real autonomy of the individual, the socio- or egocentric status of the individual in the cultural context, role expectations of the individual and the effect of the illness on these roles must be studied further and related to outcome and treatment adherence (Fig. 5.1).

In working with families to reduce EE, clinicians must take into account the role that family therapy may be seen as having in managing psychiatric illness. Some families see family therapy as intrusive and prescriptive, whereas others welcome it in order to learn more about caring for the patient in their midst and managing their illness. In this context, gender and gender-role expectations also play an important part (Box 5.2).

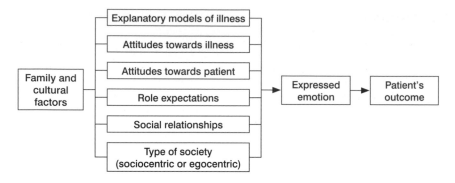

Fig. 5.1 Family and cultural characteristics that may influence patient outcome through expressed emotion.

In some settings, family structures contingent on economic inter-dependence and patriarchal norms are protective. Therefore, the normative prevalence of the components of EE should be rigorously established across different cultural groups and its constructs may have to be given different emphasis depending on cultural context.

Conclusion

Cultural variation in the degree and type of EE has to be studied carefully and understood in order to apply the principles of EE across different cultural groups and settings. Studies across cultures have not provided consistent findings, suggesting that different cultural settings have different normative rates of high EE. Clinicians and researchers must establish baseline normative data before accepting these findings and establishing family interventions.

Box 5.2 Family intervention

In family interventions, clinicians should take the following family characteristics into consideration:

- structure, e.g. nuclear or extended
- significant members
- cultural and social norms
- expectations of the patient
- knowledge of the illness
- acceptance of medical or psychological intervention
- gender-role expectations
- external support systems

References

Asarnow, J. R., Goldstein, M. J., Tompson, M., *et al* (1993) One-year outcomes of depressive disorders in child psychiatric in-patients. Evaluation of the prognostic power of a brief measure of expressed emotion. *Journal of Child Psychology and Psychiatry*, **34**, 129–137.

Asarnow, J. R., Tompson, M., Hamilton, E. B., *et al* (1994) Family expressed emotion, childhood-onset depression, and childhood-onset schizophrenia spectrum disorders. Is expressed emotion a nonspecific correlate of child psychopathology or a specific risk factor for depression? *Journal of Abnormal Child Psychology*, **22**, 129–145.

Asarnow, J. R., Tompson, M., Woo, S., *et al* (2001) Is expressed emotion a specific risk factor for depression or a nonspecific correlate of psychopathology? *Journal of Abnormal Child Psychology*, **29**, 573–583.

Baker B. L., Heller, T. L. & Henker B (2000) Expressed emotion, parenting stress and adjustment in mothers of young children with behavioural problems. *Journal of Child Psychology and Psychiatry*, **41**, 907–915.

Ball, R. E., Moore, E. & Kuipers, L. (1992) Expressed emotion in community care staff. *Social Psychiatry and Psychiatric Epidemiology*, **27**, 35–39.

Beauchaine, T. P., Gatzke-Kopp, L. & Mead, H. K. (2007) Polyvagal theory and developmental psychopathology. Emotion dysregulation and conduct problems from preschool to adolescence. *Biological Psychology*, **74**, 174–184.

Bebbington, P. & Kuipers, E. (1994) The predictive utility of expressed emotion in schizophrenia: an aggregate analysis. *Psychological Medicine*, **24**, 707–712.

Bowlby, J. (1969) *Attachment and Loss. Vol. 1: Attachment*. Hogarth Press.

Brown, G. (1959) Experiences of discharged chronic schizophrenic mental hospital patients in various types of living groups. *Millbank Memorial Fund Quarterly*, **37**, 105–131.

Brown, G. (1985) The discovery of expressed emotion: induction or deduction? In *Expressed Emotion in Families* (eds J. Leff & C. Vaughn), pp. 7–25. Guilford Press.

Brown, G., Carstairs, M. & Topping, G. (1958) Post-hospital adjustment of chronic mental patients. *Lancet*, **ii**, 685–689.

Brown, G. W., Monck, E. M., Carstairs, G. M., *et al* (1962) Influence of family life on the course of schizophrenic illness. *British Journal of Preventative and Social Medicine*, **16**, 55–68.

Brown, G. W., Birley, J. L. T. & Wing, J. K. (1972) Influence of family life on the course of schizophrenic disorders: a replication. *British Journal of Psychiatry*, **121**, 241–258.

Butzlaff, R. L. & Hooley, J. M. (1998) Expressed emotion and psychiatric relapse. A meta-analysis. *Archives of General Psychiatry*, **55**, 547–552.

Calam, R. & Peters, S. (2006) Assessing expressed emotion. Comparing Camberwell Family Interview and Five-minute Speech Sample ratings for mothers of children with behaviour problems. *International Journal of Methods in Psychiatric Research*, **15**, 107–115.

Cook, W. L., Strachan, A. M., Goldstein, M. J., *et al* (1989) Expressed emotion and reciprocal affective relationships in families of disturbed adolescents. *Family Process*, **28**, 337–348.

Halford, W. K. (1991) Beyond expressed emotion. Behavioural assessment of family interaction associated with the course of schizophrenia. *Behavioural Assessment*, **13**, 99–123.

Hashemi, A. H. & Cochrane, R. (1999) Expressed emotion and schizophrenia: a review of studies across cultures. *International Review of Psychiatry*, **11**, 219–224.

Heresco-Levy, U., Greenberg, D. & Dasberg, H. (1990) Family expressed emotion: concepts, dilemmas and Israeli perspectives. *Israeli Journal of Psychiatry and Related Sciences*, **27**, 204–215.

Hibbs, E. D., Hamburger, S. D., Lenane, M., *et al* (1991) Determinants of expressed emotion in families of disturbed and normal children. *Journal of Child Psychology and Psychiatry*, **32**, 757–770.

Hill, N. E., Bromell, L., Tyson, D. F., *et al* (2007) Ecological perspectives on parental influences during adolescence. *Journal of Clinical Child and Adolescent Psychology*, **36**, 367–377.

Hirshfeld, D. R., Biederman, J., Brody, L., *et al* (1997) Expressed emotion toward children with behavioral inhibition. Associations with maternal anxiety disorder. *Journal of the American Academy of Child and Adolescent Psychiatry*, **36**, 910–917.

Hoffman, M. L. (1983) Affective and cognitive processes in moral internalization. In *Social Cognition and Social Development: A Sociocultural Perspective* (eds E. T. Higgins, D. Ruble & W. Hartup), pp. 236–274. Cambridge University Press.

Hofstede, G. (1984) *Culture's Consequences: International Differences in Work-Related Values* (abridged edn). Sage.

Hooley, J. M. (2007) Expressed emotion and relapse of psychopathology. *Annual Review of Clinical Psychology*, **3**, 329–352.

Hooley, J. M. & Parker H. A. (2006) Measuring expressed emotion. An evaluation of the shortcuts. *Journal of Family Psychology*, **20**, 386–396.

Jacobson, C. M., Muehlenkamp, J. J., Miller, A. L., *et al* (2008) Psychiatric impairment among adolescents engaging in different types of deliberate self-harm. *Journal of Clinical Child and Adolescent Psychology*, **37**, 363–375.

Jenkins, J. (1992) Too close for comfort: schizophrenia and emotional over-involvement among Mexicano families. In *Ethnopsychiatry* (ed. A. Gaines), pp. 203–221. SUNY Press.

Kamal, A. (1995) Variables in expressed emotion associated with relapse: a comparison between depressed and schizophrenic samples in an Egyptian community. *Current Psychiatry*, **2**, 211–216.

Karno, M., Jenkins, J., Delaselva, A., *et al* (1987) Expressed emotion and schizophrenic outcome among Mexican American families. *Journal of Nervous and Mental Disease*, **175**, 143–151.

Kuipers, E. (1992) Expressed emotion in 1991. *Social Psychiatry and Psychiatric Epidemiology*, **27**, 1–3.

Kuipers, E. & Bebbington, P. (1988) Expressed emotion research in schizophrenia: theoretical and clinical implications. *Psychological Medicine*, **18**, 893–909.

Kuipers, E. & Bebbington, P. (1990) *Working in Partnership*. Heinemann Medical.

Leeb, B., Hahlweg, K., Goldstein, M. J., *et al* (1991) Cross-national reliability, concurrent validity, and stability of a brief method for assessing expressed emotion. *Psychiatry Research*, **39**, 25–31.

Leff, J. & Vaughn, C. (1985) *Expressed Emotion in Families*. Guilford Press.

Leff, J., Wig, N. N., Ghosh, A., *et al* (1987) Expressed emotion and schizophrenia in north India. III: Influence of relatives' expressed emotion on the course of schizophrenia in Chandigarh. *British Journal of Psychiatry*, **151**, 166–173.

Magaña, A. B., Goldstein, M. J., Karno, M., *et al* (1986) A brief method for assessing expressed emotion in relatives of psychiatric patients. *Psychiatric Research*, **17**, 203–212.

Magaña-Amato, A. B. (1993) *Manual for Coding Expressed Emotion from FMSS*. UCLA Family Project.

McCleary, L. & Sanford, M. (2002) Parental expressed emotion in depressed adolescents: Prediction of clinical course and relationship to comorbid disorders and social functioning. *Journal of Child Psychology and Psychiatry*, **43**, 587–595.

Miklowitz, D. J. (2004) The role of family systems in severe and recurrent psychiatric disorders. A developmental psychopathology view. *Development and Psychopathology*, **16**, 667–688.

Mino, Y., Tanaka, S., Inoue, S., *et al* (1995) Expressed emotion components in families of schizophrenic patients in Japan. *International Journal of Mental Health*, **24**, 38–49.

Moore, E. & Kuipers, E. (1999) The measurement of expressed emotion in relationships between staff and service users. The use of short speech samples. *British Journal of Clinical Psychology*, **38**, 345–356.

Moore, E., Kuipers, E. & Ball, R. (1992) Staff–patient relationships in the care of the long term mentally ill. *Social Psychiatry and Psychiatric Epidemiology*, **27**, 28–34.

Nock, M. K. & Mendes, W. B. (2008) Physiological arousal, distress tolerance, and social problem-solving deficits among adolescent self-injurers. *Journal of Consulting and Clinical Psychology*, **76**, 28–38.

Okasha, A., El-Akabawi, A., Snyder, K., *et al* (1994) Expressed emotion, perceived criticism and relapse in depression: a replication in an Egyptian community. *American Journal of Psychiatry*, **151**, 1001–1005.

Phillips, M. & Xiang, W. (1995) Expressed emotion in mainland China: Chinese families with schizophrenic patients. *International Journal of Mental Health*, **24**, 54–75.

Psychogiou, L., Daley, D. M., Thompson, M. J., *et al* (2007) Mothers' expressed emotion toward their school-aged sons. Associations with child and maternal symptoms of psychopathology. *European Child and Adolescent Psychiatry*, **16**, 458–464.

Rein, Z., Perdereau, F., Curt, F., *et al* (2006) Expressed emotion and anorexia nervosa. The validation of the Five-Minute Speech Sample in reference to the Camberwell Family Interview. *International Journal of Eating Disorders*, **39**, 217–223.

Sabbath, J. (1969) The suicidal adolescent. The expendable child. *American Journal of Child Psychiatry*, **8**, 272–289.

Schwartz, C. E., Dorer, D. J., Beardslee, W. R., *et al* (1990) Maternal expressed emotion and parental affective disorder. Risk for childhood depressive disorder, substance abuse, or conduct disorder. *Journal of Psychiatric Research*, **24**, 231–250.

Speckens, A. E. & Hawton, K. (2005) Social problem solving in adolescents with suicidal behavior. A systematic review. *Suicide and Life-Threatening Behavior*, **35**, 365–387.

Tarrier, N., Barrowclough, C., Andrews, B., *et al* (2004) Risk of non-fatal suicide ideation and behaviour in recent onset schizophrenia. The influence of clinical, social, self-esteem and demographic factors. *Social Psychiatry and Psychiatric Epidemiology*, **39**, 927–937.

Tulloch, A., Blizzard, L. & Pinkus, Z. (1997) Adolescent-parent communication in self-harm. *Journal of Adolescent Health*, **21**, 267–275.

Vaughan, K., Doyle, M., McConaghy, N., *et al* (1992) The relationship between relative's expressed emotion and schizophrenic relapse: an Australian replication. *Social Psychiatry and Psychiatric Epidemiology*, **27**, 10–15.

Vaughn, C. & Leff, J. (1976*a*) The measurement of expressed emotion in the families of psychiatric patients. *British Journal of Social and Clinical Psychology*, **15**, 157–165.

Vaughn, C. E. & Leff, J. P. (1976*b*) The influence of family and social factors on the course of psychiatric illness. A comparison of schizophrenic and depressed neurotic patients. *British Journal of Psychiatry*, **129**, 125–137.

Vostanis, P., Nicholls, J. & Harrington, R. (1994) Maternal expressed emotion in conduct and emotional disorders of childhood. *Journal of Child Psychology and Psychiatry*, **35**, 365–376.

Wearden, A. J., Tarrier, N., Barrowclough, C., *et al* (2000) A review of expressed emotion research in health care. *Clinical Psychology Review*, **20**, 633–666.

Wedig, M. M. & Nock, M. K. (2007) Parental expressed emotion and adolescent self-injury. *Journal of the American Academy of Child and Adolescent Psychiatry*, **46**, 1171–1178.

Wig, N. N., Menon, D. K., Bedi, H., *et al* (1987*a*) Expressed emotion and schizophrenia in north India. I: Cross-cultural transfer of ratings of relatives' expressed emotion. *British Journal of Psychiatry*, **151**, 156–160.

Wig, N. N., Menon, D. K., Bedi, H., *et al* (1987*b*) Expressed emotion and schizophrenia in north India. II: Distribution of expressed emotion components among relatives of schizophrenic patients in Aarhus and Chandigarh. *British Journal of Psychiatry*, **151**, 160–165.

Yates, T. M. (2004) The developmental psychopathology of self-injurious behavior. Compensatory regulation in posttraumatic adaptation. *Clinical Psychology Review*, **24**, 35–74.

CHAPTER 6

Mental illness in Black and Asian ethnic minorities: care pathways and outcomes

Kamaldeep Bhui and Dinesh Bhugra

Summary This chapter summarises the research literature on care pathways for Black and minority ethnic groups, based on a series of papers and reviews from 1999 onwards. The work contributed to the King's Fund report on London's mental health and set the foundations for important systematic reviews of the evidence and empirical studies of care pathways. Despite those initiatives, there is not much evidence that the picture is dramatically different from when the review was undertaken. Although much work is now underway on this issue, unlike when we first wrote on it for *Advances in Psychiatric Treatment* in 2002, much more service development and focused research is necessary. The chapter ends with an update on the Enhancing Pathways into Care (EPIC) project that was part of actions in the Delivering Race Equality policy, and reflections on the public health vision in mental health policy.

A substantial body of research indicates that, for people from Black and Asian[1] ethnic minorities, access to, use of and treatments prescribed by mental health services differ from those for White people (Lloyd & Moodley, 1992; for a review see Bhui, 1997). Pathways to mental healthcare are important, and the widely varying pathways taken in various societies may reflect many factors: the attractiveness and cultural appropriateness of services; attitudes towards services; previous experiences; and culturally defined lay referral systems (Goldberg, 1999). Contact with mental health services may be imposed on the individual, but people who choose to engage with services usually do so only if they think that their changed state of functioning is health-related and potentially remediable through them. In such cases, they will contact whoever they perceive to be the most

---

1. We use 'Asian' to refer to people originating from the Indian subcontinent and 'Black' to include both African–Caribbeans and Africans. The difficulties in defining and using these terms have been discussed elsewhere (Bhui, 2001).

appropriate carer, and these individuals are often not part of a national healthcare network.

The care pathway approach focuses on the point of access to care and the integration of care by culturally diverse carers. For example, if for African–Caribbean men in crisis the most common point of access to mental health services is through the police and the criminal justice system rather than through their general practitioner (GP), then the challenge is to explore the reasons for this at the interface of these agencies. Carers include the popular and folk sectors of healthcare provision as well as standard primary and secondary care services and the voluntary sector. Once the range of perceived carers for a cultural group is known, these can be considered as potential sites of case identification and intervention.

The development of a model for people in Black and Asian minority ethnic groups requires that these other access points be taken into consideration.

Goldberg & Huxley's model

Goldberg & Huxley (1980) described different levels of engagement with healthcare within community, primary and in-patient services. To reach specialist care a patient needs to pass through a series of referral filters. This model has been extremely useful, not only in understanding epidemiological findings and pathways into psychiatric care, but also as the starting point for evaluating the needs of patients with mental illness.

As UK healthcare services evolved, the model was modified. Commander *et al* (1997) added a Mental Health Act level. Moodley & Perkins (1991) tried to conceptualise the pathways taken by African–Caribbean people admitted to in-patient care and found that the police and hospital accident and emergency departments are important. The model shown in Fig. 6.1 is based on Goldberg & Huxley's original, but it includes several additional stages to reflect the appraisal, expression and presentation of distress in primary care, as well as the appraisal of community distress. It also shows the stages at which the care pathway could be strengthened by the involvement of the voluntary sector, traditional healers, specialist services or liaison with psychiatrists.

The research data that we cite relating to the experiences of patients from ethnic minorities of the care pathway are limited by the focus of the studies cited, which included mainly in-patient and psychiatric services and some primary care sites.

Community-level distress and the lay referral system

Different societies have different patterns of help-seeking, and some countries involve traditional healers in their healthcare systems (Goldberg, 1999). Indeed, Kleinman (1980) has described folk and popular sectors of

FORENSIC SERVICES

Level 6

*6b Forensic services (referral from criminal justice system)

*6a Forensic services (referral from psychiatric services)

Filter 4

PSYCHIATRIC SERVICES

Level 5

*5b In-patient admission (referral from criminal justice system or police)[†]

*5a In-patient admission (referral from psychiatric services or GP)[†]

Level 4

4b Out-patient assessment completed, leading to in-patient or out-patient treatment or discharge[†]

4a Out-patient assessment offered

Filter 3

ACTION BY GENERAL PRACTITIONER

Level 3

3d Detection: referral to specialist services

3c Detection: active management in primary care[†]

3b Detection: non-active management and non-referral[†]

3a Non-detection (although a disorder is present)

Filter 2

PRESENTATION TO GENERAL PRACTITIONER

Level 2

2b Presentation to GP after patient appraisal where help-seeking from GP was considered appropriate[†]

2a Presentation to GP, but not for subjective distress

Filter 1

APPRAISAL

Level 1

1b Community distress:
 Appraisal as needing help from GP[†]
 Appraisal as needing help from another carer[†]

1a Community distress:
 Appraisal as not needing help

*Patients presenting at these levels may be referred under a section of the Mental Health Act.
[†]Stages at which the care pathway could be augmented by involvement of voluntary sector, traditional healers, specialist services or liaison with psychiatrists.

Fig. 6.1 Care pathways: expansion of the Goldberg & Huxley (1980) model to address accessibility and service use for Black and Asian ethnic minorities.

healthcare as dominant in most societies. It might be imagined that similar patterns would emerge in immigrant communities in the UK, subject to the availability of alternative healers and the persistence of traditional pre-immigration health beliefs and illness behaviour. However, mental health professionals attend to their significance infrequently and such domains are rarely researched.

Gray (1999) has argued that the voluntary sector is the most appropriate and least stigmatising source of help for Black patients, but the voluntary sector rarely figures in the strategic development of mental health services for Black and Asian patients in the UK. The inclusion of the voluntary sector in the pathway model, together with health promotion, schools, places of worship and traditional healers, leads to a more complex but comprehensive model, matching more closely the help-seeking narratives of Black and Asian people. Another variable that is often ignored within this model is the influence of the gender of individuals on help-seeking.

Research data

Access to and use of services from community-level distress

- Cole *et al* (1995) demonstrated that for first-episode psychosis in the London borough of Haringey, compulsory admission, admission under section 136 of the Mental health Act 1983, first contact with services other than healthcare, and no GP involvement were each associated with being single rather than with ethnic group. Also, compulsory admission, admission under section 136 and police rather than GP involvement were associated with not having a supportive friend or relative. Compulsory admission was also associated with having a family of origin living outside of London.
- Koffman *et al* (1997) found that more Black patients admitted to psychiatric wards were not registered with a GP than in the White and Asian comparison group.
- Harrison *et al* (1988) records that 40% of African–Caribbeans had made contact with some helping agency in the week preceding admission, compared with 2% of the general population.
- Results from the ÆSOP study, looking into data from two UK centres over a 2-year period, suggest that GP referral to mental health services are less frequent for African–Caribbean and Black African patients than for White patients (Morgan *et al*, 2005a).

Primary care consultation rates

- Gillam *et al* (1989) studied consultation patterns in seven general practices in the London borough of Brent. Male Asians had substantially higher standardised patient consultation ratios than did other ethnic groups. Consultations for anxiety and depression were lower in all immigrant groups (72–76% of the rate for the White comparison group). White British patients more often left the surgery with a repeat appointment, prescription or sickness certificate.
- Lloyd & St Louis (1996) interviewed matched samples of Black and White women attending a GP surgery in south London. They reported that the Black women were less likely to know what they wanted from their GP (25% of the White rate), less likely to make multiple requests of their GP (23% of the White rate) and more likely to leave

a primary care consultation without a follow-up appointment. During the follow-up year, none of the White patients self-referred to accident and emergency departments, but 5% of the Black patients did. Black African women consulted their GP less frequently than other women. The Black patients were less satisfied with the consultation than the White patients, especially the Black Africans, who also were the most distressed and attended the least often.

Primary care: presentation, detection and referral to specialist services

Asians present frequently in primary care, but not with mental disorder (Gillam *et al*, 1989). Even if they do not present with physical symptoms, a significant proportion are liable to be given a physical diagnosis (Wilson & MacCarthy, 1994). Commander *et al* (1997) report that Black patients are the least likely to be recognised as having mental disorder in primary care (White patients are the most likely) and the most likely to be referred to specialist services if mental disorders are detected (Asians are the least likely to be referred). However, the findings are not consistent. Comparison of African–Caribbean and White patients by Shaw *et al* (1999) suggests that, for common mental disorders, there are few differences in detection.

It is likely that variations in local service configurations and professional practice influence detection rates as much as do the cultural origins of the patient. Asian GPs are reported to be poorer detectors of morbidity among Asian patients (Odell *et al*, 1997). Difficulties of assessment by Asian GPs may not be restricted to Asian patients (Bhui *et al*, 2001) and may reflect the fact that the cultural views of practitioners can influence the assessment and clinical management of mental disorders (Patel, 1999). The health professional's own explanatory model of illness and its influence on their practice have not received adequate attention. It is widely assumed that the uniformity of medical training across cultures leads to uniformity of skills and values regarding illness. However, in the area of mental illness there is more variation in explanatory models than might be the case with disorders that have demonstrable physical pathologies and abnormalities. Nevertheless, this explanation alone does not account for the variation in clinical management of different ethnic groups consulting the same pool of GPs. Furthermore, patients' cultural appraisal of their problems, and perhaps their preferred interventions, may differ from those of their primary care physicians, irrespective of the cultural origins of either the professionals or the patients.

Research data

Detection and referral of psychiatric morbidity

- Responses on the General Health Questionnaire (GHQ) recorded by Lloyd & St Louis (1996) in their south London study showed no statistically significant differences in the means and distributions of GHQ scores when comparing Black with White women, although within the Black group Black African women had higher scores. There were differences between scores on the Clinical Interview Schedule: GPs noted psychiatric problems in 26% of Black women and 34% of White women, all of whom had scored as cases on the GHQ.

- Li *et al* (1994) report that in Tower Hamlets (east London), 2.2% of all attendees had needs that could not be met within the district services, and that the rate of detection of conspicuous morbidity in Black patients was almost half that for White patients.
- Burnett *et al* (1999) reported that African–Caribbean people with schizophrenia were less likely than White people to have had a GP referral to mental health services.
- We found no differences in rates of detection of common mental disorders by Asian GPs in Punjabi Asian and White English patients (Bhui *et al*, 2001).

Assessment and admission in general adult services

Several authors have agreed that Black people are overrepresented in psychiatric hospitals and that their need for psychiatric help is revealed through crisis services and the Mental Health Act more often than for their White counterparts (Bhui, 1997). For example, Davies *et al* (1996) found that Mental Health Act detention for assessment and treatment was more common among Black and Asian ethnic minorities. This applied to all diagnoses and prevalent cases of psychosis. However, ethnic origin is not the only factor. For example, Black women in Hammersmith and Fulham (west London) are reported to have lower compulsory admission rates than White women, whereas in Southwark (south-east London), Black women have higher rates (Bebbington *et al*, 1991).

Falkowski *et al* (1990) showed that Black people were overrepresented among detained absconders from in-patient units. Although Black people often find services unattractive, it is likely that detained patients are more likely to perceive them as unhelpful (Parkman *et al*, 1997).

Several studies report that admission of Black patients to in-patient and forensic care more frequently follows referral from criminal justice agencies or the police. Moodley & Perkins (1991), however, report that routes into care for African–Caribbean people were not statistically significantly different from those for Whites. Cole *et al* (1995) have shown that, for all cultural groups, admission through the police is more likely if the patient does not have a confidant or GP to support them. The greater social isolation of those admitted with schizophrenia may explain their propensity to be admitted late, having failed to notice themselves to be ill.

These and subsequent data (Morgan *et al*, 2004, 2005b; Singh *et al*, 2007) suggest that stronger links with the police, courts and prisons are required. All may assist in the diversion of those with mental illness, where this is appropriate, and especially where known patients have fallen out of care and are at risk of ending up in forensic institutions (Bhui *et al*, 1998; Coid *et al*, 2000). A rapid access point for families, so that crises can be addressed quickly, is also essential. A further focus of future analysis must be decision-making processes around formal assessments. These must include consideration of attractive, safe and clinically effective alternatives to in-patient admission.

Research data

Admission rates and circumstances

- Studies in London have shown that Mental Health Act admission rates are higher for African–Caribbeans than for comparable samples of White and other ethnic groups (Bagley, 1971; Bebbington *et al*, 1991; Moodley & Perkins, 1991; Wessely *et al*, 1991; King *et al*, 1994; Callan, 1996; Davies *et al*, 1996). The magnitude of the excess varies in different parts of the city and is likely to depend on both the population and the configuration of the local service (Bebbington *et al*, 1991). A meta-analysis of 12 papers revealed that, compared with White patients, Black patients had a significantly increased risk of compulsory admission, with a pooled odds ratio of 4.31 (Bhui *et al*, 2003).

- Rates of admission with schizophrenia and affective psychoses for African–Caribbeans are 3–13 times the rates for White patients (Bebbington *et al*, 1991; Moodley & Perkins, 1991; King *et al*, 1994; van Os *et al*, 1996).

- Recent Department of Health 'experimental' data suggest continued higher rates of admission for 'mixed and Black' (18%) and 'Black British' (22%) groups; the admission rate for 'all ethnic groups' is just under 10% (Health and Social Care Information Centre, 2008).

- Once admitted, young African–Caribbean patients were more likely to be readmitted. First admissions were more likely to be young men (under 30 years) (Glover, 1989).

- Davies *et al* (1996) scrutinised hospital and community contact data relating to all prevalent cases of psychosis in London and concluded that 70% of the Black Caribbean group, 69% of the Black African group and 50% of the White group had previously been detained under the provisions of the Mental Health Act.

- The 'Count me in' annual national census of in-patients in mental health hospitals and facilities in England and Wales (Care Quality Commission, 2010) undertaken since 2005 has continued to show that minority ethnic patients are still over-represented among in-patients.

- Callan (1996) reported that African–Caribbeans had shorter readmissions than a British-born White control group, and hypothesised that a milder course exists among African–Caribbeans.

- Data from the ÆSOP study suggests that Black people also have a shorter duration of untreated psychosis (DUP). Contrary to what is commonly assumed, this study suggested that Black patients did not experience greater delay in receiving treatment (Morgan *et al*, 2006).

Forensic services

African–Caribbean men are known to be overrepresented in secure units, among remand populations and in sentenced prison populations. Coid *et al* (2000) showed that rates for first admissions to forensic units for half of England and Wales were 5.6 times higher among Black men than among White men; rates for Asian men were half those for White men. Black women's admission rates were 2.9 times higher than those of White women. Asian women had admission rates that were one-third those of White women. Patterns of offending and disposal by courts are known to vary by ethnic group (Bhui *et al*, 1998). One explanation is a lack of intervention by community mental health services early in the course of an illness (Bhui *et al*, 1998; Coid *et al*, 2000). Other possible explanations are that African–Caribbeans are actually more violent when they present with mental health problems, or that they are perceived to be so. Another explanation is failure to recognise signs of illness (by patient, family, GP or psychiatrist) until they are more severe.

The excess of contact with the criminal justice system can also result from the individual's dissatisfaction with mental health services (Parkman *et al*, 1997), or the professional's appraisal of the distress as not needing treatment (Moodley & Perkins, 1991). Another possible explanation is that Black people are less likely than White people to be actively managed and retained in primary care services. If they become distressed and their distress is not understood, it is likely to be labelled 'psychiatric' and they are referred on to specialist services (Commander *et al*, 1997).

We must conclude that either African–Caribbean groups are no different in their presentation and the risks posed but that they are assessed to carry higher risks associated with distress, or that African–Caribbeans, when distressed and developing psychoses, do present with more violence.

Research data

Prevalence

- Among patients admitted to secure units in England and Wales, roughly 20% were African–Caribbean (Jones & Berry, 1986; Coid *et al*, 2000).
- Among sentenced prisoners, the prevalence of mental illness was 6% for African–Caribbeans and 2% for the White population (Maden *et al*, 1992).

- In a sample of remanded mentally disordered offenders, 17.6% of White, 68.8% of Black Caribbean, 43.8% of Black African, 58.3% of Black British and 42.1% of other 'non-White' ethnic groups had a diagnosis of schizophrenia (Bhui *et al*, 1998). Banerjee *et al* (1995) reported a higher prevalence (51%) of schizophrenia among Black than White remanded men who were transferred to hospitals compared with the remand population as a whole. A survey examining decisions made about individuals remanded on the basis of psychiatric reports demonstrated that 37% of White defendants were granted bail and only 13% of Black defendants (National Association for the Care and Resettlement of Offenders, 1990).
- In certain areas of the UK, Black men are more likely to receive a custodial sentence than their White counterparts (National Association for the Care and Resettlement of Offenders, 1989). Black defendants received a smaller range of disposals after court appearance; three-quarters of Black defendants and half of White defendants have had previous contact with psychiatric services (National Association for the Care and Resettlement of Offenders, 1990).
- Data from the ÆSOP study suggested that African–Caribbean and Black African patients were more likely to be referred through the criminal justice system (Morgan *et al*, 2005*a*).

The effect of cultural variations on assessment

Non-recognition of mental illness by healthcare professionals may reflect a mismatch between the patient's cultural expression of distress and the signs and symptoms sought by the clinician as manifestations of particular diagnostic syndromes: for example, the visual hallucinations reported to be more common among West African patients with schizophrenia (Ndetei & Vadher, 1984). Conversely, culturally sanctioned and acceptable distress experiences may attract pathological explanations from professionals. First-rank symptoms may not have the same diagnostic significance across cultures (Chandrasena, 1987; Hickling *et al*, 1999). What psychiatrists call 'paranoid beliefs' have culturally sanctioned value among African and West Indian groups, and the assignation of pathological significance to them may therefore be flawed (Ndetei & Vadher, 1984). Paranoia and beliefs with religious content are more common among West Indians and West Africans (Littlewood & Lipsedge, 1984; Ndetei & Vadher, 1984). A study of lay perceptions of mental health problems found Bangladeshi participants to be less likely to view suspiciousness and hallucinatory behaviour as indicative of mental illness, and African–Caribbean participants to be less likely to view unusual thought content as a symptom (Pote & Orrell, 2002).

A systematic review of ethnic variations in care pathways concluded that pathways to specialist services for Black patients were more complex and more often involved crisis routes of entry (Bhui *et al*, 2003).

Box 6.1   Good practice in assessment

- Be aware of your own world view and that of your patients and their carers
- Take into account patients' explanatory models of their illness
- Assess patients' cultural appraisal of their problems
- Be aware of racialism in yourself and your patients

The care pathways approach focuses on service levels but it is professional practice that determines the outcome of consultations. Individual attitudes, professional skills and cultural awareness of norms are all influential in the patient's passage through filters and in treatment decisions (Box 6.1).

A model of engagement for African–Caribbean patients

It seems that African–Caribbean groups are the least satisfied with secure services, but are the most likely to be held in them. Parkman *et al* (1997) demonstrated that young Black men's dissatisfaction with in-patient services was directly proportional to the amount of contact they had had with such services. They describe this as the ratchet effect of consecutive contacts. This, coupled with non-detection of disorders by GPs and difficulty in managing disorders in primary care settings, increases the likelihood that such patients in crisis will come into contact with non-health-related agencies (police or forensic services).

General practitioners' diagnostic skills, knowledge about mental health, early management of mental illness and timely referral to hospital are all potential focuses for primary care intervention.

Like all patients, African–Caribbean patients too may benefit from, and prefer, management in primary care settings. This may in part be because of the less stigmatising public attitudes towards primary care than towards psychiatric hospitals. Some argue that the mental health services the Black community wants are not available, and the ones available are not particularly acceptable or helpful to that community. A trial assessing the effect on insight of cognitive–behavioural therapy for schizophrenia found that the drop-out rate for African–Caribbean and Black African participants was statistically significantly higher than for other participants. The study also found that the Black Caribbean group showed smaller change in insight (Rathod *et al*, 2005). Data on what is acceptable are less clear. Some have argued that a 'circle of fear' is responsible for the poor treatment of Black communities. Potentially fuelled by misconceptions, prejudice and racism, Black patients are mistrusting of services, while staff are wary of Black patients, not knowing how to respond. A 'systemic change' is needed, to break the cycle (Keating & Robertson, 2004).

A pathway solution here might be to improve illness recognition rates in African–Caribbean and Black African people and also to increase the skills mix of the primary care team to enable engagement with these individuals and active management of their illnesses in primary care. Another solution might be to target educational campaigns and relapse prevention strategies at the patients and their communities. Alternatively, the fundamental nature of services might be changed towards home-based care or early intervention (i.e. services delivered in public health settings rather than in psychiatric units). Such options may in themselves improve engagement, but GP surgeries and psychiatric clinics must take care to avoid the institutionalised attitudes and practices that can flourish in psychiatric hospital environments. Where competent risk assessment permits it, totally different management strategies involving family, neighbours or voluntary sector agencies might be considered as more culturally appropriate.

Partnerships between the primary care team and other pathway agencies

A study examining the incidence and outcome of schizophrenia in west London found that only 1 in 36 African–Caribbean patients with schizophrenia presented through their GPs (Bhugra *et al*, 1997). Healthcare systems in the UK are not organised in accordance with the preferred pattern of help-seeking, and do not readily lend themselves to early intervention. To ensure early intervention for African–Caribbean patients who develop a new mental illness or who relapse, there needs to be close liaison between community mental health teams and primary care teams, with agreed priority given to high-risk groups. Persistent states of distress in the absence of timely intervention can culminate in presentation in crisis, and presentation only when disorders are severe and patients' social networks and housing conditions are already compromised. Recovery times will then be longer and greater involvement of psychiatric and social services will be required to re-establish the necessary conditions for recovery and relapse prevention. If primary care teams were to become involved at an earlier stage, identifying symptoms of relapse and liaising with non-statutory agencies with which African–Caribbeans have regular contact, then this might enable early intervention. Furthermore, if culturally attractive services are identified as partners in care provision, the total package of care offered to Black and Asian people would be likely to be more attractive and more successful in engaging them in the long term (Box 6.2).

Psychiatrists can play a lead role in education and liaison with partners in care, including GPs, housing workers and voluntary agencies, that is especially useful if there is concern about unusual mental states. However, it assumes that the psychiatrist is confident that they can assess complex mental states in patients from Black and Asian ethnic minorities and that they recognise the limitations of their own skills and competencies.

Box 6.2 Primary care and other agencies

- The clinician must take the lead in identifying and maintaining liaison with primary care and other agencies
- The consultation model should ensure regular liaison with the primary care team
- Community mental health team (CMHT) members should be represented in the primary care consultation
- Where appropriate, CMHTs and trusts should use 'culture brokers' (healthcare workers trained to work with communities that have significant minority ethnic populations)
- Psychiatrists should support and educate primary care teams to engage with patients with special needs

---

Places of worship, leisure clubs, entertainment venues and culturally attractive independent services may all act as points of first contact. In one UK study, half of the Black users interviewed stated their belief that their treatment and diagnosis would (or might) have been different had they been in contact with a member of staff who understood their experiences as a Black person (a quarter felt that it would have made no difference) (Robertson *et al*, 2000).

Enhancing Pathways Into Care (EPIC)

The Enhancing Pathways Into Care (EPIC) project was designed to facilitate and evaluate change management processes within mental healthcare services. It was the first systematic assessment in the UK of a service development intervention to enhance pathways into, out of and through care, for people of Black and minority ethnic (BME) heritage. The work fills gaps in knowledge about what does and does not work in service development for BME groups; it focuses on clinical leadership to mobilise organisational systems and support the Darzi recommendations (Professor the Lord Darzi of Denham 2008). The aim was to innovate in service development to enhance the quality and effectiveness of care for people from BME groups. EPIC involved four pathways projects undertaken by the local EPIC clinical teams at four clinical sites: Easington, Sheffield, Manchester and Birmingham. Between January 2006 and March 2007 each site received coordinated support and consultancy from the national EPIC team; this provided clinical leadership and the best international research knowledge and service development skills to transform local service delivery. The four sites were part of a national learning collaborative that met at 3-month intervals. The reports and findings of the EPIC project can be found at www.wolfson.qmul.ac.uk/psychiatry/epic and are published as part of a special edition of the *International Review of Psychiatry* in 2009 (http://informahealthcare.com/toc/irp/21/5.)

Enhancing Pathways Into Care showed that substantial links with the community and with the public are essential to ensure recovery, perhaps making way for new policy that emphasises public mental health and ethnic inequalities in populations as well as in care experiences in services. How to ensure that the focus on service improvement is sustained with a policy centring on prevention and health promotion is a challenge, as is the notion that inequalities in care experiences can be eradicated by preventing inequalities in health status from occurring.

Conclusion

Goldberg & Huxley's (1980) original model is no longer sufficiently comprehensive. It requires inclusion of a wider range of agencies. Yet, the exact numbers of people passing through each level are less well described. Future research should explore the levels that we have included and the ease or resistance with which people pass from one level to another. Passage through the filter should be seen as a dynamic two-way process, and alternatives to management in psychiatric environments should be encouraged wherever possible. It is likely that patients with acute emergency presentations cannot be safely managed outside a skilled hospital environment. However, if hospitals are impoverished in terms of staffing, quality of décor, personal space and time to build therapeutic relationships, this will compound any distrust of psychiatric services.

The cultural authenticity of the voluntary and independent sectors may be essential for an engaging service, and primary care teams might usefully liaise with these sectors to maximise the opportunity to manage mental illness without referral to specialist services.

The pathways approach offers a framework within which health service research, service development and the delivery of quality care may be organised.

References

Bagley, C. (1971) The social aetiology of schizophrenia in inpatient groups. *International Journal of Social Psychiatry*, **17**, 292–304.

Banerjee, S., O'Neill-Byrne, K., Exworthy, T., *et al* (1995) The Belmarsh Scheme. A prospective study of the transfer of mentally disordered remand prisoners from prisons to psychiatric units. *British Journal of Psychiatry*, **166**, 802–805.

Bebbington, P. E., Feeney, S. T., Flannigan, C. B., *et al* (1991) Inner London collaborative audit of admissions in two health districts. II: Ethnicity and the use of the Mental Health Act. *British Journal of Psychiatry*, **165**, 743–749.

Bhugra, D., Leff, J., Mallet, R., *et al* (1997) Inception rates and one year outcome of schizophrenia in west London. *Psychological Medicine*, **27**, 791–798.

Bhui, K. (1997) London's ethnic minorities and the provision of mental health services. In *London's Mental Health* (eds S. Johnson, R. Ramsay, G. Thornicroft, *et al*). King's Fund.

Bhui, K. (2001) Epidemiology and social issues. In *Psychiatry in Multicultural Britain* (eds D. Bhugra & R. Cochrane), pp. 49–74. Gaskell.

Bhui, K., Brown, R., Hardie, T., *et al* (1998) African–Caribbean men remanded to Brixton prison. Psychiatric and forensic characteristics and outcome of final court appearance. *British Journal of Psychiatry*, **172**, 337–344.

Bhui, K., Brown, R., Bhugra, D., *et al* (2001) Common mental disorders among Punjabi and English subjects in primary care. Prevalence, detection of morbidity and pathways into care. *Psychological Medicine*, **81**, 815–825.

Bhui, K., Stansfield, S., Hull, S., *et al* (2003) Ethnic variations in pathways to and use of mental health services in the UK. A systematic review. *British Journal of Psychiatry*, **182**, 105–116.

Burnett, R., Mallett, R., Bhugra, D., *et al* (1999) The first contact of patients with schizophrenia with psychiatric services: social factors and pathways to care in a multi-ethnic population. *Psychological Medicine*, **29**, 475–483.

Callan, A. (1996) Schizophrenia in Afro-Caribbean immigrants. *Journal of the Royal Society of Medicine*, **89**, 253–256.

Care Quality Commission (2010) 'Count me in' census. CQC (http://www.cqc.org.uk/guidanceforprofessionals/healthcare/allhealthcarestaff/countmeincensus.cfm).

Chandrasena, R. (1987) Schneider's first-rank symptoms: an international and interethnic comparative study. *Acta Psychiatrica Scandinavica*, **76**, 574–578.

Coid, J. W., Kahtan, N., Gault, S., *et al* (2000) Ethnic differences in admissions to secure forensic psychiatry services. *British Journal of Psychiatry*, **177**, 241–247.

Cole, E., Leavey, G., King, A., *et al* (1995) Pathways to care for patients with a first episode of psychosis. A comparison of ethnic groups. *British Journal of Psychiatry*, **167**, 770–776.

Commander, M. J., Sashi Dharan, S. P., Odell, S. M., *et al* (1997) Access to mental health care in an inner-city health district. I: Pathways into and within specialist psychiatric services. *British Journal of Psychiatry*, **170**, 312–316.

Davies, S., Thornicroft, G., Lease, M., *et al* (1996) Ethnic differences in risk of compulsory psychiatric admission among representative cases of psychosis in London. *BMJ*, **312**, 533–537.

Falkowski, J., Watts, V., Falkowski, W., *et al* (1990) Patients leaving hospital without the knowledge or permission of staff – absconding. *British Journal of Psychiatry*, **156**, 488–490.

Gillam, S., Jarman, B., White, P., *et al* (1989) Ethnic differences in consultation rates in urban general practice. *BMJ*, **299**, 953–957.

Glover, G. (1989) The pattern of psychiatric admissions of Caribbean born immigrants in London. *Social Psychiatry and Psychiatric Epidemiology*, **24**, 49–56.

Goldberg, D. (1999) Cultural aspects of mental disorder in primary care. In *Ethnicity: An Agenda for Mental Health* (eds D. Bhugra & V. Bahl), pp. 23–28. Gaskell.

Goldberg, D. & Huxley, P. (1980) *Mental Illness in the Community*. Tavistock.

Gray, P. (1999) Voluntary organisations. In *Ethnicity: An Agenda for Mental Health* (eds D. Bhugra & V. Bahl), pp. 202–210. Gaskell.

Harrison, G., Owens, D., Holton, A., *et al* (1988) A prospective study of severe mental disorder in Afro-Caribbean people. *Psychological Medicine*, **18**, 643–657.

Health and Social Care Information Centre (2008) *Mental Health Bulletin: First Report and Experimental Statistics from Mental Health Minimum Dataset (MHMDS) Annual Returns, 2003–2007*. NHS Information Centre.

Hickling, F. W., McKenzie, K., Mullen, R., *et al* (1999) A Jamaican psychiatrist evaluates diagnoses at a London psychiatric hospital. *British Journal of Psychiatry*, **175**, 283–285.

Jones, G. & Berry, M. (1986) Regional secure units: the emerging picture. In *Current Issues in Clinical Psychology. IV* (ed. G. Edwards). Plenum Press.

Keating, F. & Robertson, D. (2004) Fear, black people and mental illness: a vicious circle? *Health and Social Care in the Community*, **12**, 439–447.

King, M., Coker, E., Leavey, G., *et al* (1994) Incidence of psychotic illness in a comparison of ethnic groups. *BMJ*, **309**, 1115–1119.

Kleinman, A. (1980) *Patients and Their Healers in the Context of Culture*. University of California Press.

Koffman, J., Fulop, N. J., Pashley, D., *et al* (1997) Ethnicity and use of acute psychiatric beds: one-day survey in north and south Thames regions. *British Journal of Psychiatry*, **171**, 238–241.

Li, P., Jones, I. & Richards, J. (1994) The collection of general practice data for psychiatric service contracts. *Journal of Public Health Medicine*, **16**, 87–92.

Littlewood, R. & Lipsedge, M. (1984) *Aliens and Alienists*. Unwin.

Lloyd, K. & St Louis, L. (1996) Common mental disorders among Africans and Caribbeans. In *Ethnicity: An Agenda for Mental Health* (eds D. Bhugra & V. Bhal), pp. 60–69. Gaskell.

Lloyd, P. & Moodley, P. (1992) Psychotropic medication and ethnicity: an inpatient survey. *Social Psychiatry and Psychiatric Epidemiology*, **27**, 95–101.

Maden, A., Swinton, M. & Gunn, J. (1992) The ethnic origins of women serving a prison sentence. *British Journal of Criminology*, **32**, 218–221.

Moodley, P. & Perkins, R. (1991) Routes to psychiatric inpatient care in an inner London borough. *Social Psychiatry and Psychiatric Epidemiology*, **26**, 47–51.

Morgan, C., Mallett, R., Hutchinson, G., *et al* (2004) Negative pathways to psychiatric care and ethnicity: the bridge between social science and psychiatry. *Social Science and Medicine*, **58**, 739–752.

Morgan, C., Mallet, R., Hutchinson, G., *et al* (2005a) Pathways to care and ethnicity. 2: Source of referral and help-seeking. Report from ÆSOP study. *British Journal of Psychiatry*, **186**, 290–296.

Morgan, C., Mallett, R., Hutchinson, G., *et al* (2005b) Pathways to care and ethnicity. 1: Sample characteristics and compulsory admission. Report from the ÆSOP study. *British Journal of Psychiatry*, **186**, 281–289.

Morgan, C., Dazzan, P., Morgan, K., *et al* (2006) First episode psychosis and ethnicity: initial findings from the ÆSOP study. *World Psychiatry*, **5**, 40–46.

National Association for the Care and Resettlement of Offenders (1989) *Race and Criminal Justice*. NACRO.

National Association for the Care and Resettlement of Offenders (1990) *Black People, Mental Health and the Courts: An Explanatory Study into the Psychiatric Remand Process as it Affects Black Defendants at Magistrates' Courts*. NACRO.

Ndetei, D. M. & Vadher, A. (1984) A cross-cultural study of the frequencies of Schneider's first rank symptoms of schizophrenia. *Acta Psychiatrica Scandinavica*, **70**, 540–544.

Odell, S. M., Surtees, P. G., Wainwright, N. W. J., *et al* (1997) Determinants of general practitioner recognition of psychological problems in a multi-ethnic inner-city health district. *British Journal of Psychiatry*, **171**, 537–541.

Parkman, S., Davies, S., Leese, M., *et al* (1997) Ethnic differences in satisfaction with mental health services among representative people with psychosis in south London: PRiSM study 4. *British Journal of Psychiatry*, **171**, 260–264.

Patel, S. (1999) General practice. In *Mental Health Service Provision for a Multi-Cultural Society* (eds K. Bhui & D. Olajide), pp. 169–180. Saunders.

Pote, H. L. & Orrell M. W. (2002) Perceptions of schizophrenia in multi-cultural Britain. *Ethnicity and Health*, **7**, 7–20.

Professor the Lord Darzi of Denham (2008) *High Quality Care for All: NHS Next Stage Review Final Report*. TSO (The Stationery Office).

Rathod, S., Kingdon, D., Smith, P., *et al* (2005) Insight into schizophrenia: the effects of cognitive behavioural therapy on the components of insight and association with socio-demographics – data on a previously published randomised controlled trial. *Schizophrenia Research*, **74**, 211–219.

Robertson, D., Sathyamoorthy, G. & Ford, R. (2000) Asking the right question. *Community Care*, **163**, 24–25.

Shaw, C. M., Creed, F., Tomenson, B., *et al* (1999) Prevalence of anxiety and depressive illness and help seeking behaviour in African Caribbeans and white Europeans. *BMJ*, **318**, 302–305.

Singh, S. P., Greenwood, N., White, S., *et al* (2007) Ethnicity and the Mental Health Act 1983. *British Journal of Psychiatry*, **191**, 99–105.

van Os, J., Castle, D. J., Takei, N., *et al* (1996) Psychotic illness in ethnic minorities: clarification from 1991 census. *Psychological Medicine*, **26**, 203–208.

Wessely, S., Castle, D., Der, G., *et al* (1991) Schizophrenia and Afro-Caribbeans. A case–control study. *British Journal of Psychiatry*, **159**, 795–801.

Wilson, M. & MacCarthy, B. (1994) General practitioner consultation as a factor in the low rate of mental health service use by Asians. *Psychological Medicine*, **24**, 113–119.

CHAPTER 7

Poverty, social inequality and mental health

Vijaya Murali and Femi Oyebode

Summary   The World Health Organization has described poverty as the greatest cause of suffering on earth. This chapter considers the direct and indirect effects of relative poverty on the development of emotional, behavioural and psychiatric problems, in the context of the growing inequality between rich and poor. The problems of children in particular are reviewed. Targets to reduce inequality have been set both nationally and internationally.

In *Bridging the Gaps*, the World Health Organization (1995) declared that 'The world's most ruthless killer and the greatest cause of suffering on earth is extreme poverty.' This statement emphasises the importance of poverty as a variable adversely influencing health. Poverty is a multidimensional phenomenon, encompassing inability to satisfy basic needs, lack of control over resources, lack of education and poor health. Poverty can be intrinsically alienating and distressing, and of particular concern are its direct and indirect effects on the development and maintenance of emotional, behavioural and psychiatric problems. The present climate of global economic recession has had a negative impact on mental health and social inequality. It has been more challenging to reduce the health inequalities and improve the mental health of the whole population, especially people from more economically disadvantaged groups.

The measurement of poverty is based on incomes or consumption levels, and people are considered poor if their consumption or income fall below the 'poverty line', which is the minimum level necessary to meet basic needs. It should be emphasised that for the analysis of poverty in a particular country, the World Bank bases the poverty line on the norms for that society.

It is a well-recognised fact that poverty has important implications for both physical and mental health. In this chapter we discuss the impact of poverty on mental health, and explore possible explanations for the relationship between the two. It is important to distinguish between absolute and relative poverty; even in countries where families generally have access to sufficient resources to maintain life, many are living in disadvantageous circumstances, with poor housing, diet and amenities that do not meet the expectations of society in general (Townsend, 1979).

Poverty and social inequality

The gulf between the poor and rich of the world is widening. In the UK, the financial gap between the wealthy and the poor is not narrowing and differences in health between social classes I and V are becoming greater (Smith *et al*, 1990). Poverty and inequality are closely linked and both have direct and indirect effects on the social, mental and physical well-being of the individual. Wilkinson (1997) believed that income inequality produces psychosocial stress, which leads to deteriorating health and higher mortality over time. One of the national targets of reducing health inequality was to increase life expectancy, and the average life expectancy for all groups in England has increased significantly over the past ten years. Nevertheless, the increase in disadvantaged groups remains slight. Those who live in deprived communities, where there is under-investment in the social and physical infrastructure, experience poor health, resulting in higher mortality for people of lower socioeconomic class. The effects of income inequality also spill over into society, causing stress, frustration and family disruption, which then increase the rates of crime, homicide and violence (Wilkinson, 1996).

There are many obstacles, deficits and threats to health inherent in poverty. It is the poor who are who are more likely to live in dangerous and unhealthy neighbourhoods, who (if employed) often have stressful, unrewarding and depersonalising work, who lack the necessities and amenities of life and who, because they are not part of the mainstream of society, are isolated from information and support. The inverse association between socioeconomic level and risk of disease is one of the most pervasive and enduring observations in public health (Kaplan *et al*, 1987). It has been known for a long time that the lowest-income groups are more likely to suffer negative effects of 'risky' health behaviours than their less poor counterparts. These 'maladaptive' behaviours are not necessarily undertaken with a harmful intent, but may be regarded as coping behaviours to provide comfort or relief from stressful lives. Moreover, people in lower socioeconomic classes by virtue of their life circumstances are exposed to more stressors, and with fewer resources to manage them and greater vulnerability to them in the first place, they are doubly victimised. Poverty is associated with many long-term problems, such as poor health and increased mortality, school failure, crime and substance misuse. The relationship between occupational class and mortality in the UK is evident from a study that compared mortality rates in the 1970s with those in the 1990s. In the 1970s the mortality rate among men aged 20–64 years was almost twice as high for those in class V as for those in class I; by the

Table 7.1 Standardised mortality rates per 100 000 for men aged 20–64 years in England and Wales: comparison of years 1970–72 and 1991–93

Social class	1970–72	1991–93
I – Professional	500	280
II – Managerial	526	300
III–N – Skilled (non-manual)	637	426
III–M – Skilled (manual)	683	493
IV – Partly skilled	721	492
V – Unskilled	897	806
All classes	624	419

Source: Drever & Bunting (1997).

early 1990s it was almost three times as high (Drever & Bunting, 1997) (Table 7.1). The 2001 population census revealed that the standardised mortality rate for working age men was 2.8 times greater for men in unskilled manual jobs than for men in higher managerial posts, compared with 2.9 times in 1991–1993 (Office for National Statistics, 2002). Hence, it is evident that there has been very little change in health inequalities since the early 1990s.

Poverty and psychiatric disorders

It is not just infectious diseases that demonstrate the powerful socio-epidemiological correlation; it is also psychiatric conditions, which not only occur at higher rates in the poorest areas, but also cluster together, usually in disintegrating inner-city communities. Money is not a guarantor of mental health, nor does its absence necessarily lead to mental illness. However, it is generally conceded that poverty can be both a determinant and a consequence of poor mental health (Langner & Michael, 1963; Wan, 2008).

The relationship between low economic status and elevated incidence and prevalence of mental illness has become increasingly apparent. Over 50 years ago the New Haven (Hollingshead & Redlich, 1958) and Midtown Manhattan (Langner & Michael, 1963) studies identified a direct relationship between the experience of poverty and a high rate of emotional disturbance, as well as differential availability and use of modes of treatment and facilities for different social classes. The socioeconomic class gradient with respect to chronic diseases can mostly be explained by differences in access to healthcare (Goudge *et al*, 2009). For many people, lack of access to a car can cause difficulties in getting to the shops or healthcare services. In 2000–2001, 11% of households without a car said they had difficulty visiting their GP, compared with 4% who had a car (Ruston, 2002: p. 7).

Table 7.2 Prevalence (%) of psychiatric disorders according to social class, with odds ratio of employment status (Meltzer *et al*, 1995)

Psychiatric disorder	I	II	III	IV	V	Employed adjusted OR	Unemployed adjusted OR (95% CI)
Mixed anxiety and depressive disorder	60	76	78	76	73	1.00	1.73** (1.34–2.24)
Generalised anxiety disorder	23	28	30	41	31	1.00	2.19** (1.53–3.10)
Depressive disorder	9	12	22	28	35	1.00	2.66** (1.73–4.10)
Phobia	2	8	8	19	13	1.00	3.11** (1.65–5.80)
Obsessive–compulsive disorder	6	13	12	11	21	1.00	2.11** (1.20–3.74)
Panic disorder	1	9	8	7	12		
Functional psychosis	4	3	4	4	17	1.00	2.98** (1.18–7.47)
Alcohol dependence	33	34	47	58	73		
Drug dependence	7	11	17	35	50	1.00	3.80** (2.55–5.60)

OR, odds ratio.
**$P<0.01$.

The complexity and interrelatedness of factors such as poverty, health and employment make it interesting to look at the relationship that prevails between them. Relationships between social status and various aspects of mental disorder have long been of interest to both clinicians and researchers, and a large body of research exists showing the importance of social status in understanding psychiatric illness and disability. Epidemiological studies throughout the world have demonstrated an inverse relationship between mental illness and social class.

The prevalence of psychiatric disorders, including neurotic disorders, functional psychoses and alcohol and drug dependence in the UK was investigated in the 1995 survey published by the Office of Population Censuses and Surveys (Meltzer *et al*, 1995). Employment status was a major factor in explaining the differences in prevalence rates of all psychiatric disorders in adults. Unemployment significantly increased the odds ratio of psychiatric disorders compared with the reference group. It almost quadrupled the odds of drug dependence after controlling for other sociodemographic variables. Unemployment also approximately trebled the odds of phobia and functional psychosis. It more than doubled the odds of depressive episode, generalised anxiety disorder and obsessive–compulsive disorder, and increased the odds of mixed anxiety and depressive disorder by more than two-thirds (Table 7.2).

The 2007 Adult Psychiatric Morbidity Survey (McManus *et al*, 2009) showed that people living in households with the lowest income were more likely to have common mental disorders such as anxiety and depression compared with those living in the highest-income households. The pattern was more marked in men than women, with men in lowest-income households three times more likely to have common mental disorders than women in those households. Of the individual disorders, depressive episodes showed the greatest difference across income groups, especially for men, rising from 0.2% of men in the highest quintile to 6.9% in the lowest. The prevalence of psychotic disorder varied significantly according to household income: the rate increased from 0.1% of adults in the highest-income quintile to 0.9% in the lowest, and again the trend was more prominent in men.

Psychoses

It is well recognised that psychoses show a relationship with social class, with the highest prevalence of psychosis in both men and women found in social class V (Argyle, 1994). However, there are controversies over whether the poor social performance and lower social class of people with schizophrenia are consequences of the illness, consequences of changes in individuals predisposed to develop schizophrenia, or due to the adverse social conditions that lead to schizophrenia. The relationship between poverty and psychosis is complex, and two explanatory hypotheses have been put forward: social causation ('breeder') and social selection ('drift'). According to the social causation theory, the greater socioeconomic adversity characteristic of lower-class living conditions precipitates psychosis in vulnerable individuals. However, this theory was challenged by Goldberg & Morrison (1963) in a study showing that the social class distribution of the fathers of patients with schizophrenia did not deviate from that of the general population. The excess of low socioeconomic status among people with schizophrenia was mainly attributable to individuals who had drifted down the occupational and social scale prior to the onset of psychosis.

It is possible that the relationship between class and schizophrenia exists because the conditions of life experienced by people of lower social class foster conceptions of social reality that are so limited and rigid as to impair their ability to deal resourcefully with problematic and stressful situations. Although such impairment does not in itself result in schizophrenia, in conjunction with genetic vulnerability and great stress it could be disabling.

The association between social inequality at birth and subsequent risk of schizophrenia is uncertain. Mulvany *et al* (2001) concluded that low social class at birth was not associated with increased risk of schizophrenia, but views remain divided on the association between social inequality and psychoses and no definite conclusion has been reached.

Brown *et al* (2000) studied the relationship between social class of origin and cardinal symptoms of schizophrenic disorders over the course of early illness. Patients whose origin was upper or middle social class, compared with those from the lower social class, had lower symptom levels of hallucinations and delusions. Patients from the lower social class were older at first contact with psychiatric services than those from the higher social classes. This might be explained by the fact that people from the lower social class find it more difficult to access services. Alternatively, people belonging to the higher social classes might be better informed about mental illness and seek treatment early. It is also possible that the beliefs and values of people in lower socioeconomic groups, such as their tolerance and acceptance of the behavioural and social aspects of the disorder, explain the observed socioeconomic inequalities.

Mood disorder

Many studies have reported that low socioeconomic status is associated with high prevalence of mood disorders (Dohrenwend *et al*, 1992). In addition, longitudinal research in Stirling County (Murphy *et al*, 1991) indicated that during the 1950s and 1960s the prevalence of depression was significantly and persistently higher among people of low socioeconomic status than among those at other socioeconomic status levels. Incidence of depression after the study began was also higher among those who were initially in the low socioeconomic status group, supporting the view that the stress of poverty may be causally related to depression. There was also a trend for prior depression to be associated with subsequent downward social mobility, supporting the view that the concentration of people with depression at the lower end of the social hierarchy may result from disabling aspects of the illness.

A positive relationship has been found between socioeconomic status and vulnerability to mood disorder, with higher rates of vulnerability found among individuals with lower educational and social achievement levels (Dohrenwend *et al*, 1992). The social causation hypothesis suggests that the stress associated with low social position, such as exposure to social adversity and lack of resources to cope with difficulty, might contribute to the development of mood disorder. The social selection hypothesis argues that genetically predisposed individuals drift down to – or fail to rise out of – such a position (Jarvis, 1971). Patients with major depressive disorder or bipolar depression were more 'downwardly mobile' than people with neurotic depression (Eisemann, 1986).

The work of Brown & Harris (1978) points strongly to the importance of supportive relationships in protecting vulnerable women from developing depression. The effect of poverty is substantially reduced when the degree of isolation from friends and family is controlled for, suggesting that social isolation mediates some of the relationships between economic status and mood disorders (Bruce & Hoff, 1994).

It has also been suggested that social class might have an influence on the psychopathological pattern of depressive symptoms. Patients who presented with somatisation and anxiety symptoms were more frequently from the lower social classes, whereas cognitive symptoms were more common among the higher classes (Lenzi *et al*, 1993). Schwab *et al* (1967) suggested that there is a relation between social class and type of depressive symptoms. However, a study by Ayuso-Gutierrez *et al* (1981) does not support this view. The amount of depression associated with economic hardship among adults may depend on age: Mirowsky & Ross (2001) found a decrease in such depression with greater age. Economic deprivation and poor marital relationships are important risk factors for the occurrence and chronicity of depression (Patel *et al*, 2002). Both depression and poverty tend to be chronic, and warrant the attention of caregivers and policy-makers.

Suicide

The National Confidential Inquiry into Suicide and Homicide by People with Mental Illness, along with many other studies, have reported that the majority of people who completed suicide were either unemployed or had a long-term illness (Appleby *et al*, 1999, 2001). Compared with the general population, people who attempt suicide belong more often to the social categories associated with social destabilisation and poverty.

Gunnell *et al* (1995) examined the relationships between suicide, parasuicide and socioeconomic deprivation. A strong association was found between suicide and parasuicide, with socioeconomic deprivation accounting for much of this relationship. Furthermore, homicide and suicide occur more frequently in highly populated deprived areas (Kennedy *et al*, 1999). This finding is also supported by Crawford & Prince (1999), who noted increasing rates of suicide in young unemployed men living in conditions of extreme social deprivation. It is also true that the mortality rates of overdoses involving cocaine and opiates are significantly associated with poverty status (Marzuk *et al*, 1997).

Alcohol and substance misuse

The relationship between alcohol and socioeconomic status is interesting. The General Household Survey 2007 shows that households classified as managerial and professional had the highest proportions of men and women who reported having had an alcoholic drink in the previous 7 days, whereas households in the 'routine and manual' classification had the lowest (Robinson & Lader, 2008). Also, the proportion of people exceeding the daily recommended intake of alcohol was greater in the 'managerial and professional' households (43%) compared with the 'routine and manual' households (31%). However, a New Zealand cohort study among young adults reported that higher socioeconomic status predicted more frequent drinking but lower amount consumed during a drinking session (Casswell *et al*, 2003). A Canadian cohort study found that recent unemployment decreases alcohol use, while longer unemployment increases it (Khan *et al*, 2002).

Social class is a risk factor for alcohol-related mortality, which is also linked to social structural factors such as poverty, disadvantage and social class (Harrison & Gardiner, 1999). Alcohol-related mortality rates are higher for men in the manual occupations than in the non-manual occupations, but the relative magnitude depends on age. Men aged 25–39 years in the unskilled manual class are 10–20 times more likely to die from alcohol-related causes than those in the professional class, whereas men aged 55–64 years in the unskilled manual class are only about 2.5–4 times more likely to die than their professional counterparts.

For women, younger women in the manual classes are more likely to die from alcohol-related causes, but among older women it is those in the professional class who have the higher mortality. Hans (1999) studied the demographic and psychosocial characteristics of substance-misusing pregnant women, and found that demographic features were related only to type of substance used, with Black women and poorer women more likely to use illicit substances, particularly cocaine, and White women and better-educated women more likely to use alcohol.

Personality disorders

The relationship between low socioeconomic status and personality disorders has not been extensively studied. However, there is some evidence that personality disorders are more frequent among single individuals from lower socioeconomic classes in inner cities (Grant *et al*, 2004).

Low family income and poor housing predict official and self-reported juvenile and adult offending (Farrington, 1995). However, the relationship between poverty and criminality is complex and continuous. The interaction between impulsivity and neighbourhood on criminal activities indicates that the effects of impulsivity are stronger in poorer neighbourhoods than in better-off ones (Lynam *et al*, 2000). In severely disadvantaged settings, even quite young children may be directly exposed to community violence (Osofsky, 1995).

In the Cambridge Study in Delinquent Development, which followed up a group of south London males from age 8 to age 32, an unstable job record at 18 years of age was an important independent predictor of young men's convictions between the ages of 21 and 25 (Farrington, 1995). In addition, having an unskilled manual job at the age of 18 was an independent predictor of adult social dysfunction and antisocial personality at the age of 32. Between the ages of 15 and 18, the young males in this study were convicted at a higher rate when they were unemployed than when they were employed, suggesting that unemployment is associated with crime. It seems likely that financial need is an important link in the causal chain between unemployment and crime.

Personality disorder or criminality?

It is interesting to note that the major criticism of the DSM–III–R criteria for antisocial personality disorder (American Psychiatric Association, 1987) was that personality traits or symptoms of psychopathy were neglected and that the disorder was conceptualised as synonymous with criminality. However, the criteria for the disorder in DSM–IV (American Psychiatric Association, 1994), and also in ICD–10 (World Health Organization, 1992), reflect personality traits more than overt criminal behaviour.

Effect of poverty on children

Psychiatric disorders of childhood result from the interplay between genetic and environmental factors. The link between adverse experiences and childhood disorder is complex and involves reciprocal effects from the children, as they are not just passive recipients of experience. A growing body of research relating to poverty and health indicates that low income combined with disruptive demographic factors and poor external support generate the stress and life crises that put children at risk, and may precipitate psychiatric disorders in childhood.

Children in the poorest households are three times more likely to have a mental illness than children in the best-off households (Department of Health, 1999). Poverty and social disadvantage are most strongly associated with deficits in children's cognitive skills and educational achievements (Duncan & Brooks-Gunn, 1997). In the behavioural domain, conduct disorder and attention-deficit hyperactivity disorder show links with family poverty, and this is most marked for children in families facing persistent economic stress. The relationship between poverty and childhood disruptive behaviour appears to be more marked for boys than for girls, and seems to be stronger in childhood than in adolescence. Rates of childhood disorders such as emotional disorder and conduct disorder vary in different neighbourhoods and communities. An early study showed that the risks of developing such disorders in inner-city areas were twice those in small towns (Rutter *et al*, 1975). More recently, it has been reported that children living below the poverty line, whose parents had low levels of education and who lived in single-parent families or with a step-mother or step-father showed more behavioural problems and poor social competence (Assis *et al*, 2009)

It is well recognised that conduct disorder is three to four times more common in children who live in socioeconomically deprived families with low income, or who live in a poor neighbourhood. A household survey carried out in England, Scotland and Wales in 1999 by the Office for National Statistics (Meltzer *et al*, 2000) revealed that children in families of social class V (14%) were more likely to have a mental disorder, including conduct disorder, hyperkinetic disorder, emotional disorders, than those in social class I families (5%). The highest rate was found among children in the small group of families where no parent had ever worked (21%).

With regard to economic disadvantage, persistent poverty should be distinguished from current poverty: persistent poverty significantly predicts internalising symptoms such as childhood depression, whereas just current poverty predicts externalising symptoms such as childhood behavioural disorders (McLeod & Shanahan, 1993). It is likely that poverty imposes stress on parents and that this inhibits family processes of informal social control, in turn increasing the risks of harsh parenting and reducing parents' emotional availability to meet their children's needs.

Kaplan *et al* (2001) studied childhood socioeconomic status and cognitive function in adulthood and concluded that both higher socioeconomic status in childhood and greater educational attainment are associated with higher cognitive function in adulthood, with mothers and fathers each contributing to their offspring's formative cognitive development and later-life cognitive ability. Improvements in both parental socioeconomic circumstances and the educational attainment of their offspring could possibly enhance cognitive function and decrease the risk of dementia later in life.

Erratic, threatening and harsh discipline, lack of supervision and weak parent–child attachments mediate the effects of poverty and other structural factors on delinquency. In the Cambridge Study in Delinquent Development, one of the most important childhood predictors of delinquency was poverty (Farrington, 1995). Poverty was also found to have an effect on both academic failure and extreme delinquency when maternal education and early childhood behaviour were controlled for (Pagani *et al*, 1999). In a literature review examining the developmental outcome of drug-exposed infants during the first 2 years of life, Eyler & Behnke (1999) concluded that the effects of drugs appear to be exacerbated in children living in poverty. Among methadone-exposed infants, Marcus *et al* (1984) reported poorer motor coordination only in those from families with poorer resources, including low socioeconomic status.

Health inequalities – explanatory models

We have argued that economic distress has significant effects on health indicators. How might such effects be mediated? The Black Report (Townsend *et al*, 1992) highlights various explanations for existing health inequalities, dividing them into four categories: the artefact theory; theories of natural or social selection; materialist or structuralist explanations; and cultural and behavioural explanations.

Artefact theory

The artefact theory suggests that both class and health are artificial variables, and that the relationship between them may itself be an artefact. It is believed that the failure to reduce the gap between classes has been counterbalanced by the shrinkage in the relative size of the lower socioeconomic classes themselves.

Natural or social selection

Theories of natural or social selection relegate occupational class to the status of dependent variable, and health acquires the greater degree of causal significance. This explanation suggests that social class I has the lowest rate of premature mortality because it is made up of the strongest and most robust men and women in the population, and that class V has the weakest people. It puts forward the idea that poor health carries low social worth as well as low economic reward, but that these factors do not do not cause the high mortality.

Materialist and structuralist theories

Materialist or structuralist explanations emphasise the role of economic and associated sociostructural factors in the distribution of health. It is difficult to ascribe the premature mortality in the lower socioeconomic class to subsistence poverty. Social class and the characteristics associated with belonging to a particular class have health implications. As poverty is a relative concept, people belonging to a low socioeconomic class may be relatively disadvantaged in relation to the risks of illness or accident, or to the factors that promote a healthy lifestyle.

Behavioural and cultural theories

The behavioural and cultural explanations of the distribution of health suggest that its unequal distribution in modern industrial society is the result of incautious lifestyles, wherein people harm themselves or their children by their excessive consumption of harmful commodities and refined foods, and by their underutilisation of preventive healthcare and contraception. It is implied that there are subcultural lifestyles, rooted in personal character- istics and level of education, that govern behaviour. According to the 'culture of poverty' view of Oscar Lewis (1967), human existence in any given environment involves a process of biological and social adaptation, which gives rise to the elaboration of a structure of norms, ideas and behaviours. Over time, this 'culture of poverty' seems to help individuals to cope with their environment. This view firmly ascribes poor health to the behaviour of people themselves, and by implication makes them fully responsible for the untoward outcomes. The implication that the poor are in some respects a homogeneous group has caused this view to be widely criticised by British social scientists (Rutter & Madge, 1976; Holman, 1978; Townsend, 1979).

Discussion

Social inequality and poverty have demonstrable adverse effects on health. These effects are, in our view, amenable to remediation. In the UK, the National Health Service has several interlinked responsibilities in relation to health inequalities, one of which is the provision of equity of access to effective healthcare. A recommendation of the Independent Inquiry into Inequalities in Health (Acheson, 1998) was that, as part of health impact assessment, all policies likely to have a direct or indirect effect on health should be evaluated in terms of their impact on health inequalities. These policies should be formulated in such a way that, by favouring those who are less well-off, they should ultimately reduce such inequalities. In the consultation document *Tackling Health Inequalities* (Department of Health, 2001), the government set national targets for doing this (Box 7.1).

Tackling Health Inequalities: 10 Years On (Department of Health, 2009) summarises improvements in the health of the population as measured by life expectancy and infant mortality. It shows that the targets set relating to infant mortality, life expectancy, smoking and teenage pregnancy in particular are being addressed vigorously. The average life expectancy increased significantly, for males by an extra 3.1 years and for females by an extra 2.1 years between 1995/1997 and 2005/2007. Infant mortality fell from 5.6 infant deaths per 1000 live births in 1995/1997 to 4.7 per 1000 live births in 2005/2007. The previous upward trend of teenage pregnancy has been reversed and the rate reduced by 10.7%. Having identified smoking as a major contributory factor in major illness (Department of Health, 1998), the government announced several action plans to reduce smoking. These included a ban on tobacco advertising, the introduction of nicotine replacement products and provision of NHS smoking cessation services. On 1 July 2007, all enclosed workplaces and public places in England became smoke-free. Although the target to reduce child poverty by a quarter set between

---

Box 7.1   National targets for reducing health inequalities

Infant mortality   Starting with children under 1 year old, by 2010 to reduce by at least 10% the gap in mortality between manual groups and the population as a whole

Life expectancy   Starting with health authorities, by 2010 to reduce by at least 10% the gap between the fifth of areas with lowest life expectancy at birth and the population as a whole

Child poverty   To work towards the eradication of child poverty by reducing the number of children living in poverty by a quarter by 2004

Smoking   To reduce smoking rates among manual groups from 32% in 1998 to 26% by 2010, so that we can narrow the gap between manual and non-manual groups

Teenage pregnancy   By achieving agreed local conception reduction targets, to reduce the national under-18 conception rate by 15% by 2004 and 50% by 2010

(Department of Health, 2001)

Box 7.2 Responding to poverty

Poverty can be fought by:

- improving the distribution of income and wealth and, more importantly, learning about the impact of policies on income distribution
- accelerating social development, which includes education of girls and women, provision of safe water and sanitation, child immunisation and the setting up of safety nets to protect the most vulnerable
- international agencies that support countries showing a determination to take up the challenges of the goals for the 21st century
- international agencies that work with low- and middle-income countries to strengthen each country's capacity to monitor its progress on outcomes
- accelerating economic growth, which will require policies that encourage macroeconomic stability, shift resources to more efficient sectors, and integrate with the global economy

(World Bank Group, 2004)

1998/1999 and 2004/2005 was missed, taking 60% of median income in 1998/1999 as the definition of poverty, the proportion of children living in poverty fell from 26% in 1998/1999 to 22% in 2006/07. This represents 600 000 children taken out of poverty, before housing costs are deducted.

At a global level, the Development Assistance Committee of the Organisation for Economic Co-operation and Development has called for a global partnership to pursue a new development strategy focused on poverty and social goals (Development Assistance Committee, 1996), and the World Bank suggests various ways of responding to poverty (Box 7.2). The poverty goal is to halve the proportion of people in extreme poverty by 2015. This is expected to be achieved by accelerating economic growth and by improving the distribution of income and wealth. The social goals include making progress towards gender equality by 2005 and, by 2015, reducing infant mortality by two-thirds, achieving universal primary education in all countries and providing access to reproductive health services for all. To achieve these goals, international agencies must support countries that show interest and determination to take up the challenges of the goals for the 21st century, and must strengthen their capacity to monitor progress. In order to build a successful economy, new challenges have to be met with resilience, fresh thinking and courage. This will enable us to make long-term decisions and progress towards a better world.

References

Acheson, D. (1998) *Independent Inquiry into Inequalities in Health: Report*. TSO (The Stationery Office).

American Psychiatric Association (1987) *Diagnostic and Statistical Manual of Mental Disorders (3rd edn, revised) (DSM–III–R)*. APA.

American Psychiatric Association (1994) *Diagnostic and Statistical Manual of Mental Disorders (4th edn) (DSM–IV)*. APA.

Appleby, L., Shaw, J., Amos, T., et al (1999) *Safer Services: Report of the National Confidential Inquiry into Suicide and Homicide by People with Mental Illness*. TSO (The Stationery Office).

Appleby L., Shaw J., Sherratt J., et al (2001) *Safety First. Five Year Report of the National Confidential Inquiry into Suicide and Homicide by People with Mental Illness*. TSO (The Stationery Office).

Argyle, M. (1994) *The Psychology of Social Class*. Routledge.

Assis, S. G., Avanci, J. Q., de Vasconcellors, R., et al (2009) Socioeconomic inequalities and child mental health. *Revista de Saúde Pública*, **43** (suppl 1), 92–100.

Ayuso-Gutierrez, J. A., Montefo-Iglesias, L., Ros-Brieva, J. A. (1981) Social class and depressive symptomatology. *International Journal Social Psychiatry*, **27**, 297–299.

Brown, A. S., Susser, E. S., Jandorf, L., et al (2000) Social class of origin and cardinal symptoms of schizophrenic disorders over the early illness course. *Social Psychiatry and Psychiatric Epidemiology*, **35**, 53–60.

Brown, G. W. & Harris, T. (1978) *Social Origins of Depression: A Study of Psychiatric Disorders in Women*. Tavistock.

Bruce, M. L. & Hoff, R. A. (1994) Social and physical health risk factors for first-onset major depressive disorder in a community sample. *Social Psychiatry and Psychiatric Epidemiology*, **29**, 165–171.

Casswell, S., Pledger, M. & Hooper, R. (2003) Socioeconomic status and drinking patterns in young adults. *Addiction*, **98**, 601–610.

Crawford, M. J. & Prince, M. (1999) Increasing rates of suicide in young men in England during the 1980s: the importance of social context. *Social Science and Medicine*, **49**, 1419–1423.

Department of Health (1998) *Smoking Kills: A White Paper On Tobacco*. TSO (The Stationery Office).

Department of Health (1999) *Saving Lives: Our Healthier Nation*. TSO (The Stationery Office).

Department of Health (2001) *Tackling Health Inequalities: Consultation on a Plan for Delivery*. Department of Health.

Department of Health (2009) *Tackling Health Inequalities: 10 Years On. A Review of Developments in Tackling Health Inequalities in England over the Last 10 Years*. TSO (The Stationery Office).

Development Assistance Committee (1996) *Shaping the 21st Century: The Contribution of Development Co-operation*. Organisation for Economic Co-operation and Development.

Dohrenwend, B. P., Levav, I., Shrout, P. E., et al (1992) Socioeconomic status and psychiatric disorders: the causation-selection issue. *Science*, **255**, 946–952.

Drever, F. & Bunting, J. (1997) Patterns and trends in male mortality. In *Health Inequalities: Decennial Supplement no. 15* (eds F. Drever & M. Whitehead), pp. 95–107. TSO (The Stationery Office).

Duncan, G. J. & Brooks-Gunn, J. (eds) (1997) *Consequences of Growing Up Poor*. Russell Sage.

Eisemann, M. (1986) Social class and social mobility in depressed patients. *Acta Psychiatrica Scandinavica*, **73**, 399–402.

Eyler, F. D. & Behnke, M. (1999) Early development of infants exposed to drugs prenatally. *Clinical Perinatology*, **26**, 107–150.

Farrington, D. P. (1995) The development of offending and antisocial behaviour from childhood: key finding from the Cambridge Study in Delinquent Development. *Journal of Child Psychology and Psychiatry*, **36**, 929–964.

Goldberg, E. M. & Morrison, S. L. (1963) Schizophrenia and social class. *British Journal of Psychiatry*, **109**, 785–802.

Goudge, J., Gilson, L., Russell, S., et al (2009) Affordability, availability and acceptability barriers to health care for the chronically ill: Longitudinal case studies from South Africa. *BMC Health Services Research*, **9**, 75.

Grant, B. F., Hasin, D. S., Stinson, F. S., *et al* (2004) Prevalence, correlates, and disability of personality disorders in the United States: results from the national epidemiologic survey on alcohol and related conditions. *Journal of Clinical Psychiatry*, **65**, 948–958.

Gunnell, D. J., Peters, T. J., Kammerling, R. M., *et al* (1995) Relation between parasuicide, suicide, psychiatric admissions and socioeconomic deprivation. *BMJ*, **311**, 226–230.

Hans, S. L. (1999) Demographic and psychosocial characteristics of substance-abusing pregnant women. *Clinical Perinatology*, **26**, 55–74.

Harrison, L. & Gardiner, E. (1999) Do the rich really die young? Alcohol-related mortality and social class in Great Britain, 1988–94. *Addiction*, **94**, 1871–1880.

Hollingshead, A. B. & Redlich, F. C. (1958) *Social Class and Mental Illness: A Community Study*. John Wiley.

Holman, R. T. (1978) *Poverty: Explanations of Social Deprivation*. Robertson.

Jarvis, E. (1971) *Insanity and Idiosy in Massachusetts: Report of the Commission of Lunacy, 1855*. Harvard University Press.

Kaplan, G. A., Haan, M. N, Syme, S., *et al* (1987) Socio-economic status and health. In *Closing the Gap: The Burden of Unnecessary Illness* (eds R. W. Amler & H. B. Dull), pp. 125–129. Oxford University Press.

Kaplan, G. A., Turrell, G., Lynch, J. W., *et al* (2001) Childhood socioeconomic position and cognitive function in adulthood. *International Journal of Epidemiology*, **30**, 256–263.

Kennedy, H. G, Iveson, R. C. & Hill, O. (1999) Violence, homicide and suicide: strong correlation and wide variation across districts. *British Journal of Psychiatry*, **175**, 462–466.

Khan, S., Murray, R. P. & Barnes, G. E. (2002) A structural equation model of the effect of poverty and unemployment on alcohol abuse. *Addiction Behavior*, **27**, 405–423.

Langner, T. S. & Michael, S. T. (1963) *Life Stress and Mental Health*. Collier-Macmillan.

Lewis, O. (1967) *The Children of Sanchez*. Random House.

Lenzi, A., Lazzerini, F., Marazziti, D., *et al* (1993) Social class and mood disorders: clinical features. *Social Psychiatry and Psychiatric Epidemiology*, **28**, 56–59.

Lynam, D. R., Caspi, A., Moffitt, T. E, *et al* (2000) The interaction between impulsivity and neighbourhood context on offending: the effects of impulsivity are stronger in poorer neighbourhoods. *Journal of Abnormal Psychology*, **109**, 563–574.

Marcus, J., Hans, S. L. & Jeremy, R. J. (1984) A longitudinal study of offspring born to methadone-maintained women. Effects of multiple risk factors on development at 4, 8, and 12 months. *American Journal of Drug and Alcohol Abuse*, **10**, 195–207,

Marzuk, P. M., Tardiff, K., Leon, A. C., *et al* (1997) Poverty and fatal accidental drug overdoses of cocaine and opiates in New York City: an ecological study. *American Journal of Drug and Alcohol Abuse*, **23**, 221–228.

McLeod, J. D. & Shanahan, M. J. (1993) Poverty, parenting, and children's mental health. *American Sociological Review*, **58**, 351–366.

McManus, S., Meltzer, H., Brugha, T., *et al* (eds) (2009) *Adult Psychiatric Morbidity in England, 2007: Results of a Household Survey*. NHS Information Centre for Health and Social Care.

Meltzer, H., Gill, B., Petticrew, M., *et al* (1995) *OPCS Surveys of Psychiatric Morbidity in Great Britain: 1995*. TSO (The Stationery Office).

Meltzer, H., Gatward, R., Goodman, R., *et al* (2000) *The Mental health of Children and Adolescents in Great Britain*. TSO (The Stationery Office).

Mirowsky, J. & Ross, C. E. (2001) Age and the effect of economic hardship on depression. *Journal of Health and Social Behaviour*, **42**, 132–150.

Mulvany, F., O'Callaghan, E., Takei, N., *et al* (2001) Effect of social class at birth on risk and presentation of schizophrenia: case–control study. *BMJ*, **323**, 1398–1401.

Murphy, J. M., Oliver, D. C., Monson, R. R., *et al* (1991) Depression and anxiety in relation to social status: a perspective epidemiological study. *Archives of General Psychiatry*, **48**, 223–229.

Office for National Statistics (2002) *2001 Census, Mid-year Population Estimates, Death Registrations. ONS Longitudinal Study*. ONS.

Osofsky, J. D. (1995) The effects of exposure to violence on young children. *American Psychologist*, **50**, 782–788.

Pagani, L., Boulerice, B., Vitaro, F., *et al* (1999) Effects of poverty on academic failure and delinquency in boys: a change and process model approach. *Journal of Child Psychology and Psychiatry*, **40**, 1209–1219.

Patel, V., Rodrigues, M. & DeSouza, N. (2002) Gender, poverty, and postnatal depression: a study of mothers in Goa, India. *American Journal of Psychiatry*, **159**, 43–47.

Robinson, S & Lader, D. (2008) *General Household Survey 2007: Smoking and Drinking among Adults, 2007*. Office for National Statistics (http://www.statistics.gov.uk/Statbase/Product.asp?vlnk=5756).

Ruston, D. (2002) *Difficulty in Accessing Key Services*. Office for National Statistics (http://www.statistics.gov.uk/downloads/theme_social/access_key_services/access_to_services.pdf).

Rutter, M. & Madge, N. (1976) *Cycles of Disadvantage*. Heinemann.

Rutter, M., Yule, B., Quinton, D., *et al* (1975) Attainment and adjustment in two geographical areas. III: Some factors accounting for area differences. *British Journal of Psychiatry*, **126**, 520–533.

Schwab, J. J., Bialow, M., Holzer, C. E., *et al* (1967) Sociocultural aspects of depression in medical inpatients. I. Frequency and social variables. *Archives of General Psychiatry*, **17**, 533–538.

Smith, G. D., Bartly, M. & Blane, D. (1990) The Black Report on socioeconomic inequalities in health: 10 years on. *BMJ*, **301**, 373–377.

Townsend, P. (1979) *Poverty in the United Kingdom*. Penguin.

Townsend, P., Davidson, N. & Whitehead, M. (eds) (1992) *The Black Report and the Health Divide: Inequalities in Health* (2nd edn). Penguin.

Wan, K. W. (2008) Mental health and poverty. *Journal of the Royal Society for the Promotion of Health*, **128**, 108–109.

Wilkinson, R. G. (1996) *Unhealthy Societies: The Afflictions of Inequality*. Routledge.

Wilkinson, R. G. (1997) Health inequalities: relative or absolute material standards. *BMJ*, **314**, 591–595.

World Bank Group (2004) *Responding to Poverty: How to Move forward in Achieving the Millennium Development Goals?* World Bank Group (http://www.worldbank.org/poverty/mission/rp1.htm).

World Health Organization (1992) *Tenth Revision of the International Classification of Diseases and Related Health Problems (ICD–10)*. WHO.

World Health Organization (1995) *Bridging the Gaps*. WHO.

Part 2
Specific mental health conditions across cultures

CHAPTER 8

Schizophrenia in African–Caribbeans: contributing factors

Dinesh Bhugra and Kamaldeep Bhui

Summary Studies over the past half-century using various methods and assessment tools have consistently reported higher than expected rates of schizophrenia among people of African–Caribbean descent compared with other minority ethnic groups and White British. These rates have varied from twofold to sixteenfold. The reasons for such a discrepancy are not clear, although various hypotheses have been put forward. There are undoubtedly methodological problems in determining accurate rates. Both biological and social factors have been proposed as potential aetiological factors. In this chapter we give an overview of the evidence and make suggestions for improved assessment and management.

The epidemiology and management of schizophrenia have been well studied over the past few decades. In the UK, key findings that have emerged time and again are the excess prevalence and incidence rates of schizophrenia among people of African–Caribbean origin. The reasons for this excess and its implications are many. The findings may reflect a true excess or a methodological artefact related to errors in the estimation of numerator and denominator data. The findings have been increasingly accepted as better-designed studies have emerged, but these still do not fully address concerns about the nature of schizophrenia in other cultural groups and in societies in which industrialisation and the economic productivity of the individual are not considered to be as crucial to an individual's sense of belonging in a community. Implications include individual and family distress related to the loss of hopes and expectations and being seen as belonging to a group at high risk for a condition that carries stigma. In addition, there is economic burden on the individual, family and society if unemployment and disability diminish financial security. There are also significant implications for service providers and planners, who are required to meet the health and social care needs of patient, family and community in order to maximise the chances of a functional recovery at each of these levels.

Problems in studying rates

There are several problems in studying rates of schizophrenia in any ethnic group. First, the heterogeneity of ethnic groups and limitations of ethnic group definitions are not fully appreciated, but they must be understood for meaningful interpretation of prevalence and incidence studies. Second, the definition of schizophrenia has been criticised for adopting a disease model and for universal application of a Western concept that may not have validity as an illness, disease or disability in other societies. The existence of schizophrenia is deduced on the basis of clinical diagnostic practice, which varies within and across cultures, societies and economic systems. For example, the syndrome of 'sluggish schizophrenia' in the former USSR demonstrated how diagnostic criteria are permeable to value judgements that promote a society's moral and political ideology. Diagnostic formulation may also emphasise as pathological symptoms phenomena that are prominent in non-schizophrenic psychoses and in culturally sanctioned states of distress.

Thus, studies generally have looked at incidence cases of a syndromal diagnosis without attention to local contexts, and this leads to the interpretation of data in isolation from cultural, social and historical biographies. Depending on the position one takes – universalist or relativist, not to mention psychiatrist as physician or psychiatrist as shaper of social conditions – these data will be interpreted in markedly different ways. Although methodological and interpretive flaws in studies have received increasing attention as the data have been gathered, they are often defined from within the same closed system of thinking. Cross-fertilisation between different systems of research method is rarely witnessed, but is necessary for a more global interpretation of the data, rather than a psychiatric and purely medical research-oriented interpretation that is founded on assumptions that are not easy to question from within the closed system. Therefore, a fuller and more complete appreciation of the true position requires that one interpret the data with and without these assumptions. In this chapter, however, we assume the research data to reflect a truly higher incidence and prevalence of schizophrenia. We consider the possible explanations for these findings, with an emphasis on sociocultural perspectives.

Over the years, the terms used in the literature to describe the group of Caribbean people of Black African descent have included 'African– Caribbeans', 'Afro-Caribbeans', 'West Indians', 'Blacks' and 'Negros'. Such etymological use illustrates difficulties in identifying both the denominator and the numerator when ascertaining rates of illness. Here, we first present American studies on samples that are now identified as African–Americans; then we present UK studies on people commonly identified as African– Caribbeans. We compare the two groups, drawing out similarities and differences.

American studies

American studies have not specifically identified Caribbean populations, although these might have been included in their data. Hence, direct comparisons between the studies in the USA and the UK are not valid. Rates of mental illness among the 'Negro' cohort were 17.5 per 100 000 population in 1850, but had shot up to 91.2 per 100 000 within 30 years (Babcock, 1895). This increase was attributed by Babcock to emancipation of the slaves: slaves did not get excited because they did not indulge in political discussions, did not participate in religious activities and did not have any anxieties. It is possible that some of the increase was indeed the result of the release of slaves with mental illnesses, who then ended up in asylums, whereas previously they may have remained on the plantations. Green (1914) reported that in 1914 it was a 6:1 ratio of White:Black; between 1870 and 1880 it was 1:4 White:Black; and by 1882 it was 1:2.2 White:Black. Drugs and toxic psychosis were said to be more common in Whites, whereas Blacks had higher levels of senile psychosis, general paralysis, dementia praecox and manic–depressive psychosis (bipolar disorder with psychotic symptoms). Chasson (1963), reporting on first admissions to a psychiatric hospital in Washington, DC, between 1950 and 1957, showed that White males were more likely to be discharged than White females, who in turn were more likely to be discharged than Black males. Black females had the lowest discharge rates. Discharge from hospital depended on a number of factors. However, Chasson argued that the hardships endured by Blacks intensified the psychopathology. Crawford *et al* (1960) set out to test whether rates of mental illness differed between Blacks and Whites, using ethnically matched interviewers. The rates based on known cases were similar in both groups. The Black samples saw mental illness as a problem that people brought on themselves. The authors postulated that, because Blacks lived in a minority culture, when problems became extremely difficult to control they 'invited' dominant White authorities to intercede.

Early studies gave varying differential rates of mental illness among Blacks and Whites (Table 8.1). This variation has been attributed to confusion between prevalence and incidence and definitions of schizophrenia. It also reflects changes in diagnoses and in data collection. Jaco (1960) was the only author to show that rates of psychosis were highest in Anglo-Americans, followed by 'non-Whites' and finally Spanish Americans, who had the lowest rates. Marital status was an important factor. Snowden & Cheung (1990) reported that for all types of in-patient care schizophrenia was diagnosed consistently more often for Blacks (56.3%) than for Whites (31.5%). Some authors (e.g. Mukherjee *et al*, 1983) have suggested that auditory hallucinations are subject to pathoplastic cultural influences and may therefore be interpreted wrongly, undue emphasis being given to pathological explanations leading to misdiagnosis (see Racism below).

Table 8.1 Summary of early studies from the USA

Study	Admission rates		Admission rates for schizophrenia		
	Blacks	Whites	Blacks	Whites	Ratio
McLean (1949)	173	110			1.6:1
Frumkin (1954)	80	43	19	8	2.3:1
Faris & Dunham (1960)	41	33			1.3:1
Jaco (1960)	53	80	31	38	0.68:1
Malzberg (1963)	340	174	112	49	2.2:1
Klee et al (1967)	1950	1650	–	–	1.18:1
Wilson & Lantz (1957)	105	48	22	7	3:1

Misdiagnosis has indeed become a more important issue, of which patients, carers and some mental health professionals complain. Misdiagnosis can arise from ignorance of cultural variability in expressions of distress, or because psychopathological phenomena have differing significance across cultures, or because cross-cultural stereotyping (by patient and doctor) lead to difficulties in obtaining a sufficiently detailed history. However, misdiagnosis alone cannot explain all the findings in both the USA and the UK. Although misdiagnosis in this context is assumed to mean overdiagnosis, interpreting the behaviour of Black adolescents from low socioeconomic urban dwellings as normative has also caused professionals to miss or ignore underlying psychiatric disorders. This institutional practice leads to poorer outcomes for Black people. In any assessments the clinician must be aware of the basic principles outlined in Box 8.1.

Box 8.1 Good practice points in assessing a case of schizophrenia

- Take a careful history
- Understand delusional phenomena in their cultural context
- Understand hallucinatory experience in its cultural context
- Check thought disorder in the patient's primary language
- Ascertain abnormal mood states
- Ascertain passivity phenomena
- Carry out a physical and neurological examination
- Carry out physical investigations
- Check third-party information, including cultural identity

UK studies

Since the late 1960s, a number of comparative studies of psychosis have been carried out in the UK. Apart from the above-mentioned problems of incidence and prevalence, their authors often relied on denominators that were not entirely accurate because under-enumeration in census data was particularly prevalent among Black and minority ethnic groups. We have divided the studies into two periods – before and after 1980 – largely because the more recent studies are more epidemiologically sound.

Before 1980

Hemsi (1967), using data from the Camberwell Psychiatric Case Register, reported that the rates of case-note diagnosis of schizophrenia among patients attending their general practitioner (GP) were 4.5 times higher in African–Caribbeans than in the White population. Organic psychosis, alcoholism and drug dependence, however, were absent in the African–Caribbean population. Kiev (1965) found higher prevalence rates of mental illness among Blacks attending a GP surgery in south London compared with Whites. Rwegellera (1977) too used the Camberwell Psychiatric Case Register, but over a 3-year period, and calculated that inception rates (rates of first contact) for schizophrenia were 0.92 per 1000 among West Indians compared with 0.12 per 1000 among Whites and 4.18 per 1000 among West Africans. Using age-standardised data for 15- to 24-year-olds, the West Indian rates were 1.40 per 1000 compared with 0.16 per 1000 for Whites; for 25- to 44-year-olds, these rates were 0.80 per 1000 and 0.17 per 1000 respectively for the two groups. Ethnicity was determined using country of birth. In all three studies, however, small numbers of base population and the use of admissions case-note data provided indicators at psychiatric service contact level only, rather than a population-based picture in which help-seekers and only help-seekers would be included. The rates were based on admissions.

After 1980

Carpenter & Brockington (1980) found from hospital case notes in Manchester that rates of schizophrenia among West Indians were five times higher than those among Whites. Dean *et al* (1981), in south London, reported that rates of schizophrenia were five times higher in African–Caribbeans compared with their White counterparts (Table 8.2).

Littlewood & Lipsedge (1981) interviewed 36 patients who had presented to an east London hospital with symptoms of a religious fervour. Of these, 20 were African–Caribbeans, 4 were West Africans and 8 were White. Among the first two groups, 70% of the sample were female. The symptoms were of gross excitement, violence and hostile irritability. There was no doubt about the diagnosis of psychosis, but doubt existed about its exact type.

Table 8.2 Rates of schizophrenia in African–Caribbeans in the UK (per 1000) (modified from Bhugra, 2001)

Study	Location	Diagnosis	Age std	White	A–C	Ratio[a]
Hemsi (1967)	Camberwell (London)	Case notes	Yes	3.0	13.0	4.0
Cochrane (1977)	England & Wales	MHE data	Yes	(m) 8.7 (f) 8.7	29.0 32.3	3.3 3.7
Carpenter & Brockington (1980)	Manchester	Hospital	Yes	2.0	11.0	5.5
Dean et al (1981)	South East England	Own	Yes	(m) 1.1 (f) 1.0	5.5 5.3	5.0 5.3
Littlewood & Lipsedge (1981)	Hackney (London)	Own	Yes	2.0	5.0	2.5
McGovern & Cope (1987)	Birmingham	Hospital	Yes	(16–29 y) 1.4 (30–64 y) 1.1	11.7 4.7	8.4 4.3
Harrison et al (1988)	Nottingham	Own	Yes	(16–29 y) 2.0 (30–44 y) 1.6	29.1 19.7	14.6 12.3
Cochrane & Bal (1989)	England & Wales	MHE data	Yes	(m) 1.2 (f) 1.2	3.9 3.3	3.3 2.8
Castle et al (1991)	London	Case notes	1965–69[b] 1970–74[b] 1980–84[b]	0.88 0.98 1.20	4.6 7.9 5.08	5.3 8.2 4.0
Thomas et al (1993)	Manchester	Hospital	Yes	3.5	32.5	9.2
Harrison et al (1997)	Nottingham	Own	Yes	5.7	46.7	8.2
Bhugra et al (1997)	London	PSE	Yes	7.5	14.7	2.0

A–C, African–Caribbean; MHE, Mental Health Enquiry; PSE, Present State Examination; std, standardised.
a. African–Caribbeans:Whites.
b. Years in which data were collected.

Harrison et al (1988), using the rigid criteria previously used for World Health Organization studies over 2 years, identified cases of first-onset schizophrenia and observed that the mean annual incidence among African–Caribbeans aged 15–54 years was 13.5 per 100000, 10 times that reported in the White population. Mean annual rates for ages 16–29 years was 36.4 per 100000, 18 times the rate in general populations. A key problem remained in calculations of the denominator; also, they compared their data with White populations for whom the sample had been collected a few years previously.

McGovern & Cope (1987) collected data from case notes of admissions to a Birmingham hospital and found that first admission rates for 16- to 29-year-olds were 53.8 per 1000 for Whites, 360.2 per 1000 for African–Caribbean immigrants and 246.0 per 1000 for African–Caribbeans born in the UK. The rates among females in the two African–Caribbean groups were broadly similar. Harvey *et al* (1990) reported that admission rates for 15- to 24-year-olds in south London were 186 per 100 000 for all African–Caribbeans (both immigrant and UK-born), compared with 58 per 100 000 for Whites. Three-quarters of the African–Caribbean patients were unemployed, compared with just over half (56%) of the Whites. The relative risk was slightly lower for their older sample.

In the early 1990s, a number of prospective studies were set up. King *et al* (1994), in north London, reported that rates of schizophrenia were 1.2 per 10 000 for Whites, 4.6 per 10 000 for Black groups (5.3 for Black Caribbeans) and 15.3 per 10 000 for Pakistanis. The last group had only two patients, as did some other groups, making generalisation a problem. Cases of psychosis among African–Caribbeans, Asians and Whites identified in two London health districts over a 1–2 year period showed rates for Whites of 3.0 per 10 000, compared with 3.6 per 10 000 for Asians and 5.9 per 10 000 for African–Caribbeans (Bhugra *et al*, 1997). When age-standardised for 18- to 29-year-olds, the rates were 14.7 per 10 000 for African–Caribbeans and 7.5 per 10 000 for Whites. The African–Caribbean group had more males, and rates of unemployment were 82%, compared with 22% in the general population and 55% among Whites. One-third of the African–Caribbeans were living alone and logistic modelling showed that ethnicity, age and gender were key factors in association with schizophrenia. Harrison *et al* (1997), in a study from Nottingham, reported that the standardised incidence rate for all psychotic disorders was higher in the African–Caribbean groups. For schizophrenia, the age-standardised rate ratio between the African–Caribbean and the White sample was 8.1, with standardised incidence rates of 46.7 per 100 000 and 5.7 per 100 000 for the two groups respectively. The majority of the African–Caribbeans (81%) were born in the UK (the rest in the Caribbean), suggesting that those who are born in this country still have considerably higher rates. The most recent study looking at rates of psychoses in populations from three centres in England (the ÆSOP study) has shown that African–Caribbeans had incidence rate ratios (IRRs) of 9.1 for schizophrenia and 8.0 for manic psychosis, compared with 5.8 and 6.2 respectively for Africans (Fearon *et al*, 2006).

In one of the few community-based prevalence studies, Nazroo (1997) observed that the annual prevalence of non-affective psychotic disorders was higher for African–Caribbeans than for Whites (13 per 1000 *v.* 8 per 1000).

From our review, some common themes start to emerge, the first being that, bearing in mind the caveats discussed above, incidence rates for schizophrenia are consistently higher among African–Caribbeans, especially the younger age groups. The aetiological factors of schizophrenia are many and it would appear that ethnicity alone may not be able to explain such a variation.

Hypotheses for high rates

Many explanations for differential incidence rates of schizophrenia have been hypothesised (Box 8.2). These hypotheses must be considered in the context of heterogeneity of the African–Caribbean samples. Using Mental Health Inquiry data on psychiatric admissions and ethnicity in London, Glover (1989) was able to demonstrate that annual rates of admissions over a 3-year period were highest among Jamaicans, at 6.82 per 1000 for men and 6.33 per 1000 for women, compared with 4.19 per 1000 for men and 4.47 per 1000 for women born in Barbados and 3.61 per 1000 for men and 4.08 per 1000 for women born in Trinidad and Tobago. However, for schizophrenia, Jamaican men and Barbados-born men had similar rates and Trinidad-born were the lowest, whereas for mania, Trinidad-born men had the highest rates. This is a rare study that makes a distinction between different Caribbean islands, thus showing the importance of defining cultural groups with some precision. The severity of economic conditions in the Caribbean, as in other countries, is a key factor in genesis of ill health. Bearing in mind this heterogeneity of population, the problems of data collection and diagnosis and the varying socioeconomic factors, the following hypotheses for explaining high rates are put forward.

Genetic factors

Rates of strictly and narrowly defined schizophrenia show less variation across different cultures and different nations when compared with rates of broadly defined schizophrenia. Studies have shown that among White

---

Box 8.2   Hypotheses for high rates

- Genetic factors
- Pregnancy and birth complications
- Social factors:
    - social inequality
    - economic status
    - discrimination
- Racism:
    - harassment
    - racial life events
    - population density

---

populations genetic factors contribute to the risk of schizophrenia. If the increased incidence of schizophrenia among UK-resident African–Caribbeans were due to a special genetic vulnerability (for example, an inherited polymorphism) that showed linkage to genes coding for physical (racial) appearance, and this conferred a greater risk among African–Caribbeans than exists among Whites in the UK, we would expect similar and higher incidence rates in all African–Caribbean populations. Incidence rates among African–Caribbeans in Jamaica are the same as those among Whites in the UK. The incidence rate among British-born African–Caribbeans is higher than among Caribbean-born African–Caribbeans. The lifetime risk of schizophrenia increases tenfold among siblings of an affected individual and is almost 50% for identical twins. Sugarman & Craufurd (1994) reported that siblings of people with schizophrenia in the African–Caribbean groups were at significantly higher risk than any other group of relatives. These findings were replicated by Hutchinson *et al* (1996), who found that siblings of second-generation schizophrenia probands had a morbid risk of schizophrenia four times higher than that of their White counterparts. The overall conclusion is that the excess incidence of schizophrenia among African–Caribbean people cannot be explained by genetic vulnerability alone. McKenzie *et al* (1995) found that UK-resident African–Caribbean people with schizophrenia had a better prognosis and suggested this finding to be more compatible with psychosocial and environmental risk factors than with genetic aetiology. Data obtained from the ÆSOP first-episode psychosis study were analysed for evidence of grey matter correlates of minor physical anomaly in ethnic groups categorised as White, African–Caribbean and Other. A higher level of anomaly was found in all three groups and was identified as a non-specific risk factor for psychosis (Dean *et al*, 2007). The same group (Dean *et al*, 2006) also demonstrated that minor physical abnormalities are associated with regional grey matter changes in the brain. Increase in the AAT-triplet repeat of the *CNR1* cannabinoid receptor gene in African–Caribbean males was found to be associated with cocaine dependence, with or without schizophrenia, but it was not identified as a specific risk for schizophrenia (Ballon *et al*, 2006).

Pregnancy and birth complications

Some researchers have shown that pregnancy and birth complications are associated with schizophrenia (McGrath & Murray, 1995), although this has been challenged (Kendell *et al*, 2000). We have observed that, in Trinidad, with normal rates of schizophrenia, pregnancy and birth complications were actually lower than those reported for the African–Caribbean populations in the UK. As the number of studies is so limited, this causative factor cannot be ruled out entirely, but certainly such observations, if replicated in Jamaican and Barbadian samples, would rule out these complications as a possible cause in this group. Related to pregnancy and birth complications

111

are other neurodevelopmental delays and factors, such as those mentioned in the previous section (Dean *et al*, 2006, 2007). There has been some research looking into the possible impact of low maternal and neonatal 25-hydroxy vitamin D_3 levels in Black (and possibly White) mothers and infants as a potential risk factor for several conditions, including schizophrenia (Bodnar *et al*, 2007). This study was carried out in Pittsburgh in the USA, but it is possible that these low levels contribute to higher incidence of several conditions in the African–Caribbean population in temperate countries, although this has not yet been proven.

Social factors

The effects of social environment and social factors such as life events on the genesis and outcome of schizophrenia are well known. The differences between immigrants and their children may well be related to a number of social factors. (It is not entirely acceptable to use terms such as 'second generation', but the alternatives are cumbersome and even less palatable.) Although new arrivals have their own problems, they also share problems with those who have been settled in the country for a considerable time.

Two hypotheses have been proposed to explain the relationship between migration and psychopathology – selection and stress. The selection hypothesis posits that those who are vulnerable to mental illness (or already ill) tend to migrate. In contrast, the stress hypothesis proposes that psychosocial stressors related to migration are implicated in mental illness. A key aspect of this stress is related to social isolation and loss of social status and social networks, and it is further complicated by acculturative processes. History of migration (foreign birth or foreign birth of at least one parent) has been associated with a relative risk of 2 for psychosis in a cross-sectional survey of children in The Netherlands (Patino *et al*, 2005).

Goal-striving and additional high expectations may be shattered by various social stressors and economic factors, thereby lowering the individual's self-esteem and intensifying stress. Once living in the host country, immigrant groups are exposed to stressful experiences similar to those faced by majority groups, but their responses may vary owing to migratory stressors (pre- and post-migration), personality, past experiences, social networks, family support and other vulnerability and protective factors. Certain social factors appear to be significant in the impact of stressors on an individual's well-being – these include housing, employment, socioeconomic status and social networks. There is little doubt that unemployed people are more likely to have poor self-esteem, low socioeconomic status and perhaps less than ideal social networks. Poor physical and mental health, poverty and poor housing are related to aetiological factors in the onset of schizophrenia (Reininghaus *et al*, 2008).

Work on social capital, defined as social cohesion and trust at a community level, shows that it is associated with psychosocial risk (Wilkinson, 1999). Analysing data from the ÆSOP first-episode psychosis study, Kirkbride *et al* (2008) found that ethnic density and social capital (measured by proxy through voter turnout) in the south London sample were both independently associated with a 5% reduced risk of non-affective psychosis. Social status and affiliations, and inequalities of power, income and status, are considered risk factors (and supportive social relations protective) for a number of health and social problems. For example, they operate on the risk of mortality and community crime, including murder. They may be seen as manifestations of extreme community distress and, if operative for African–Caribbean groups in the UK, might explain some of their vulnerability. It is known that early childhood environments and the quality of peer and attachment relationships are predictive of adult risks of ill health (Wilkinson, 1999). If African–Caribbean people born in Britain are exposed to a social environment in which they suffer exclusion, low social status, an internalised sense of inferiority and disadvantage in adulthood, then such influences might explain the higher risk of adult psychological distress. There are few data directly linking the risk of schizophrenia to social capital or to the childhood experience of relationships, attachment and identity, other than data showing that Black children internalise projected prejudicial stereotypes. However, the ÆSOP study offers some support for the theory that a disrupted childhood relationship with parents is associated with increased risk of psychosis. Separation from or death of a parent before 16 was associated with a two- to threefold increase in the risk of psychosis in both Black Caribbean and White British (but not Black African) individuals. Separation from (but not death of) a parent was more common among the Black Caribbean than the White British controls, perhaps contributing to the excess of psychosis among African–Caribbeans (Morgan *et al*, 2007). The question of why second- and third-generation African–Caribbean people rather than other immigrant minority groups are especially at risk also requires more research. Long periods of separation from one or both parents may also lead to problems in adult attachment that affect patients' engagement with and adherence to treatment (Bhugra *et al*, 1999).

As noted above, Bhugra *et al* (1997) found that rates of unemployment were much higher among African–Caribbean patients compared with African–Caribbeans in the general population and with White patients. They were also more likely to have been living alone, with low social support and poor confiding. African–Caribbean males were more likely to have been separated from their fathers for longer than 4 years. More recently, from their analysis of data from the ÆSOP study, Reininghaus *et al* (2008) reported that the increased association of non-affective psychosis and unemployment was moderated by 'social contact'. People with 'high social contact' no longer had a significant association between unemployment and non-affective psychosis. These findings appear to fit with the social capital literature, but any assertions need careful empirical work. Without it, as historical experience shows, stereotypes may be reinforced, to the detriment of African–Caribbean groups.

Racism

Racism and psychiatry have been associated in the minds of ethnic minorities as well as the majority public largely because psychiatry and psychiatrists are seen as controlling and oppressive. Misdiagnosis, as well as mismanagement, are perceived to explain the increased rates of both schizophrenia and detention under compulsory orders. This equating of misdiagnosis with racism requires careful analysis. Racism can be an institutional practice that disadvantages particular groups, or it can consist of the damaging ignorance or prejudicial attitudes of individuals. At one level, all forms of disadvantage due to professional intervention among African–Caribbean groups can, if racism is defined by a detrimental outcome, be considered racist. Institutional practices can lead to both over- and underdiagnosis. The problem of only invoking racism (individual or institutional) is that scrutiny is not given to the precise relationships, motivations and practices that should be explored further. Direct racism in the form of racial harassment or traumatic life events that are linked to the sufferer's racial, ethnic or cultural origins do not, of course, cause schizophrenia, but they are serious life events that are, by definition, experienced by Black and other ethnic minorities. Life events are known to increase the risk of relapse, and they can be compounded by the stresses of poor social situation, housing or unemployment. In a survey of employed White UK, Bangladeshi and African–Caribbean individuals, the African–Caribbeans reported more stress at work. In female African–Caribbean respondents, reported racial discrimination was associated with increased work stress and higher levels of psychological distress (Wadsworth *et al*, 2007). Analysis of data collected from the ÆSOP study revealed that 'perceived disadvantage' was associated with higher incidence of psychosis after controlling for other factors. Interestingly, Black respondents from the 'non-psychotic' group attributed their disadvantage to racism, whereas Black people with psychosis attributed it to their own situation (Cooper *et al*, 2008).

All mental health institutions should endeavour to understand institutional racism, as it may be an added burden that African–Caribbean people with schizophrenia have to bear. It is likely that racist assumptions and behaviours affect some vulnerable individuals more than others, and exploring these in a clinical assessment of cultural, identity and self-esteem-related factors will help us develop an aetiological and conceptual model of schizophrenia better suited to African–Caribbean groups.

Population density

As discussed in Chapter 2 (p. 22) one explanation for differential rates of schizophrenia may be ethnic density. We believe that, rather than the size alone of a particular immigrant group, it is population density on the one hand and social isolation, trust in the community and low self-esteem on the other that contribute to the aetiology of psychosis. Faris & Dunham (1960) showed that individuals with schizophrenia were more likely to be living alone with smaller numbers of people from their own ethnic background around them. It is possible that individuals from cultures and societies that are largely sociocentric who find themselves living alone, isolated from their own culture, may develop phenomena in response to distress that a psychiatrist considers to be psychosis; in individuals living in proximity to others from their culture, the distress might be mediated by their peers and manifest in a non-psychotic form. Furthermore, low self-esteem may act as an intermediary factor in affecting the individual's self-concept, adding to a sense of loneliness and isolation.

Conclusion

The literature leaves little doubt that rates of schizophrenia diagnosed among African–Caribbeans in the UK are much higher than among the White population, although findings on comparison with other minority ethnic groups are equivocal. Some of the increase can be explained by poor housing, high rates of unemployment and social isolation. Schizophrenia surely has a multifactorial aetiology. In different populations, some factors seem to be more loaded and therefore more significant than others, and ethnicity and implicit racism may play a role in this. This interactional factorial model remains hypothetical and needs to be confirmed in large multicentre studies involving a wide range of ethnic groups. The factors themselves, both environmental and psychological, must be identified and explored (Fig. 8.1). The sequence in which they operate and the relative contribution they make to the total risk of schizophrenia requires more research.

For African–Caribbeans, living in Britain can generate distress by influencing self-esteem, identity and chances of success. Schizophrenia, although understood as a predominantly genetic condition among Whites, is the label we give to the same syndromal pattern African–Caribbeans, but we believe that it has different aetiological factors and prognosis in this group.

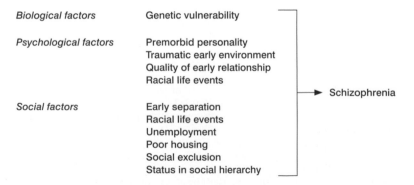

Fig. 8.1 Aetiological factors requiring empirical evaluation.

115

References

Babcock, J. W. (1895) The colored insane. *Alienist and Neurologist*, **16**, 423–447.

Ballon, N., Leroy, S., Roy, C., *et al* (2006) (AAT)n repeat in the cannabinoid receptor gene (CNR1): association with cocaine addiction in an African–Caribbean population. *Pharmacogenomics Journal*, **6**, 126–130.

Bhugra, D. (2001) Migration and schizophrenia. *Acta Psychiatrica Scandinavica Supplementum*, **407**, 68–73.

Bhugra, D., Leff, J., Mallett, R., *et al* (1997) Incidence and outcome of schizophrenia in Whites, African–Caribbeans and Asians in London. *Psychological Medicine*, **27**, 791–798.

Bhugra, D., Mallett, R. & Leff, J. (1999) Schizophrenia and African–Caribbeans: a conceptual model of aetiology. *International Review of Psychiatry*, **11**, 145–152.

Bodnar, L., Simhan, H., Powers, R., *et al* (2007) High prevalence of vitamin D insufficiency in black and white pregnant women residing in the Northern United States and their neonates. *Journal of Nutrition*, **137**, 447–452.

Carpenter, L. & Brockington, I. F. (1980) A study of mental illness in Asians, West Indians and Africans living in Manchester. *British Journal of Psychiatry*, **137**, 201–205.

Castle, D., Wessely, S., Der, G., *et al* (1991) The incidence of operationally defined schizophrenia in Camberwell, 1965–84. *British Journal of Psychiatry*, **159**, 790–794.

Chasson, J. B. (1963) Race, age and sex in discharge probabilities of first admissions to a psychiatric hospital. *Psychiatry*, **26**, 391–393.

Cochrane, R. (1977) Mental illness in immigrants in England and Wales. *Social Psychiatry*, **12**, 25–35.

Cochrane, R. & Bal, S. S. (1989) Mental hospital admission rates of immigrants to England. *Social Psychiatry and Psychiatric Epidemiology*, **24**, 2–11.

Cooper, C., Morgan, C., Byrne, M., *et al* (2008) Perceptions of disadvantage, ethnicity and psychosis. *British Journal of Psychiatry*, **192**, 185–190.

Crawford, F., Rollins, G. & Sutherland, R. (1960) Variation between Negroes and whites in concepts of mental illness and its treatment. *Annals of the New York Academy of Sciences*, **84**, 918–937.

Dean, G., Walsh, D., Downing, H., *et al* (1981) First admissions of native-born and immigrants to psychiatric hospitals in South-East England 1976. *British Journal of Psychiatry*, **139**, 506–512.

Dean, K., Fearon, P., Morgan, K., *et al* (2006) Grey matter correlates of minor physical anomalies in the ÆSOP first-episode psychosis study. *British Journal of Psychiatry*, **189**, 221–228.

Dean, K., Dazzan, P., Lloyd, T., *et al* (2007) Minor physical anomalies across ethnic groups in a first episode psychosis sample. *Schizophrenia Research*, **89**, 86–90.

Faris, R. & Dunham, W. (1960) *Mental Disorders in Urban Areas*. University of Chicago Press.

Fearon, P., Kirkbride, J. B., Morgan, C., *et al* (2006) Incidence of schizophrenia and other psychoses in ethnic minorty groups: results from the MRC ÆSOP study. *Psychological Medicine*, **36**, 1541–1550.

Frumkin, R. (1954) Race and major mental disorders. *Journal of Negro Education*, **23**, 97–98.

Glover, G. (1989) Differences in psychiatric admission patterns between Caribbeans from different islands. *Social Psychiatry*, **24**, 209–211.

Green, E. M. (1914) Psychosis among Negroes. A comparative study. *Journal of Neurones and Mental Disease*, **41**, 697–708.

Harrison, G., Owens, D., Holton, A., *et al* (1988) A prospective study of severe mental disorder in Afro-Caribbean patients. *Psychological Medicine*, **18**, 643–657.

Harrison, G., Glazebrook, C., Brewin, J., *et al* (1997) Increased incidence of psychotic disorders in migrants from the Caribbean in the UK. *Psychological Medicine*, **27**, 799–806.

Harvey, I., William, M., McGuffin, P., et al (1990) The functional psychoses in Afro-Caribbeans. British Journal of Psychiatry, **157**, 515–522.

Hemsi, L. K. (1967) Psychiatric morbidity of West Indian immigrants. Social Psychiatry, **2**, 95–100.

Hutchinson, G., Takei, N., Fahy, T. A., et al (1996) Morbid risk of schizophrenia in first-degree relatives of white and African–Caribbean patients with psychosis. British Journal of Psychiatry, **169**, 776–780.

Jaco, E. G. (1960) The Social Epidemiology of Mental Disorders. Russell Sage Foundation.

Kendell, R. E., McInneny, K., Juszczack, E., et al (2000) Obstetric complications and schizophrenia. Two case–control studies based on structured obstetric records. British Journal of Psychiatry, **176**, 516–522.

Kiev, A. (1965) Psychiatric morbidity of West Indian immigrants in an urban general practice. British Journal of Psychiatry, **111**, 51–56.

King, M., Cole, E., Leavy, G., et al (1994) Incidence of psychotic illness in London. BMJ, **309**, 1115–1119.

Kirkbride, J. B., Boydell, J., Ploubidis, G. B., et al (2008) Testing the association between the incidence of schizophrenia and social capital in an urban area. Psychological Medicine, **38**, 1083–1094.

Klee, G. D., Spiro, E., Bahm, E., et al (1967) An ecological analysis of diagnosed mental illness in Baltimore. In Psychiatric Epidemiology and Mental Health Planning (eds R. R. Monroe, G. D. Klee & E. B. Brody). American Psychiatric Association.

Littlewood, R. & Lipsedge, M. (1981) Some social phenomenological characteristics of psychotic immigrants. Psychological Medicine, **11**, 289–302.

Malzberg, B. (1963) Mental disorders in the US. In Encyclopaedia of Mental Health (ed. M. A. Deutsch). Vol. 5. Franklin Watts.

McGovern, D. & Cope, R. (1987) First admission rates of first and second generation Afro-Caribbeans. Social Psychiatry, **22**, 139–148.

McGrath, J. & Murray, R. (1995) Risk factors for schizophrenia from conception to birth. In Schizophrenia (eds S. R. Hirsch & D. Weinberger). Blackwell Science.

McKenzie, K., van Os, J., Fahy, T., et al (1995) Psychosis with good prognosis in Afro-Caribbean people now living in the United Kingdom. BMJ, **311**, 1325–1328.

McLean, H. U. (1949) The emotional health of Negroes. Journal of Negro Education, **18**, 283–290.

Morgan, C., Kirkbridge, J., Leff, J., et al (2007) Parental separation, loss and psychosis in different ethnic groups: a case–control study. Psychological Medicine, **37**, 495–503.

Mukherjee, S., Shukla, S., Woodle, J., et al (1983) Misdiagnosis of schizophrenia in bipolar patients. American Journal of Psychiatry, **140**, 1571–1574.

Nazroo, J. Y. (1997) Ethnicity and Mental Health. PSI Press.

Patino, L. R., Selten, J.-P., Van Engeland, H. V., et al (2005) Migration, family dysfunction and psychotic symptoms in children and adolescents. British Journal of Psychiatry, **186**, 442–443.

Reininghaus, U. A., Morgan, C., Simpson, J., et al (2008) Unemployment, social isolation, achievement–expectation mismatch and psychosis: findings from the ÆSOP study. Social Psychiatry and Psychiatric Epidemiology, **43**, 743–751.

Rwegellera, G. G. C. (1977) Psychiatric morbidity among West Africans and West Indians living in London. Psychological Medicine, **7**, 317–329.

Snowden, L. & Cheung, F. (1990) Use of inpatient mental health services by members of ethnic minority groups. American Psychologist, **45**, 347–355.

Sugarman, P. A. & Craufurd, D. (1994) Schizophrenia in the Afro-Caribbean community. British Journal of Psychiatry, **164**, 474–480.

Thomas, C. S., Stone, K., Osborn, M., et al (1993) Psychiatric morbidity and compulsory admission among UK-born Europeans, Afro-Caribbeans and Asians in central Manchester. British Journal of Psychiatry, **163**, 91–99.

Wadsworth, E., Dhillon, K., Shaw, C., et al (2007) Racial discrimination, ethnicity and work stress. Occupational Medicine, **57**, 18–24.

Wilson, D. & Lantz, E. (1957) The effect of culture change of the Negro race in Virginia as indicated by a study of state hospital admissions. *American Journal of Psychiatry*, **114**, 25–32.

Wilkinson, R. G. (1999) Income inequality, social cohesion and health: clarifying the theory. A reply to Muntaner and Lynch. *International Journal of Health Services*, **29**, 525–543.

CHAPTER 9

Depression in immigrants and ethnic minorities

Dinesh Bhugra and Oyedeji Ayonrinde

Summary   Migration and its associated processes can be a considerable stress for those who are migrating as well as those around them. Depression should be a common sequela of the process, but is not consistently found to be so. This chapter reviews the literature and suggests that various vulnerability factors, including culture shock and changed cultural identity, can play a role in the genesis of depression. Clinicians must be aware of patterns of migration and resilience factors in order to plan any intervention strategies. Stresses due to political and economic factors will have differing influences on the mental state of individuals. One possible contribution may be a discrepancy between aspiration and achievement, which can result in poor self-esteem, leading to depression.

Migration, whatever its cause or purpose, can place the individual under considerable stress. However, the process can be made more manageable and less traumatic by factors such as adequate preparation and social support, along with acceptance by the new culture. Whether individuals travel alone or with family, how the new country welcomes them, their legal status and economic factors all play a role in their adjustment to migration.

People moving within the same culture, for example those moving from rural hamlets to large cities, can also experience stress and feelings of alienation. The resulting changes in environment and social support can act as pathogens and the stress (following the stress diathesis model) can increase the likelihood of mental illness. The ideological commitments of individuals to the migration as well as their personality traits need to be understood (see Chapter 2, this volume). Coupled with personality traits are beliefs and attitudes related to the individuals' own culture and their individual aspirations and role performance.

Personality factors lead to a number of stress-related illnesses. Eysenck (1990) noted that there is sufficient evidence to show that personality factors and stress can lead to feelings of helplessness and hopelessness and finally to depression. It has been argued that schizotypal personality disorder is associated with migration and subsequent psychosis, but no similar model has been identified for depression in immigrants. It is possible that some personality types are more vulnerable to dealing poorly with loss, and in such individuals it may produce depression.

Symptoms of depression such as guilt, shame and loss of libido vary across cultures (for an overview see Bhugra, 1996). Murphy *et al* (1967) reported that psychiatrists in 30 countries found varying prevalence of depressive symptoms such as fatigue, loss of appetite, loss of sexual interest, weight loss and self-accusatory ideas. These symptoms are largely biological, whereas a five-centre cross-cultural study by Jablensky *et al* (1981) reported the core symptoms of depression to be predominantly psychological: sadness, joylessness, anxiety, tension, lack of energy, loss of interest, poor concentration and ideas of insufficiency, inadequacy and worthlessness. Since the presence and expression of guilt, somatic symptoms and shame in migrants can depend on their culture of origin, depressive manifestations can be overlooked (Bhugra, 2003).

Prevalence of depression

Most epidemiological studies have used European or North American assessment instruments, which might not identify depression if it does not appear in the standard Western form. Consequently, the findings of such studies among immigrant groups are equivocal, to say the least. Some have demonstrated high rates of common mental disorders in immigrants (Krupinski, 1967; Kimura *et al*, 1975), whereas others (e.g. Nazroo, 1997) have shown low rates in some immigrant communities.. Cochrane (1977) reported that rates of admission to psychiatric hospitals in England and Wales were nearly twice as high among immigrants compared with native groups. After standardisation for age and gender, studies showed much higher admission rates for Irish and West Indian immigrants than for those from India and Pakistan.

Cochrane (1983) subsequently attributed some of the discrepancy in rates across immigrants to selective migration, ambivalent relationships and adjustment to culture. Kuo (1976), from the USA, recommended that the role of social isolation, culture shock, goal-striving stress and culture change must be understood in the aetiology of psychological distress in immigrants. Data on increased rates of common mental disorders among foreign students prompted Ward (1967) to propose a 'foreign student syndrome', which is characterised by non-specific somatic complaints, a passive withdrawn interaction style and an unkempt appearance. He further suggested that students presenting with the syndrome were more likely to seek help for physical complaints. Others have reported similar findings (Schild, 1962; Hopkins *et al*, 1975; Still (1961), cited in Furnham, 1988). Although these findings are old, they are still important. In a study of higher education students in the UK published in 1961 and cited by Furnham (1988), Still observed that only 14% of British students had psychological problems, compared with 28% of Iraqi, Iranian and Nigerian students, 22% of Turkish and Egyptian students and 18% of students from the Indian subcontinent. Babiker *et al* (1980) noted that increased rates of medical consultations and symptoms were associated with greater distance from country or culture of origin, and they reported that students who were 'culturally distant' used health services as an approachable haven.

Subsequent studies have confirmed some, but not all, of these findings. The variations in results may be due to different or better methods and may also reflect different interactions between immigrants and their new community. In a community sample of 'native' White people and immigrant groups in Britain, Nazroo (1997) observed the following weekly prevalence rates of depressive neurosis (men/women: 'native' White 2.7%/4.8%; Irish 5.8%/6.8%; African–Caribbean 5.6%/6.4%; Indian 2.5%/3.2%; Pakistani 3.8%/2.9%; Bangladeshi 1.6%/2.2%. These diagnoses were made using the Clinical Interview Schedule – Revised Version. Immigrants who were fluent in English reported the same rates as their British counterparts. If fluency in English were taken as a proxy measure for acculturation, it would appear that morbidity among immigrants with fluent English was at the same level as in the White British community. The data thus show mixed results. It would appear that migration produces stresses, but that as time goes by the stresses of the act of migration are replaced by the stresses of living in an alien culture. Therefore, the stage at which data are collected can affect results.

Data from the EMPIRIC study (Sproston & Nazroo, 2002), which focused on the main ethnic groups in England, showed that the Irish group had the highest prevalence of common mental disorders (although only 10% of Irish men with any ICD–10 diagnosis met criteria for a depressive episode) and that the differences across ethnic groups were not statistically significant. Among the Indian and Pakistani groups, common mental disorders were more prevalent in the women than in the men. However, rates were also high among those who were born in England or migrated here at an early age; this might be related to the problems of culture conflict (see Acculturation below).

One further meta-analysis reported that there is no conclusive evidence for a large increase in the risk of mood disorders associated with migration. However, it acknowledged that few studies were available solely focusing on unipolar depression (Swinnen & Selten, 2007).

The three stages of migration (pre-migration, the migration itself and post-migration), although discrete in theory, are not always so in practice. The pre- and post-migration stages last for varying periods. The key pathoprotective or pathoprovocative factors in the genesis of depression and other common mental disorders are listed in Box 9.1.

Bochner (1986) suggests that two modes of cultural contact govern the reaction of people to unfamiliar cultures: adjustment to and reflective learning of the new culture. Individuals exposed to another culture (be it

---

Box 9.1 Aetiological model of common mental disorders in immigrants

Vulnerability factors

Pre-migration:
- Biological and psychological factors
- Social skills deficit
- Forced migration
- Persecution

Migration:
- Negative life events
- Bereavement

Post-migration:
- Culture shock
- Culture conflict
- Cultural bereavement
- Discrepancy between achievement and expectation

Protective factors

Pre-migration:
- Psychological factors such as resilience
- Higher socioeconomic status
- Voluntary migration
- Adequate preparation and run-in time

Migration:
- Strong cultural and ethnic identity
- Social support and social networks

Post-migration:
- Resilience
- Social support

---

by cross-border or within-country migration) may reject their culture of origin, reject the new culture and militantly retreat into their own culture (exaggerated deculturation) or vacillate between the two cultures (marginal syndrome). Furthermore, they might not adhere rigidly to a single option. It might be hypothesised that there would be exaggerated levels of depression among those who are marginalised, but data for this observation are lacking. Taft (1986) recommends that adjustments, national identity, cultural competence, social absorption and role socialisation all need to be identified and studied in immigrant populations.

Aetiological factors

Furnham & Bochner (1986) highlighted eight theoretical constructs for adjustment following the process of migration: movement as loss; fatalism; selective migration; expectations; negative life events; social support; social skills deficit; and a clash of values with the new culture. Some of these might cause depression (e.g. loss, negative life events), whereas others (e.g. social skills deficit) might simply be associated with depression. We do not propose to discuss them all here. Theoretically, immigrants who have lost a number of support factors might be more prone to depression, but the data are not very robust.

Acculturation

Acculturation is the process by which a minority group assimilates cultural values and beliefs of a majority community. The minority group's adaptation to the majority culture's customs, values and language can be voluntary or forced. Acculturation can arouse strong feelings, especially if it is forced. In addition, the contact between the two groups can lead to assimilation, integration, rejection or deculturation. Each of these can have different effects on individuals' personal and social functioning.

Culture shock might be defined as sudden unpleasant feelings that violate an individual's expectations of the new culture and cause them to value their own culture negatively. Oberg (1960) identified six aspects of culture shock: strain; a sense of loss or feelings of deprivation; rejection by members of the new culture; role expectation and role confusion; surprise, anxiety and indignation; and feelings of impotence. Furnham (1988) points out that, although others have emphasised different aspects, these six are useful core concepts. Bock (1970) defines culture shock as an emotional reaction to an inability to understand, control and predict behaviour, which appears to be a basic human need. This lack of familiarity may extend to other aspects of functioning such as language, etiquette, food, clothes and climate.

Culture shock can thus be seen as a stress reaction arising from the uncertainty of important physical and psychological rewards. Immigrants may therefore remain confused, anxious, apathetic or angry until a level of adjustment is reached. Culture shock may be seen as a transitional experience and also as essential for self-development and personal growth. However, journalists, business executives and film stars with several places of residence around the globe and ease of movement are less likely to experience culture shock than are economic migrants. Thus, social class and having a financial 'cushion' might also influence stress responses.

Culture conflict refers to the sense of tension experienced by people from a minority culture. This is much more common for the children of immigrant parents, when the parents' culture and values compete with those of the majority culture in which the children spend a significant part of the day. This conflict can contribute to a further sense of alienation and isolation, where the children find themselves 'belonging' to neither the majority nor the minority culture.

Both culture shock and culture conflict can cause depression in immigrants, probably by interacting with the personality traits of individuals.

Clinicians should be aware of culture shock and have ready a strategy for dealing with it. This might include a focused psychotherapeutic intervention to address the aftermath of the experience. After investigating an individual's cultural identity, the clinician should have an idea of that person's resilience, social support and other protective factors that can be used in treatment planning.

Cognitions

The cognitive schemas of depression in immigrants and ethnic minorities require study. The standard model of the depressive triad – 'I am a failure, the world is a horrible place and the future is bleak' – might not apply universally. Notions of the self and 'I-ness' too will vary across cultures. In sociocentric societies, the individual self may be subsumed in the kinship, family and society. Migration might cause individuals to reconsider, and even change, their notions of self, which might cause additional stress.

If the individual's model of depression is non-medical or non-psychological it might not fit with standard Western diagnostic models or classificatory categories. The cognitive schema of refugees and political asylum-seekers may contain realistic components of persecution. Such paranoid or persecutory thoughts might further contribute to social withdrawal and a sense of despair and alienation. Time elapsed since migration is another factor that should be taken into consideration. The period immediately after migration is likely to prove a vulnerable time, as is the period 5–7 years later, when individuals have settled down but not fulfilled their aspirations (Bhugra, 2003).

Gilbert & Allan (1998) propose that social rank, defeat and a sense of entrapment (which is linked with learned helplessness) are important cognitive factors for depression. If the pathway to flight is blocked for social or personal reasons, the sense of entrapment may be more significant in the aetiology of depression. Arrested flight involves suppression of explorative behaviour, submissive postures, isolation and severely restricted movement, all of which can be experienced by immigrants at various times.

More recent intra-country migration studies, in which concepts such as acculturation may interpreted as less powerful, are also available. China has seen a significant rural to urban migration occur over the past two decades. Li et al (2007) reported no significant increases in depression and hypothesised that this was due to the positive aspects of such migration, including increased upward economic mobility, improved opportunities and high social capital in the immigrant communities.

Having an external locus of control (when the individual feels that external forces or events such as chance, fate or the stars are causing their behaviour or actions) has been shown to be related to poor mental health and a lack of adaptation (Furnham & Bochner, 1986). However, it is likely that individuals who accept their 'fate' also accept their stresses. This might explain lower than expected rates of reported mental distress among immigrants from the Indian subcontinent, among whom belief in karma, fate or the stars is quite prevalent.

Selective migration

The hypothesis of selective migration of vulnerable individuals predicts that those who are prone to depression tend to migrate. Although studies have shown a wide variation in prevalence rates of depression in different countries (Simon *et al*, 2002), it is unlikely that current strict immigration laws allow vulnerable individuals to move freely.

Achievements and expectations

Mismatched aspirations and achievements can also produce stress, which can be related to the onset or genesis of depression. Expectations of the new country in terms of both personal and social gains (prestige in particular) must be matched by achievement if the individual is to function well. If achievements do not match aspirations, individuals are open to low mood, a sense of alienation and, more importantly, a sense of failure – all of which can trigger depression. It is possible that economic migrants will have heightened expectations of social mobility, which are more likely to contribute to a striving for success that might not be matched by achievement. The discrepancy might contribute to poor self-esteem, which in itself might not cause depression but joins cumulative stressors such as racial discrimination.

More recent studies from China again add to the literature. In a study of forced migration due to the construction of the Three Gorges Dam, Hwang *et al* (2007) concluded that anticipation of involuntary migration is a robust predictor of mental distress. Anticipation of forced migration elevates depression (Center for Epidemiologic Studies Depression Scale score) not only directly, but also indirectly by weakening the social and psychological resources (i.e., social support and mastery) that safeguard the mental well-being of immigrants. However, the results show much less support for the hypothesis that resources moderate harmful effects of forced migration overall.

In assessing the presence of depression in immigrants (Box 9.2) it is important that clinicians establish whether mismatched aspirations and achievements might be creating stress (Box 9.3).

Box 9.2 Assessing depression in immigrants

- Assess sadness, joylessness, hopelessness, lack of energy, poor concentration
- Look for biological symptoms, e.g. loss of sleep and libido, change in appetite
- Assess the reasons for migration, preparation and the migration itself
- Ascertain aspirations and achievements
- Ascertain social support and peer group contacts
- Assess negative life events, feelings of loss and grief
- Assess self-esteem and self-confidence
- Assess whether any social skills deficit is present
- Assess the degree of culture shock
- Assess cultural identity

Box 9.3 Aspirations and achievements

The following questions determine patients' aspirations and achievements:

- What had you achieved before you migrated?
- What level did you think you would reach in the field of ...?
- Have you done so?
- If not, how far do you think you have to go?
- Do you feel let down that you have not done so?
- Do you feel content that you have done so?

The clinician can address the discrepancy between a patient's aspirations and achievements by encouraging the individual to look at these in different ways, for example by looking at realistic situations and thinking of even small achievements in a positive light.

Conclusion

Not all immigrants develop depression. Both personal vulnerabilities and the experiences of migration contribute to its genesis and perpetuation. Culture shock and cultural identity are both involved. Clinicians must be aware of the reasons for migration, social support, models or explanations of depression and how help is sought. Immigrants may give different emphasis to different symptoms. The clinician must take into account social, cultural and individual factors. Causative and associative factors of depression should be assessed in the context of the migration itself. Our discussion of the factors that can affect depression in migrants is not exhaustive: see Bhugra (2003) for a fuller consideration. However, we have highlighted areas in the lives of minority ethnic and migrant groups that we believe to be of significance.

References

Babiker, I., Cox, J. & Miller, P. (1980) The measurement of cultural distance and its relationship to medical consultations, symptomatology and examination performance of overseas students at Edinburgh University. *Social Psychiatry and Psychiatric Epidemiology*, **15**, 109–116.

Bhugra, D. (1996) Depression across cultures. *Primary Care Psychiatry*, **2**, 153–165.

Bhugra, D. (2003) Migration and depression. *Acta Psychiatrica Scandinavica Supplementum*, **418**, 67–73.

Bochner, S. (1986) Coping with unfamiliar cultures. *Australian Journal of Psychology*, **38**, 347–358.

Bock, P. (ed.) (1970) *Culture Shock: A Reader in Modern Cultural Anthropology*. Knopf.

Cochrane, R. (1977) Mental illness in immigrants to England and Wales. *Social Psychiatry*, **12**, 25–35.

Cochrane, R. (1983) *The Social Causation of Mental Illness*. Longman.

Eysenck, H. (1990) The prediction of death from cancer by means of personality stress questionnaire. *Perceptual and Motor Skills*, **72**, 216–218.

Furnham, A. (1988) Adjustment of sojourners. In *Cross-Cultural Adaptation* (eds Y. Y. Kim & W. B. Gudykunst). Sage.

Furnham, A. & Bochner, S. (1986) *Culture Shock*. Routledge.

Gilbert, P. & Allan, S. (1998) The role of defeat and entrapment (arrested flight) in depression: an exploration of an evolutionary view. *Psychological Medicine*, **28**, 585–598.

Hopkins, J., Malleson, N. & Sarroff, I. (1975) Some non-intellectual correlates of success and failure among university students. *British Journal of Sociology*, **9**, 25–36.

Hwang, S.-S., Xi, J., Cao, Y., *et al* (2007) Anticipation of migration and psychological stress and the Three Gorges Dam project, China. *Social Science and Medicine*, **65**, 1012–1024.

Jablensky, A., Sartorius, N., Gulbinat, W., *et al* (1981) Characteristics of depressive patients contacting psychiatric services in four cultures. A report from the WHO collaborative study on the assessment of depressive disorders. *Acta Psychiatrica Scandinavica*, **63**, 367–383.

Kimura, S. D., Mikolashek, P. & Kirk, S. (1975) Madness in paradise: psychiatric crises among newcomers in Honolulu. *Hawaii Medical Journal*, **34**, 275–278.

Krupinski, J. (1967) Sociological aspects of mental ill health in migrants. *Social Science and Medicine*, **1**, 267–281.

Kuo, W. (1976) Theories of migration and mental health. *Social Science and Medicine*, **10**, 297–306.

Li, L., Wang, H., Ye, X., *et al* (2007) The mental health status of Chinese rural–urban migrant workers. Comparison with permanent urban and rural dwellers. *Social Psychiatry and Psychiatric Epidemiology*, **42**, 716–722.

Murphy, H. B. M., Wittkower, E. D. & Chance, N. (1967) Crosscultural inquiry into the symptomatology of depression: preliminary report. *International Journal of Social Psychiatry*, **13**, 6–15.

Nazroo, J. (1997) *Ethnicity and Mental Health*. PSI.

Oberg, K. (1960) Culture shock: adjustment to new culture environments. *Practical Anthropology*, **7**, 177–182.

Schild, E. (1962) The foreign student, as a stranger, learning the norms of host cultures. *Journal of Social Issues*, **18**, 41–54.

Simon, G., Goldberg, D., Vonkorff, M., *et al* (2002) Understanding cross-national differences in depression prevalence. *Psychological Medicine*, **32**, 585–594.

Sproston, K. & Nazroo, J. (eds) (2002) *Ethnic Minority Psychiatric Illness Rates in the Community (EMPIRIC)*. TSO (The Stationery Office).

Swinnen, S. G. H. A. & Selten, J.-P. (2007) Mood disorders and migration. Meta-analysis. *British Journal of Psychiatry*, **190**, 6–10.

Taft, R. (1986) Methodological considerations in the study of immigrant adaptations in Australia. *Australian Journal of Psychology*, **38**, 339–346.

Ward, E. (1967) Some observations of the underlying dynamics of conflict in a foreign student. *Journal of the American College of Health*, **10**, 430–440.

CHAPTER 10

Attempted suicide among South Asian women

Dinesh Bhugra and Manisha Desai

Summary In this chapter we illustrate epidemiological findings on attempted suicide in South Asian people in their countries of origin and in the UK and compare social and cultural factors across the two settings. There is considerable evidence to suggest that rates of attempted suicide are elevated in South Asian women. The causes of this increase are not clearly understood. In this chapter we explore some of the underlying reasons and differences between adolescent and young adult women of South Asian descent.

Humans have attempted and successfully completed suicide since time immemorial. The reasons for killing or harming oneself vary with cultures and societies and in urban and rural settings. In ancient European cultures, suicide was common, usually by hanging among women and by self-harm with various tools among men. Ancient Hindu texts allowed individuals to kill themselves, but in later Upanishadic periods suicide was generally condemned, although it was acceptable for holy men, especially if they had reached the stage in their life where they had gained insight into life's problems. Suicide was permitted on religious grounds, as death was seen as the beginning of another life. Somasundaram *et al* (1989) report that the *Purananuru*, a great 11th-century Tamil collection of poems includes references to self-immolation by a widow on the death of her husband. There is also mention of suicide by starvation or fasting. The authors conclude that, irrespective of race, religion, culture and location of the civilisation, there was almost identical motivation for suicidal behaviour. In most countries cited in the World Health Organization's statistics on suicide rates in 2004, the rate for men is two to four times higher than that for women. China and India are the exceptions, where rates across genders are comparable. In both of these countries, conflict with family or in-laws is often cited as a major contributing factor (Bhugra *et al*, 1999*a*; Zhang *et al*, 2004).

Parasuicide, attempted suicide and self-harm may be suicidal gestures, manipulative attempts to seek help or unsuccessful attempts to die.

Generally, the act is non-habitual and may be influenced by single or multiple crises. Although methods of psychological autopsy often suggest an association between suicide and psychiatric morbidity (Pouliot & DeLeo, 2006), in countries with high suicide rates such as China (Zhang *et al*, 2002) and Sri Lanka (Marecek, 1998) local psychiatrists often do not subscribe to the view that suicide is related to mental illness.

The Indian subcontinent

Most reported data have been collected from general hospitals. One of the key problems in identifying rates of attempted suicide is that of defining the act. A second problem is that, particularly in countries such as India, where suicide is legally proscribed, individuals or their families give false reasons for their behaviour and hide problems rather than admit to suicidal thoughts or acts.

In Madurai in South India, the number of patients presenting with attempted suicide trebled between 1974 and 1978. Of the 114 suicide attempts studied in 1965, 65 were by men and this male dominance persisted in data collected 2 years later. The dominant feelings of those attempting suicide were depression, anger, spite, jealousy and a desire for attention. At 10-year follow-up of those who repeated a suicide attempt, 19 of the 35 individuals were men. The clinician described 20 of the 35 as 'hysterical' with an inadequate or immature personality; of the rest, 8 had schizophrenia, 3 were dependent on drugs, 2 had a stammer, 1 had epilepsy and 1 had a toxic psychosis. The absence of depression is striking (Rao & Chennian, 1972).

When differentiating between suicide and attempted suicide on the basis of psychological factors, Rao (1992) cautions that suicide does not result from a single cause. He suggests that attempted suicide should be linked with personality disorders and argues that social isolation contributes to increased rates of suicide and attempted suicide.

Quarrels with in-laws and problems in interpersonal relationships appear to be extremely common causes of attempted suicide (Ponnudurai *et al*, 1986; Bannerjee *et al*, 1990).

Repeat attempts are linked with alcohol misuse and poor personal relationships. In a 2-year follow-up of 86 patients in Madras, Ponnudurai *et al* (1991) found that a sizeable minority of participants could not be traced at the address given. Of those who were traced, 14% continued to have suicidal intent and men were three times more likely to show this than women. For women, their husbands' unemployment and alcohol misuse were relevant factors in suicidal thought and intent. Ponnudurai *et al*'s original (1986) study of these patients found that in 10% of cases alcohol had played a significant role and that more than one-third of patients (38%) had made a suicide attempt using organophosphorus compounds. Males were more likely to attempt suicide than were females, with those aged 15–20 years being the most vulnerable. This confirmed the findings of earlier studies (Rao, 1965; Sathyavathi, 1971). Interpersonal difficulties and arguments had led to suicide attempts in 25% of patients. Unemployment and alcohol misuse were also important factors.

Khan & Reza (1998), reporting from Karachi, found that women were more likely to attempt suicide than men and the causative factors included family conflicts, problems with their mothers-in-law and domestic violence.

In Sri Lanka, it has been suggested that an increase in the suicide rate could be linked to the easy access to poisonous agricultural chemicals (Gunesvaran et al, 1984). Marecek (1998) found that, when asked about suicide using a case vignette, a Sri Lankan sample suggested causes that included academic failure and interpersonal difficulties, especially disappointments in love. This sample attributed disturbed feelings and actions to planetary influences. A psychological autopsy of suicide cases in Sri Lanka found moderate to severe depression in 37% of individuals, but alcohol dependence in about 50% of the males and only 2.5% of the females (Abeyasinghe & Gunnell, 2008).

Women admitted with puerperal psychosis in India were found to have high rates (38%) of suicidal ideation (Babu et al, 2008). A study of suicidal ideation in patients with depression (Chakraborty & Chatterjee, 2007) reported that individuals who attempted suicide during the current episode had significantly more past suicide attempts, suicidal ideation, early and middle insomnia, and total Hamilton Depression Rating Scale score. Multivariate logistic regression analysis showed severity of suicidal ideation to be the most significant predictor of suicide attempts.

Dramatic and public suicide is a way of political protest, and in 1990 Indian newspaper articles described a series of public deaths, many by self-immolation, triggered by a government decision on employment of the lower castes (Bhugra, 1991). Kumar et al (1995) reported on 50 consecutive suicide attempts and found that 90% of patients had a psychiatric diagnosis and that the risk of suicide was linked with this. However, their findings are not universal.

South Asian immigrant populations

We now compare these rates with those reported among South Asian populations originating from the Indian subcontinent that have settled in other countries around the world.

Several studies have indicated that rates of attempted and completed suicide are high among South Asians around the world. In a study from a hill resort in Malaysia, where three-quarters of attempted suicides were by Indians, most of whom were of Tamil origin, Maniam (1988) hypothesised that the ambivalent attitudes of the Hindu religion towards suicide may account for part of the increased rates of suicide and attempted suicide. The study showed that younger Asian females had higher suicide and attempted suicide rates than older females and males of all ages and ethnicity, and the most common method they used was poisonous agricultural chemicals. Common precipitating factors included interpersonal difficulties and family conflicts, especially intercaste love problems.

The young married women from the Indian diaspora in South Africa were found to have higher suicide rates in Durban (Meer, 1976). People of Indian origin in Penang Malayasia were found to be more likely to use 'chemical poisoning' and had a higher mortality rate compared with people of Malay or Chinese origin (Fathelrahman *et al*, 2001).

In Fiji, Haynes (1984) reported that rates of suicide were higher among older men and young women of Indian origin than among the native Fijian population. She argued that the Indians were probably particularly vulnerable to attempted suicide, because of their historical low status and stereotyping and because they were a political minority, underrepresented in government and the professional classes.

Similar findings have been reported in Trinidad (Mahy, 1993). Studies there too have shown that interracial relationships and marriages play a very important role in precipitating suicide attempts. Paraquat was reported to be one of the key substances used by Trinidadian Asians.

The UK

There have been very few studies of attempted suicide in minority ethnic groups in the UK. An early study was a retrospective case note study of Asian immigrants in the West Midlands city of Birmingham (Burke, 1976). This reported that crude adjusted suicide rates were twice as high among females than males, although repeat attempts were infrequent. Agricultural chemicals were rarely taken. Overall, the number of suicide attempts was low among Asians when compared with the base population. More than half (58%) attributed their attempt to interpersonal problems, and a quarter gave no reason. The crude adjusted rates for the immigrants were in the middle of the range reported for natives in India and natives in Edinburgh.

In a prospective study from Birmingham nearly a decade later, Merrill & Owens (1986) reported that the picture was beginning to change. All cases of individuals admitted to a hospital following attempted suicide were studied over a 2-year period. Of 196 Asian patients recruited, 139 had been born on the Indian subcontinent, 52 had been born in the UK and a few had been born in East Africa. Females were almost three times as likely to present with attempted suicide and were of a younger age group. Females of Asian origin reported marital problems significantly more frequently and many of these problems were due to cultural conflicts. Arranged marriages, rejection of arranged marriages and associated marital problems were reported as contributory factors by the Asian female sample. Since the researchers were White and male, they acknowledge that they may have missed some important and relevant information.

In a subsequent study, Merrill & Owens (1988) compared attempted suicide in four immigrant groups (Asian, West Indian, Irish and Scottish) and in an English-born sample. The annual rates of self-poisoning in the immigrant groups exceeded rates in their countries of origin. Among the Asians and West Indians, males and older females were underrepresented but young females had rates similar to those of the English-born group. Interesting issues are raised by considering whether this is explained by Cochrane's selection hypothesis (Cochrane, 1977, 1983) that if migration is easy, less-stable individuals may self-select to migrate. Furthermore, reasons for migration and associated stress may need to be studied under these circumstances to explain why suicide is attempted rather than how.

Glover et al (1989) analysed the records of patients aged 10–24 years presenting with self-poisoning to the two casualty departments at the London Hospital between 1980 and 1984. There were no reported suicides, but Asian females showed an excessive rate of attempted suicide compared with the base population. Wright et al (1981) also found high rates of attempted suicide in young Asian women in Birmingham.

In our study of attempted suicide in a west London sample (Bhugra et al, 1999a), we included all cases except for primary presentations of habitual self-mutilation and alcohol misuse. Efforts were made in the first instance to gauge as accurately as possible the inception rates of attempted suicide over a 1-year period. The rates among South Asian women aged 18–24 were higher than those for White women in the same age group.

A systemic review of research into self-harm in different ethnic groups in the UK confirmed some of the findings already discussed (Bhui et al, 2007). It found a higher rate of self-harm among South Asian women, compared with South Asian men and White women. In a pooled estimate from two studies, Asian women were more likely to self-harm and Asian men were less likely to self-harm compared with their White counterparts. Some studies concluded that South Asian adults self-harm impulsively in response to life events rather than in association with a psychiatric illness. However, data in this field are not always consistent. A study of suicide rates in England and Wales in 1999–2003 (McKenzie et al, 2008) found that the age-standardised rate for men of South Asian origin was lower than that for other men, whereas the rate for women of South Asian origin was marginally raised. In aggregated data for the period, the age-specific rate for young women of South Asian origin was lower than that for other women. However, among those over 65, the rate among women of South Asian origin was double that of other women. The reason for the discrepancy needs further investigation and might be related to attempted suicide as opposed to completed suicide.

Adolescents

It has been suggested that an increase in the rates of attempted and completed suicide among adolescents in Europe might be attributable to the interplay of three sets of factors: the socialisation of a specific repertoire of problem-solving behaviour; socioeconomic conditions; and attitudes towards suicide (Diekstra, 1985). Certainly, these factors will be equally applicable to adolescents of Asian and other minority ethnic extraction.

Hawton *et al* (1982*a*) found that adolescents in the UK who take an overdose tend to have problems in their relationship with their parents. In a consecutive sample of 50 (White) adolescents admitted to hospital, 45 were girls (Hawton *et al*, 1982*b*). The most common difficulties identified were problems in relationships with parents and boyfriends, or at school. Problems at school and in relationships cross ethnic boundaries.

Goldberg & Hodes (1992) highlighted the relationship between racism in schools and self-poisoning among adolescents. They saw in overdosing a reproduction as an attack on the self of the racist attack on the individual. They hypothesised that racism is bound to influence the family life cycle as well as the internal family organisation. An important issue is the view taken by the family and the adolescents involved of the severity of the external threat related to racism. The responses of each member of the family have to be understood in context.

Several small retrospective studies of Asian adolescents in Coventry and Barnsley showed no differences in rates of attempted suicide when compared with White adolescents (Biswas, 1990; Handy *et al*, 1991).

Handy *et al* (1991) reported on adolescents who had taken an overdose and found that social and parental relationships were a key cause of isolation and attempted suicide. Asian adolescents were less likely than their White peers to be in contact with their friends, saw them less frequently and for shorter periods, and their relationships with their parents did not compensate for this. Most Indian communities maintain their traditional cultural identity and uphold the importance placed on academic and economic success, the stigma attached to failure, the overriding authority of elders and an unquestioning compliance of the younger members.

In a case note study of adolescents, we observed that inception rates for attempted suicide among teenaged Asians were no different from those among their White counterparts; neither was the method used in the attempts or the associated sociocultural factors (Bhugra *et al*, 2002). Nearly one-quarter of both the Asian and the White adolescents had conduct problems and a similar proportion had acknowledged a communication problem. The Asian girls were marginally more likely to report a family history of suicide and, not surprisingly, more likely to acknowledge cultural conflict. The Asians of both genders were more likely to admit that their attempt was impulsive, were less likely to express regret after the attempt and were more likely to be at risk of attempts in the future.

Social and cultural factors

As well as establishing the rates of attempted suicide, our west London study also assessed the influence of social and cultural factors (Bhugra *et al*, 1999*b*). South Asian women who had attempted suicide and agreed to be interviewed in detail about their cultural identity and life events were age-matched with an equal number of South Asian women attending a GP's surgery in the same catchment area and also with nearly twice the number of White women who had presented with self-harm.

The comparison between the two Asian groups showed that those in the attempted suicide group were significantly more likely to have a history of psychiatric disorder, more likely to have had repeated attempts and more likely to be in an interracial relationship. They were also more approving if their children wanted to have an interracial relationship or choose their marriage partner themselves. Those in the control group were more likely to see arranged marriage as good and were less likely to approve of cohabitation before marriage. Those who had attempted suicide were more likely to have changed their religion and to spend less total time with their families. Interestingly, one-quarter of each group acknowledged having experienced a racial life event in the previous 6 months. This is defined as an event that the individual identifies as having a racial component, such as rejection of a mortgage loan application on racial rather than financial grounds. Thus, a racial life event in itself is not likely to lead to self-harm (see Chapter 4, this volume).

Interesting differences emerged from our comparison of the Asian women who had attempted suicide and the White women who had done so. The Asian women were more likely to have no psychiatric disorder, were less likely to have used alcohol as part of the suicide attempt and were more likely to have been assaulted physically or verbally. The methods of attempted suicide for each group were broadly similar but Asians took a smaller number of tablets. Serious intent to take their life and regret that their attempt was unsuccessful were more common in the Asian sample. The findings need to be interpreted with caution as only a small number of individuals were interviewed.

At 16–17 years of age, the White and Asian girls had broadly similar adjustment reactions, alcohol and drug use, peer and relationship problems. However, the attempted suicide rate for Asian women aged 18–24 was higher than that for White women of the same age, suggesting that they came under more stress, possibly owing to social and cultural factors such as those listed in Box 10.1. Indeed, a qualitative review of self-harm among South Asian women in the UK found specific cultural factors such as level of acculturation, cultural conflicts, stigma and interpersonal relationships to be strongly associated with distress and resilience (Ahmed *et al*, 2007). However, more research is needed, particularly into the influence on suicide and self-harm of gender-role expectations, family conflict, domestic violence and alcohol use by males in the families of Asian women.

Box 10.1   Social and cultural factors that influence rates of self-harm in South Asian women

- Gender: self-harm is more likely in females
- Gender-role expectations
- Alienation from culture, especially one's own but also from that of the majority population
- Family conflict, e.g. with parents, partner
- Domestic violence: by male members
- Alcohol use in the family: by male members
- Cultural conflict: liberal views *v.* traditional setting
- Psychological distress expressed in the individual's alienation and rejection of cultural values
- Poor self-esteem

(Bhugra *et al*, 1999*b*)

Assessing suicide risk in Asians

General risk factors for suicide in any population are: past psychiatric history and present psychiatric symptoms such as depression, schizophrenia, alcohol dependency and psychopathic personality disorder; social factors such as social isolation and unemployment; physical illness; previous suicide attempts; and labile mood. Risk factors for suicide attempts include: recent previous attempts, especially if these were premeditated; precautions taken to avoid discovery and intervention by others; social isolation; prior communication of suicidal intent; the completion of final acts in anticipation of death, such as writing a will or a suicide note; violent methods; acts perceived to be lethal and irreversible; regrets on surviving the attempt; and taking no action to get help after the act. Formation of a suicide plan, an inclination to deal with internal conflict and recent experience of failure and rejection are also important factors. Asian women are more likely to repeat overdoses, which suggests that adequate preventive strategies may be successful (Bhugra *et al*, 1999*b*). As a significant proportion of attempted suicides by Asian females are impulsive, any assessment and intervention should also take impulsive acts into account.

The process of assessing suicide risk in Asians is basically the same as that for other groups (Box 10.2). However, additional information, especially on social and cultural alienation, social support, family structures and expectations, as well as such factors as less-traditional thinking, must be explored as a key part of the assessment (Box 10.3).

It is important that clinicians determine precipitating events, motives for the act, consequences of the act, precautions taken against discovery, preparatory acts and symptoms of depression, as well as the family's reactions and attitudes, and that an examination of the patient's physical and mental state is carried out as indicated.

135

Box 10.2   Assessing a recent suicide attempt

- Was the act impulsive?
- Was any action taken to prevent outsider intervention?
- Was the risk of discovery minimised?
- Had suicidal intent been communicated verbally or otherwise and to whom?
- What was the chosen suicide method?
- Did the individual believe that the act would be fatal?
- Does the individual regret surviving the attempt?
- Did the individual attempt to seek help after the act?
- Does the individual have a history of previous attempts? Ascertain details of the act

---

Clinicians assessing self-harm should use non-directive, open questions and a primary language that the patient is happy speaking. They should take into account the cultural values and beliefs of the individual, including their religious views. If interpreters are needed, these should be independent rather than family members.

Conclusion

An individual's ethnicity and cultural group remain useful starting points for understanding the motives behind attempted suicide as well as for assessing the probability that the attempt will be repeated. The impact of migration and socioeconomic and political disadvantages may well contribute to a sense of chronic ongoing difficulty and act as potential stressors. When these are combined with a sense of alienation from their own culture, this may well reduce people's sense of belonging and acceptance and influence

---

Box 10.3   Additional factors for assessing Asians

Assess the following:

- Migration (if indicated) and associated stressors and social support
- Cultural identity and cultural alienation
- Gender-role expectations
- Type of family network, e.g. extended, nuclear
- Social support and confidants
- Cultural idioms of distress and expectations
- Any prior racial life events

Note that suicidal motivation may be interpreted by the attempter in terms of cultural expectations of behaviour

---

their self-esteem, producing an affective reaction. It is also possible in society-centred cultures and groups that if the density of individuals from the same ethnic group is great, there will be an inordinate pressure on individuals to conform. Under the circumstances, any vulnerable individual in conflict with their own culture may choose to take the route of self-harm to avoid dealing with that conflict.

Definitions of the self differ and are influenced by culture and society. Hence, it becomes important that the individuals' perceptions of self are identified in the context of their culture. Clinicians must also be aware of the differences between those who consider suicide, those who attempt it and those who complete it. The association between these three groups and their relationship with other factors needs to be further clarified. Suicidal behaviour needs to be studied across the life cycle in relation to gender roles and cultural and social expectations. There is only emerging literature on suicide from native South Asia. There is very little on suicidal behaviour of people of South Asian origin across the globe. The Indian diaspora has also been studied in a few countries. However, the most extensive research in this field has possibly been in the UK.

References

Abeyasinghe, R. & Gunnell, D. (2008) Psychological autopsy study of suicide in three rural and semi-rural districts of Sri Lanka. *Social Psychiatry and Psychiatric Epidemiology*, **43**, 280–285.

Ahmed, K., Mohan, R. A. & Bhugra, D. (2007) Self-harm in South Asian women: a literature review informed approach to assessment and formulation. *American Journal of Psychotherapy*, **61**, 71–81

Babu, G. N., Subbakrishna, D. K. & Chandra, P. S. (2008) Prevalence and correlates of suicidality among Indian women with post-partum psychosis in an inpatient setting. *Australian and New Zealand Journal of Psychiatry*, **42**, 1440–1614.

Bannerjee, G., Nandi, D., Nandi, S., *et al* (1990) The vulnerability of Indian women to suicide. *Indian Journal of Psychiatry*, **32**, 305–308.

Bhugra, D. (1991) Politically motivated suicides. *British Journal of Psychiatry*, **159**, 594–595.

Bhugra, D., Desai, M. & Baldwin, D. (1999a) Attempted suicide in West London. I: Inception rates. *Psychiatric Medicine*, **29**, 1125–1130.

Bhugra, D., Baldwin, D., Desai, M., *et al* (1999b) Attempted suicide in West London. II: Social and cultural factors. *Psychiatric Medicine*, **29**, 1131–1139.

Bhugra, D., Singh, J., Fellow-Smith, E., *et al* (2002) Deliberate self-harm in adolescents: a case study among two ethnic groups. *European Journal of Psychiatry*, **16**, 145–151.

Bhui, K., McKenzie, K. & Rasul, F. (2007) Rates, risk factors and methods of self harm among minority ethnic groups in the UK: a systematic review. *BMC Public Health*, **7**, 336.

Biswas, S. (1990) Ethnic differences in self-poisoning. *Journal of Adolescence*, **13**, 189–193.

Burke, A. W. (1976) Attempted suicide among Asian immigrants in Birmingham. *British Journal of Psychiatry*, **128**, 528–533.

Chakraborty, R. & Chatterjee, A. (2007) Predictors of suicide attempt among those with depression in an Indian sample. A brief report. *Internet Journal of Mental Health*, 4 (2).

Cochrane, R. (1977) Mental illness in immigrants to England and Wales. *Social Psychiatry*, **12**, 25–35.

Cochrane, R. (1983) *The Social Creation of Mental Illness.* Longman.

Diekstra, R. F. (1985) Suicide and suicide attempts in the European Economic Community: an analysis of trends, with special emphasis upon trends among the young. *Suicide and Life Threatening Behaviour,* **15**, 27–42.

Fathelrahman, A. I., Ab Rahman, A. F. & Mohd Zain, Z. (2001) Self-poisoning by drugs and chemicals: variations in demographics, associated factors and final outcomes. *General Hospital Psychiatry,* **30(5)**, 467–470.

Glover, G., Marks, F. & Nowers, M. (1989) Parasuicide in young Asian women. *British Journal of Psychiatry,* **154**, 271–272.

Goldberg, D. & Hodes, M. (1992) The poison of racism and the self poisoning of adolescents. *Journal of Family Therapy,* **14**, 51–67.

Gunesvaran, T., Subramaniam, S. & Mahadeva, N. K. (1984) Suicide in a northern town in Sri Lanka. *Acta Psychiatrica Scandinavica,* **69**, 420–425.

Handy, S., Chithiramohan, R., Vallard, C., *et al* (1991) Ethnic differences in adolescent self poisoning: a comparison of Asian and Caucasian groups. *Journal of Adolescence,* **14**, 157–162.

Hawton, K., Osborn, M., O'Grady, J., *et al* (1982*a*) Classification of adolescents who take overdoses. *British Journal of Psychiatry,* **140**, 124–131.

Hawton, K., O'Grady, J., Osborn, M., *et al* (1982*b*) Adolescents who take overdoses: their characteristics, problems and contacts with helping agencies. *British Journal of Psychiatry,* **140**, 118–123.

Haynes, R. H. (1984) Suicide in Fiji: a preliminary study. *British Journal of Psychiatry,* **145**, 433–438.

Khan, M. M. & Reza, H. (1998) Attempted suicide in Karachi, Pakistan. *Suicide and Life Threatening Behaviour,* **28**, 54–60.

Kumar, P. N. S., Kuruvilla, K., Dutta, S., *et al* (1995) Psychosocial aspects of attempted suicide: study from a medical intensive care unit. *Indian Journal of Psychological Medicine,* **18**, 32–42.

Mahy, G. (1993) Suicide behaviour in the Caribbean. *International Review of Psychiatry,* **5**, 261–269.

Maniam, T. (1988) Suicide and parasuicide in a hill resort in Malaysia. *British Journal of Psychiatry,* **153**, 222–225.

Marecek, J. (1998) Culture, gender and suicidal behaviour in Sri Lanka. *Suicide and Life Threatening Behaviour,* **28**, 69–81.

McKenzie, K., Bhui, K., Nanchahal, K., *et al* (2008) Suicide rates in people of South Asian origin in England and Wales: 1993–2003. *British Journal of Psychiatry,* **193**, 406–409.

Meer, F. (1976) *Race and Suicide in South Africa.* International Library of Sociology.

Merrill, J. & Owens, J. (1986) Ethnic differences in self-poisoning: a comparison of Asian and white groups. *British Journal of Psychiatry,* **148**, 708–712.

Merrill, J. & Owens, J. (1988) Self-poisoning among four immigrant groups. *Acta Psychiatrica Scandinavica,* **77**, 77–80.

Ponnudurai, R., Jeyakar, J. & Saraswathy, M. (1986) Attempted suicide in Madras. *Indian Journal of Psychiatry,* **28**, 59–62.

Ponnudurai, R., Vivekanathan, V., Raju, B., *et al* (1991) Attempted suicide: two year follow up study. *Indian Journal of Psychiatry,* **33**, 291–292.

Pouliot, L. & DeLeo, D. (2006) Critical issues in psychological autopsy studies: the need for a standardization. *Suicide and Life Threatening Behaviour,* **36**, 491–510.

Rao, A. V. (1965) Attempted suicide. *Indian Journal of Psychiatry,* **7**, 253–259.

Rao, A.V. (1992) Parasuicide and suicide: some psychological considerations. *Indian Journal of Social Psychiatry,* **8**, 3–7.

Rao, A. V. & Chennian, R. (1972) Attempted suicide and suicide in students in Madurai. *Indian Journal of Psychiatry,* **14**, 389–396.

Sathyavathi, K. (1971) Attempted suicide in psychiatric patients. *Indian Journal of Psychiatry,* **13**, 37–42.

Somasundaram, O. S., Babu, C. K. & Geelthayan, I. A. (1989) Suicide behaviour in ancient civilization with special reference to the families. *Indian Journal of Psychiatry*, **31**, 208–212.

Wright, N., Trethowan, W. & Owens, J. (1981) Ethnic differences in self poisoning. *Postgraduate Medical Journal*, **57**, 792–793.

Zhang, J., Jia, S., Wieczorek, W. F., *et al* (2002) An overview of suicide research in China. *Archives of Suicide Research*, **6**, 167–184.

Zhang, J., Conwell, Y., Zhou, L., *et al* (2004) Culture, risk factor and suicide in rural China. A psychological Autopsy case–control study. *Acta Psychiatrica Scandinavica*, **110**, 430–437.

CHAPTER 11

Mental health of the ageing immigrant population

Gill Livingston, Sati Sembhi and Rahul Bhattacharya

Summary   More than 8% of people aged 65 and over in the UK are immigrants. Concentrated in deprived inner-city areas, their numbers are rising rapidly, with the ageing of those arriving after the Second World War. Cultural, language and educational differences cause problems in studying this group's mental health. Idioms of distress may affect presentation, help-seeking behaviour and acceptability of treatment. Older people from Black and minority ethnic groups may be vulnerable to depression because of socioeconomic deprivation, immigrant status and old age, but studies are contradictory and may use inappropriate screening instruments. Relatively few consider immigrant status and dementia. Uncontrolled hypertension could relate to higher dementia rates in Black immigrants which are not reflected in the country of origin. No genetic risk has been found. There is potential for prevention in this population.

This chapter concerns the mental health of people aged 65 and over who have moved from their country of birth – the older immigrant population. In the UK, although the absolute numbers of older people from Black and minority ethnic groups are relatively small, there is a greater concentration in deprived inner-city areas. Numbers are also increasing rapidly, as those who immigrated to the UK after the Second World War reach retirement age. This is evident from the exponential increase, particularly in England and Wales, of people over 65 who come from an ethnic minority, from 3% in the 1991 census to 8.2% in 2001 (Shah *et al*, 2005). Estimates based on 2004 data suggest that 11 860 individuals from Black and minority ethnic groups in the UK have dementia (King's College London & London School of Economics, 2007), and between 33 559 and 52 980 have depression (Shah, 2008). The prevalence of dementia and depression in older people is generally similar or higher in those from minority ethnic groups than in the indigenous population (Bhatnagar & Frank, 1997). A systematic review of dementia in African–Caribbean people living in Britain found an excess prevalence in comparison with White British peers. Of the 11 papers assessed, all except one found a statistically significant increase in prevalence in the African–Caribbean population (Adelman *et al*, 2009).

Box 11.1   Difficulties in studying immigrant populations

Misinterpretation of responses because of cultural differences, language and levels of education

Idioms of distress may affect presentation, help-seeking behaviour, likelihood of diagnosis and acceptability of treatment

Unjustifiable assumption of homogeneity of people from a single large geographical area

Varying reasons for immigration, e.g. to improve education, seek asylum, find employment

---

In 2001 the Royal College of Psychiatrists concluded that services for older people from Black and minority ethnic groups had received little attention: this continues to be an issue of concern (Oommen *et al*, 2009).

It is important to be aware of immigrant groups, not only for adequate and culturally appropriate provision of services, but also because immigrant status can hold important clues to the aetiology of illnesses. It has been hypothesised that relative socioeconomic deprivation, ageing and immigrant status – the 'triple whammy' – confer a particular vulnerability to mental illness (Rait *et al*, 1996). Although there have been more studies of older immigrants in recent years, there is a relative lack of research.

Pitfalls of studying immigrant people

There are considerable difficulties in studying immigrant and minority ethnic populations. In addition to personal factors intrinsic to being a new immigrant (Box 11.1), we should consider the effect of the new country of residence on immigrants. There is little explicit consideration of the changes that occur when immigrants live in a new culture. It is often assumed that they remain unaffected by the experience. In fact, immigrants interact and adapt to their new environment, undergoing a degree of acculturation and sometimes assimilation. Furthermore, the meaning of the move, the welcome (or lack of it) on arrival, and the age and stage of life at which people move make for different experiences, even when people originate from the same culture. Much of the research into the effect of immigration focuses on increased vulnerability rather than on the resilience and protection that may be afforded by, for example, close social groups.

Defining race and ethnicity

The definition of race and ethnicity (Box 11.2) as research variables is contentious. An 'ethnic group' may share geographical origins, culture, religious traditions and language. 'Culture' is the network of shared ideas,

---

Box 11.2   Defining race and ethnicity

Race

- The term often implies genetic homogeneity
- Racial distinctions are often made on the basis of appearance, particularly skin colour

Ethnicity

- This is self-described, on the basis of shared origins, culture, religion and language
- Self-description of ethnicity is not fixed
- Forced choice of ethnic category (e.g. as in the 1991 UK census) may lead to oversimplification and falsification

---

meaning and rules, a lens through which a person perceives and understands the world (Helman, 2000: p. 2). 'Ethnicity' in this context therefore refers to a self-described identity. As people see themselves in different ways at different times, it is not a fixed concept. When immigrants' children are subjects of research, the study of ethnicity becomes more difficult, as classification becomes even less clear. People from ethnic minorities are also increasingly likely to marry people from the indigenous population or those from a different ethnic minority. Ethnicity can also refer to imposed categories such as those in the 1991 UK census, which has been used for much of the UK research but did not allow a mixed ethnicity category. Many people found it difficult to classify themselves. 'Race' is a term implying genetic homogeneity, and racial distinctions are generally based on physical appearance – largely skin colour. It gives little information about immigrant status or ethnic group.

As immigrant groups establish themselves, they may wish to continue a lifestyle based on cultural or religious traditions from their country of origin and hope to pass this on to the next generation. Tensions may arise if children do not want to adopt the way of life preferred by their parents. This can become particularly apparent at important times in the life cycle, such as marriage and childbirth, which are traditionally times when families come together. There may also be problems as older immigrants become more frail and dependent.

Assessing dementia

Cross-cultural assessment of dementia in older people (Box 11.3) has specific pitfalls related to language and literacy skills. In particular, the use of culturally biased screening instruments that rely on language recognition and familiarity with test situations may be inappropriate or misleading for people with cognitive impairment (Lindesay, 1998). Culturally appropriate

> **Box 11.3**   Key learning points: dementia
>
> Relatively few studies consider immigrant status as a risk factor for dementia
>
> Recent studies suggest that dementia may be increased in Black immigrants
>
> Increased rates of dementia in Black immigrants do not appear to reflect increased rates in the country of origin
>
> Excess of hypertension in African–Caribbean populations in the West is well documented
>
> Excess of dementia may be related to uncontrolled hypertension and diabetes
>
> There is potential for primary and secondary prevention in this population
>
> ApoE4 allele frequency does not seem to vary between populations but expression may be decreased in African and Hispanic Americans

norms are also important in the evaluation of dementia. Immigrants may be literate in a different language or functionally illiterate. Recent immigrants from rural areas may have had little need for the concept of complex maps and exact dates. As a result, interpreting cognitive testing without a knowledge of education and background is likely to lead to errors in diagnosis. It may be important, therefore, to validate and modify instruments for examining cognitive function in different ethnic groups. One report of validation of the Mini-Mental State Examination (MMSE) in South Asians in the UK found that cut-offs varied when judged against a diagnostic instrument for the detection of dementia (Rait *et al*, 2000). A new normative test battery for cognitive function in African–Caribbean elders in the UK shows that, compared with normative data for the African American population, scores on verbal fluency were lower but scores on memory tests were comparable (Stewart *et al*, 2001b). Following the judiciary challenge of its amended guidance on donepezil, galantamine, rivastigmine and memantine for treatment of Alzheimer's disease, the National Institute for Health and Clinical Excellence (2009) now acknowledges potential scenarios in which MMSE scores cannot be relied on in particular patient groups (such as in people whose first language is not English). There are several diagnostic challenges of identifying dementia in people from minority ethnic groups. Apart from the cultural bias of neuropsychometric tests, there is a lack of normative data applicable to the unique population. Bilingual immigrants often tend to lose English quicker than their mother tongue, leading to the over-estimation of impairment. There is also a dearth of validated tests for assessment of premorbid IQ for non-English speaking people.

Owing to cultural beliefs in the community, the person as well as their carer might attribute impairment related to dementia as a mere sign of ageing and hence not seek medical consultation, especially in the early stages.

The need for specially tailored information for, approaches to and training about dementia in Black and minority ethnic groups has been identified in the National Dementia Strategy (Department of Health, 2009).

Despite these caveats, a 1-year follow-up of a multicultural community sample of people with a diagnosis of dementia found that stability of diagnosis did not vary according to ethnic background (Schofield *et al*, 1995). Similarly, a small study of Gujarati people diagnosed with dementia found that the diagnosis was stable at follow-up (Shah *et al*, 1998).

Assessing depression

Depression may present with different patterns of symptoms in different cultures. People of some cultures commonly present with predominant symptoms of sadness and low mood during depression, whereas others present with pain and somatic symptoms. The language of distress used, for example, by African Americans differs from that on which structured diagnoses are made and may lead to an underestimate of distress and anxiety levels. When screening for depression in older people, lower cut-offs have been found to be appropriate for older Black people living in the UK (Abas *et al*, 1998).

Another challenge in assessing depression in elderly immigrants is the lack of validated screening tools for this population (Box 11.4). The Geriatric Depression Scale can give high levels of 'false positives' in elderly Indian (Ganguli *et al*, 1996) and elderly Chinese populations (Mui, 1996).

Current research evidence

Much of our current knowledge of mental illness in immigrant elders relies on research carried out in the USA, where the experience of immigration may differ from that in the UK. The USA sees itself as a melting pot and it is proud of the idea that economic migrants come to strive for, and find, success. In contrast, the term 'economic migrant' is used in the UK as a term of abuse, with implications in parts of the media that people are coming here to live off the state. Conversely, African Americans are descendants of an extremely oppressed population, subject to overt racism. The studies from the USA are therefore of a population that is different from that in the UK, and comparable studies between the two countries may have different results.

Dementia in older immigrants

Prevalence of dementia

The overall worldwide prevalence of dementia is usually found to be between 5% and 6% of those aged 65 years and above, living at home. Meta-analysis (Jorm *et al*, 1987) has shown that the prevalence doubles with every

5-year increase in age band up to around 90 years of age. Most studies have found that education is protective against both the development and the progression of dementia. Immigrant groups with relative socioeconomic deprivation, often associated with less education, might therefore be expected to be more vulnerable to dementia. The relative youth of the ageing immigrant population compared with the ageing indigenous population would then decrease the overall prevalence.

Few studies consider whether ethnicity or immigrant status are risk factors for dementia and most that do are small and lack concurrent controls. For example, one comparison of Black with White community residents found that, out of a total of 26 people with dementia, Black older people were significantly more likely to have dementia than White (16% v. 3%) and that there was an excess history of stroke, diabetes and hypertension in the Black population (Heyman et al, 1991).

Another small study (14 people in the total sample had dementia) surveyed English-speaking Black and White retired people in the USA (Perkins et al, 1997). The age-adjusted prevalence of dementia among the Black men was found to be almost twice that among White men (4.8% v. 2.4%), although the difference was not statistically significant.

In the UK, 418 elderly people from Black and minority ethnic groups living in Liverpool were interviewed (McCracken et al, 1997). There was a high prevalence of dementia in the sample as a whole, particularly among the Black Africans, when compared with an earlier study using the same instruments. The authors concluded that these results could be attributed to the effects of participants' age, gender and the inability of some to speak English and that there was no true increase in community prevalence in the minority ethnic population. Another UK study examined elderly South Asians and found an increased rate of dementia compared with similar but not directly comparable populations using the same instrument, although again no direct comparisons were made (Bhatnagar & Frank, 1997). Language difficulties may have affected the results of this study, as participants were interviewed in Hindi, although this was not necessarily their first language. This may account for the fact that the concordance of the diagnosis from the study with psychiatric diagnosis was very low.

A more recent UK pilot study, however, suggested a higher rate of dementia in African–Caribbeans than in age- and gender-matched White people (Richards et al, 2000). Our own study, in the London borough of Islington, found that the prevalence of dementia was raised in immigrant African–Caribbeans compared with White and minority ethnic UK-born individuals, despite the fact that those of African–Caribbean origin were significantly younger (Livingston et al, 2001a). Our result did not appear to be related to language artefacts or differing education.

The excess of hypertension in the African–Caribbean population in the West is well documented, as is an increased mortality in this group from cerebrovascular disease. Nevertheless, we did not find an excess of self-reported hypertension or of people taking antihypertensive medication, although there was an excess of self-reported diabetes (e.g. Chaturvedi *et al*, 1993). In a small study in north London (a follow-up from the Islington study) the combined African and Black Caribbean group had nearly double the proportion of vascular dementia (Stevens *et al*, 2004).

A comparison of the prevalence of dementia in community-dwelling people living in Nigeria and in African Americans living in Indianapolis, USA, found a significantly lower rate in Nigeria (2.3% *v.* 4.8%) (Hendrie *et al*, 1995). A follow-up study compared the incidence rates of dementia in the two populations: the Yoruba in Nigeria and age-standardised African Americans. The Yoruba group showed a significantly lower incidence of both Alzheimer's disease (1.2% *v.* 2.5%) and dementia (1.4% *v.* 3.2%) (Hendrie *et al*, 2001). This suggests that the development of dementia is influenced by changes associated with moving from Nigeria to live in the USA.

Dementia and the ApoE4 allele

Most studies have found that the strongest genetic risk factor for the development of Alzheimer's disease is the possession of the apolipoprotein E (ApoE) 4 allele. The allele frequency does not vary between Black Americans, Hispanic Americans and White Americans. Possession of the allele has, however, been found to have a weaker association with Alzheimer's disease in some populations, including African Americans, Caribbean–Hispanics in the USA and native Spanish people, although not in Indians (Ganguli *et al*, 2000). In a comparison of rural community samples in Ballabgarh, India, and Pennsylvania, USA, the prevalence rates for Alzheimer's disease among those aged 70–79 years was 0.7% *v.* 3.1%. The American sample had higher rates of the ApoE4 allele and rates of the Alzheimer's disease diagnosis among those with this allele did not differ.

One meta-analysis of studies found that, overall, the association between possession of the ApoE4 allele and the development of Alzheimer's disease was lower for African and Hispanic Americans than for Whites but higher for Japanese people (Farrer *et al*, 1997). As the individual studies reported a heterogeneous effect of the allele, in particular with regard to African Americans, the true effect requires further clarification.

Dementia ACE gene polymorphism, interleukin-6, plasma homocysteine levels

Although no direct association has been demonstrated between the genotypes, the angiotensin converting enzyme (ACE) DD genotype in a British African–Caribbean sample appeared to have a facilitator effect on strengthening the association between age and cognitive decline (Stewart *et al*, 2004). In the same cohort, raised plasma interleukin-6 (IL-6) levels were associated with cognitive decline over 3 years (Jordanova *et al*, 2007). High levels (highest quartile of the population) of plasma homocysteine together with poor educational attainment was associated with cognitive impairment (Stewart *et al*, 2002).

Pattern, presentation and course of dementia

As we have already discussed, sociocultural factors such as education and language may influence the time of presentation and pattern of symptoms in dementia.

We recently compared in a quantitative systematic review and meta-analysis of 33 articles the use of health and social services, treatments for dementia and dementia research between different ethnic groups. We found consistent evidence, mostly from the USA, that minority ethnic people accessed diagnostic services later in their illness and, once they had received a diagnosis, were less likely to access antidementia medication, research trials and 24-hour care. Increasing community engagement and specific recruitment strategies for minority ethnic groups might help address inequalities, and these need to be evaluated. More research is also needed to evaluate access of minority ethnic outside the USA to dementia services (Cooper *et al*, 2010).

A systematic review of barriers and facilitators to accessing specialist help for dementia found that barriers included: not conceptualising dementia as an illness; believing dementia to be a normal consequence of ageing; thinking dementia has spiritual, psychological, physical health or social causes; feeling that caring for the person with dementia is a personal or family responsibility; experiences of shame and stigma within the community; believing there is nothing that can be done to help; and negative experiences of healthcare services (Mukadeen *et al*, 2010). Recognition of dementia as an illness and knowledge about dementia improved rates of access to help.

The meaning of memory difficulties and dependency may differ in different cultures, so that if older people are expected to be less independent, the symptoms of early dementia may not be regarded as pathological. Those who are supported by their families and communities may present relatively early, as change is noticed in them. Those without social support may present late. The lack of insight, apathy and decreased ability to express and organise experienced by people with dementia mean that they lack their own voice and require advocates.

A study comparing Black and White Americans with Alzheimer's disease found that Black patients had fewer years of education, were more likely to have hypertension and reported shorter duration of illness at the time of presentation but had lower MMSE scores (Hargrave *et al*, 1998). They also reported more insomnia but less anxiety. However, a study of consecutive admissions of older African American and White people with dementia found no difference in behavioural disturbance or response to treatment between the two groups (Akpaffiong *et al*, 1999). Ethnic differences have been found to have little effect on mortality rates (Jolley & Baxter, 1997).

Depression (Box 11.4)

In most studies of older adults in the USA, Black and White people show no difference in rates of depression (e.g. Blazer *et al*, 1996). In the UK, rates of depression and anxiety have been found to be the same (e.g. Lindesay *et al*, 1997) or slightly higher in Black African elders (McCracken *et al*, 1997). The latter study found that Black Africans with depression were less likely to see relatives, and the authors considered that this was significantly associated with depression. In east London, older people of Bengali and Somalian ethnicity were found to have a surprisingly high but varying prevalence of depression (77% and 25%, respectively) compared with two different control populations of White people (5% and 25%) (Silveira & Ebrahim, 1998*a*,*b*). However, the populations were sampled in very different ways: the Somali population was from a lunch club, the Whites from an age–gender register. The same study found that Gujaratis had a lower prevalence of depression (2%). When adjusted for age, income, physical health and social problems, ethnicity was no longer a significant risk factor for high depression scores.

Another study of older people of South Asian origin estimated a 20% prevalence of depression (Bhatnagar & Frank, 1997). A study in north London showed that the mental health of Hindu grandmothers was associated with family structure, with those coming from nuclear rather than extended families being more susceptible to depression (Guglani *et al*, 2000).

For African–Caribbean elders, in particular, rates based on community screening using instruments with cut-offs validated on predominantly White populations have been found to be underestimates (Abas *et al*, 1998). Irish immigrants in general, although not older Irish immigrants

---

Box 11.4   Key learning points: depression

Older people in immigrant communities are thought to be particularly vulnerable to depression because of risk factors of socioeconomic deprivation, immigrant status and old age

The results of studies are contradictory

Most studies do not describe potential confounders such as physical ill health, living alone and social class

Screening instruments validated in a mainly White older population may not be valid for other populations

The vascular hypothesis suggests that depression in old age is caused by vascular pathology but recent studies suggest an association with stroke but not vascular risk factors

in particular, have been shown to have poorer mental and physical health than other minority ethnic groups. They have the highest rates of hospital admissions for mental illness and high rates of suicide and attempted suicide (Merril & Owens, 1988).

Our own study of older immigrants found an excess of depression in Cypriots but not in other groups, including African–Caribbean and Irish groups. This excess occurred despite the fact that they were less likely to live alone and were no more likely to be physically ill. They did, however, have increased subjective ill health and were much less likely to speak English or have had a secondary education and so were possibly less able to access help when required (Livingston *et al*, 2002). Cypriots with depression were likely to present to many services but not to complain of psychological symptoms. They often presented with prominent somatic symptoms. This is likely to be due to a different idiom of distress. Similar patterns of presentation were found in a study of immigrants to Israel from the former USSR, with somatisation being more common in those who were older, currently single and female.

The vascular hypothesis of depression suggests that new depression in older people may be caused by cerebrovascular pathology (Hickie & Scott, 1998) and therefore might be increased in the African–Caribbean population in the West. Older African–Caribbean people living in the West might therefore represent a population particularly at risk of depression from vascular causes and stroke. One study of older African–Caribbean people living in south London found an expected association of depression with stroke but no association with vascular risk factors in those who had not had a stroke (Stewart *et al*, 2001a). The conclusion was that it is stroke itself that causes depression rather than experiencing vascular risk factors.

There is little research in the field of spirituality and its impact on mental health in the ageing immigrant population in UK. However, one such study reported that participation in religious activities appeared to have a protective effect against developing depression in Taiwanese Korean immigrants (Hahn *et al*, 2004). At this stage it is not clear whether these effects are generalisable in other immigrant populations.

The wide variation in rates of depression in people from the Indian subcontinent might reflect a complex picture. The wide variation in the incidence of depression in South Asians may be related to variations in presentation, which might lead to diagnostic inconsistencies. It has been suggested that depression should be considered in presentations with symptoms of body ache and 'abdominal gas' in people from the Indian subcontinent (Bhatnagar, 1997). A relatively recent review concluded that somatic symptoms accompany the presentation of depression across the world (Bhugra & Mastrogianni, 2004). Any increased rates may be a result of comparing populations that differ in important confounding characteristics, such as physical ill health and social disadvantage. It might also be related to the use of inappropriate screening instruments. The results in studies on the prevalence of depressive disorders are therefore unsurprisingly inconsistent and inconclusive.

Psychosis

The issue of the over-representation in hospitals of younger Black people with a diagnosis of schizophrenia has been studied extensively. This contrasts with the situation for older people, partly because there is less literature on psychosis and schizophrenia in this group. Depression and dementia in people over 65 are more common and more studied than is schizophrenia. One study of paranoid symptoms in older people in the community reported that being Black is a risk factor (Blazer *et al*, 1996) but we did not find this in our study (Livingston *et al*, 2001*b*).

Suicide

Despite the high rate of completed suicide in older people, in particular older men, there has been little research considering the role of immigration and ethnicity as risk factors. Existing evidence is contradictory. In the UK, one study of suicide rates according to age and ethnicity found that all suicides in the over-75 age group were of Asian women and Whites of either gender and that there were no suicides from any other ethnic group (Neeleman *et al*, 1997). This contrasts with another report from the UK showing that suicide rates in elderly first-generation immigrants from the Indian subcontinent are low compared with those of the indigenous elderly population (Soni Raleigh *et al*, 1990). Although younger Asian women are more likely to self-harm than their White counterparts, this is clearly not so for the older Asian population (Bhugra *et al*, 1999). In the USA, the highest suicide rates were found to be among elderly White men (Cattell, 2000). It has been suggested that older African Americans have surmounted more threats to their self-esteem than older Whites and are thereby better adapted to new challenges associated with ageing. However, older immigrants in Sweden have an increased rate of suicide (Johansson *et al*, 1997).

Service utilisation

The factors that influence service utilisation are complex and include accessibility, perception of usefulness, availability of alternative help, stigma and beliefs about racism. Thus, it is unclear how immigration will affect the use of services.

Studies of immigrant Asian and Black elders showed that, in general, they were more likely to consult their general practitioner than their British-born counterparts. This contrasts with the picture of consultation in social service and secondary care. In general, studies report findings on small numbers of older people and they are based on referrals. In the main (e.g. Shah & Dighe-Deo, 1997), they suggest that ethnic elders are referred less to secondary care health and social services, in particular psychiatric services, than their White UK-born counterparts (or have increased untreated morbidity). Subsequent studies, one comparing Asian and White referral to secondary care and one comparing service use by community-dwelling older people from Black and minority ethnic groups and their White counterparts, were unable to confirm this (e.g. Odutoye & Shah, 1999; Livingston *et al*, 2002).

A variety of reasons has been suggested for lack of service use, for example interpreting symptoms as a spiritual problem rather than as a depressive or physical illness. In addition, there have been reports of a reluctance in ethnic elders to accept referral to secondary mental health services (Shah *et al*, 1998) and of perceptions by Black people of racism in health workers (Hutchinson & Gilvarry, 1998). It might be that the medical profession is less able to recognise the presentation of psychological distress by people from other cultures.

A qualitative study in London compared Black older people with and without depression with White counterparts. They found that Black elders often chose not to use medical services, as they perceived them to be irrelevant and stigmatising. However, there was little evidence of perceived racism (Marwaha & Livingston, 2003).

As part of the 2006 Count Me In survey (Commission for Healthcare Audit and Inspection, 2007), in-patient bed use in mental health and learning (intellectual) disability services was assessed in England and Wales. Compared with the national average, standardised admission rates for people over 65 years of age were higher for the White Irish, Other White, Other Asian, Black African, Black Caribbean and Other Black ethnic groups, but not significantly different for the Indian, Pakistani and Bangladeshi population; the White British and Chinese populations had below average rates of in-patient admission. To improve services in line with the Royal College of Psychiatrists' (2007) Race Equality Action Plan, members of Black and minority ethnic users' and carers' groups should be consulted and research in this area promoted. To promote inclusion, it has been suggested that 'cultural capability' should be incorporated in the core training of clinicians (Oommen *et al*, 2009).

Caring for people with dementia is stressful and associated with distress and depression, particularly in female and spouse caregivers. The meaning of caring and ways of coping may vary between ethnic and immigrant groups although the demands may be similar. Immigrants may have left their families and therefore their traditional sources of support. A review of 12 US studies comparing caregivers of people with dementia showed that Black and Hispanic caregivers were less likely to be a spouse and more likely to be an adult child, friend or other family member than White caregivers. Black and Hispanic caregivers reported lower levels of caregiver stress, burden and depression. They endorsed more strongly held beliefs about filial support and were more likely to use prayer, faith or religion as a coping mechanism (Connell & Gibson, 1997). This contrasts with a US study comparing Hispanic and White non-Hispanic primary caregivers for dementia. This found that Hispanic caregivers were more likely to have depression, but the most robust risk factors were female gender and spouse status (Harwood et al, 1998).

References

Abas, M. A., Phillips, C., Carter, J., et al (1998) Culturally sensitive validation of screening questionnaires for depression in older African–Caribbean people living in south London. British Journal of Psychiatry, 173, 249–254.

Adelman, S., Blanchard, M. & Livingston, G. (2009) A systematic review of the prevalence and covariates of dementia or relative cognitive impairment in the older African–Caribbean population in Britain. International Journal of Geriatric Psychiatry, 24, 657–665.

Akpaffiong, M., Kunik, M., Hale, D., et al (1999) Cross-cultural differences in demented geropsychiatric inpatients with behavioural disturbances. International Journal of Geriatric Psychiatry, 14, 845–850.

Bhatnagar, K. (1997) Depression in South Asian elders. Geriatric Medicine, February, 55–56.

Bhatnagar, K. & Frank, J. (1997) Psychiatric disorders in elderly from the Indian subcontinent living in Bradford. International Journal of Geriatric Psychiatry, 12, 907–912.

Bhugra, D. & Mastrogianni, A. (2004) Globalisation and mental disorders. Overview with relation to depression. British Journal of Psychiatry, 184, 10–20.

Bhugra, D., Desai, M. & Baldwin, D. S. (1999) Attempted suicide in west London. I: Rates across ethnic communities. Psychological Medicine, 5, 1125–1130.

Blazer, D. G., Hays, J. C. & Salive, M. C. (1996) Factors associated with paranoid symptoms in a community sample of older adults. Gerontologist, 36, 70–75.

Cattell, H. (2000) Suicide in the elderly. Advances in Psychiatric Treatment, 6, 102–108.

Commission for Healthcare Audit and Inspection (2007) Count Me In. Results of the 2006 National Census of Inpatients in Mental Health and Learning Disability Services in England and Wales. Commission for Healthcare Audit and Inspection.

Chaturvedi, N., McKeigue, P. M. & Marmot, M. G. (1993) Resting and ambulatory blood pressure differences in Afro-Caribbeans and Europeans. Hypertension, 22, 90–96.

Connell, C. & Gibson, G. (1997) Racial, ethnic and cultural differences in dementia caregiving: review and analysis. Gerontologist, 37, 355–364.

Cooper, C., Tandy, A., Balamurali, T., et al (2010) A systematic review and metaanalysis of ethnic differences in access to dementia treatment, care and research. American Journal of Geriatric Psychiatry, doi: 10.1097/JGP.0b013e3181bf9caf.

Department of Health (2009) Living Well with Dementia: A National Dementia Strategy. Department of Health.

Farrer, L. A., Cupples, L. A., Haines, J. L., et al (1997) Effects of age, sex and ethnicity on the association between apolipoprotein E genotype and Alzheimer disease. A meta-analysis. JAMA, 278, 1349–1356.

Ganguli, M., Chandra, V., Gilby, J. E. et al (1996) Cognitive test performance in a community based non-demented sample in rural India: the Indo–US cross-national epidemiology study. International Psychogeriatrics, 8, 507–524.

Ganguli, M., Chandra, V., Kamboh, M. I., et al (2000) Apolipoprotein E polymorphism and Alzheimer disease: the Indo–US cross-national dementia study. Archives of Neurology, 57, 824–830.

Guglani, S., Coleman, P. & Sonuga-Barke, E. J. S. (2000) Mental health of elderly Asians in Britain: a comparison of Hindus from nuclear and extended families of differing cultural identities. *International Journal of Geriatric Psychiatry*, **15**, 1046–1053.

Hahn, C. Y., Yang, M. S., Yang, M. J., *et al* (2004) Religious attendance and depressive symptoms among community dwelling elderly in Taiwan. *International Journal of Geriatric Psychiatry*, **19**, 1148–1154.

Hargrave, R., Stoeklin, M., Haan, M., *et al* (1998) Clinical aspects of Alzheimer's disease in Black and White patients. *Journal of the National Medical Association*, **90**, 78–84.

Harwood, D., Barker, W., Cantillon, M., *et al* (1998) Depressive symptomatology in first-degree family caregivers of Alzheimer's disease patients: a cross-ethnic comparison. *Alzheimer Disease and Associated Disorders*, **12**, 340–346.

Helman, C. G. (2000) *Culture, Health and Illness*. Butterworth-Heinemann.

Hendrie, H. C., Osuntokun, B. O., Hall, K. S., et al (1995) The prevalence of Alzheimer's disease and dementia in two communities: Nigerian Africans and African Americans. *American Journal of Psychiatry*, **152**, 1485–1492.

Hendrie, H. C., Ogunniyi, A., Hall, K. S., *et al* (2001) Incidence of dementia and Alzheimer disease in two communities: Yoruba residing in Ibadan, Nigeria, and African Americans residing in Indianapolis, Indiana. *JAMA*, **285**, 739–747.

Heyman, A., Fillenbaum, G., Prosnitz, B., *et al* (1991) Estimated prevalence of dementia among elderly Black and White community residents. *Archives of Neurology*, **48**, 594–598.

Hickie, I. & Scott, E. (1998) Late-onset depressive disorders: a preventable variant of cerebrovascular disease? *Psychological Medicine*, **28**, 1007–1013.

Hutchinson, G. & Gilvarry, C. (1998) Ethnicity and dissatisfaction with mental health services. *British Journal of Psychiatry*, **172**, 95c–96c.

Johansson, L. M., Sundquist, J., Johansson, S. E., *et al* (1997) Suicide among foreign-born minorities and native Swedes: an epidemiological follow-up study of a defined population. *Social Science and Medicine*, **44**, 181–187.

Jolley, D. & Baxter, D. (1997) Mortality in elderly patients with organic brain disorder enrolled on the Salford psychiatric case register. *International Journal of Geriatric Psychiatry*, **12**, 1174–1181.

Jordanova, V., Stewart, R., Davies, E., *et al* (2007) Markers of Inflammation and cognitive decline in an African–Caribbean population. *International Journal of Geriatric Psychiatry*, **22**, 966–973.

Jorm, A. F., Korten, A. E. & Henderson, A. S. (1987) The prevalence of dementia: a quantitative integration of the literature. *Acta Psychiatrica Scandinavica*, **76**, 465–479.

King's College London & London School of Economics (2007) *Dementia UK. The Full Report*. Alzheimer's Society.

Lindesay, J. (1998) Diagnosis of mental illness in elderly people from ethnic minorities. *Advances in Psychiatric Treatment*, **4**, 219–226.

Lindesay, J., Jagger, C., Hibbett, M. J., *et al* (1997) Knowledge, uptake and availability of health and social services among Asian Gujarati and White elders. *Ethnicity and Health*, **2**, 59–69.

Livingston, G., Leavey, G., Kitchen, G., *et al* (2001a) Mental health of migrant elders – the Islington study. *British Journal of Psychiatry*, **179**, 361–366.

Livingston, G., Kitchen, G., Manela, M., *et al* (2001b) Persecutory symptoms and perceptual disturbance in a community sample of older people: the Islington study. *International Journal of Geriatric Psychiatry*, **16**, 462–468.

Livingston, G., Leavey, G., Kitchen, G., *et al* (2002) Accessibility of health and social services to immigrant elders: the Islington study. *British Journal of Psychiatry*, **180**, 369–373.

Marwaha, S. & Livingston, G. (2003) Stigma, racism or choice. Why do depressed ethnic elders avoid psychiatrists? *Journal of Affective Disorders*, **72**, 257–265.

McCracken, C. F. M., Boneham, M. A., Copeland, J. R. M., *et al* (1997) Prevalence of dementia and depression among elderly people in Black and ethnic minorities. *British Journal of Psychiatry*, **171**, 269–273.

Merril, J. & Owens, J. (1988) Self-poisoning among four immigrant groups. *Acta Psychiatrica Scandinavica*, **77**, 77–80.

Mui, A.C. (1996) Geriatric Depression Scale as a community screening instrument for elderly Chinese community. *International Psychogeriatrics*, **8**, 445–458.

Mukadeen, N., Cooper, C. & Livingston, G. (2010) A systematic review of ethnicity and pathways to care in dementia. *International Journal of Geriatric Psychiatry*, in press.

National Institute for Health and Clinical Excellence (2009) *Donepezil, Galantamine, Rivastigmine (Review) and Memantine for the Treatment of Alzheimer's Disease (Amended)*. NICE Technology Appraisal Guidance 111 (Amended September 2007, August 2009). NICE.

Neeleman, J., Mak, V. & Wessely, S. (1997) Suicide by age, ethnic group, coroners' verdicts and country of birth. A three-year survey in inner London. *British Journal of Psychiatry*, **171**, 463–467.

Odutoye, K. & Shah, A. (1999) The characteristics of Indian subcontinent origin elders newly referred to a psychogeriatric service. *International Journal of Geriatric Psychiatry*, **14**, 446–453.

Oommen, G., Bashford, J &, Shah, A. (2009) Ageing, ethnicity and psychiatric services. *Psychiatric Bulletin*, **33**, 30–34.

Perkins, P., Annegers, J. F., Doody, R. S., *et al* (1997) Incidence and prevalence of dementia in a multiethnic cohort of municipal retirees. *Neurology*, **49**, 44–50.

Rait, G., Burns, A. & Chew, C. (1996) Age, ethnicity and mental illness: a triple whammy. *BMJ*, **313**, 1347.

Rait, G., Burns, A., Baldwin, R., *et al* (2000) Validating screening instruments for cognitive impairment in older South Asians in the United Kingdom. *International Journal of Geriatric Psychiatry*, **15**, 54–62.

Richards, M., Brayne, C., Dening, T., *et al* (2000) Cognitive function in UK community-dwelling African Caribbean and white elders: a pilot study. *International Journal of Geriatric Psychiatry*, **15**, 621–630.

Royal College of Psychiatrists (2001) *Psychiatric Services for Black and Minority Ethnic Older People* (College Report CR103). Royal College of Psychiatrists.

Royal College of Psychiatrists (2007) *Race Equality Action Plan. Guidance for Chairs of College Policy Working Groups/Authors of College Reports*. Royal College of Psychiatrists.

Schofield, P. W., Tang, M., Marder, K., *et al* (1995) Consistency of clinical diagnosis in a community based longitudinal study of dementia and Alzheimer's Disease. *Neurology*, **45**, 2159–2164.

Shah, A. K. (2008) Estimating the absolute number of cases of dementia and depression in the black and minority ethnic elderly population in the United Kingdom. *International Journal of Migration, Health and Social Care*, **4** (2), 4–15.

Shah, A. K. & Dighe-Deo, D. (1997) Elderly Gujaratis and psychogeriatrics in a London psychogeriatric service. *Bulletin of the International Psychogeriatric Association*, **14**, 12–13.

Shah, A., Lindesay, J. & Jagger, C. (1998) Is the diagnosis of dementia stable over time in elderly immigrant Gujaratis in the UK (Leicester)? *International Journal of Geriatric Psychiatry*, **7**, 440–444.

Shah, A. K., Oommen, G. & Wuntakal, B. (2005) Cross-cultural aspects of dementia. *Psychiatry*, **4**, 103–106.

Silveira, E. & Ebrahim, S. (1998*a*) A comparison of mental health among minority ethnic elders and Whites in East and North London. *Age and Ageing*, **27**, 375–383.

Silveira, E. & Ebrahim, S. (1998*b*) Social determinants of psychiatric morbidity and well-being in immigrant elders and Whites in east London. *International Journal of Geriatric Psychiatry*, **13**, 801–812.

Soni Raleigh, V., Bulusu, L. & Balarajan, R. (1990) Suicides among immigrants from the Indian subcontinent. *British Journal of Psychiatry*, **156**, 46–50.

Stevens, T., Leavey, G. & Livingston, G. (2004) Dementia and hypertension in African/Caribbean elders. *Age and Ageing*, **33**, 193–195.

Stewart, R., Prince, M., Mann, A., *et al* (2001*a*) Stroke, vascular risk factors and depression. Cross-sectional study in a UK Caribbean-born population. *British Journal of Psychiatry*, **178**, 23–28.

Stewart, R., Richards, M., Brayne, C., *et al* (2001*b*) Cognitive function in UK community-dwelling African Caribbean elders: normative data for a test battery. *International Journal of Geriatric Psychiatry*, **16**, 518–527.

Stewart, R., Asonganyi, B. & Sherwood, R., (2002) Plasma Homocysteine and cognitive impairment in an older British Afro-Caribbean population. *Journal of American Geriatrics Society*, **50**, 1227–1232.

Stewart, R., Powell, J., Prince, M., et al (2004) ACE genotype and cognitive decline in an African Caribbean population. *Neurobiology of Aging*, **25**, 1369–1375.

CHAPTER 12

Intellectual disability and ethnicity: achieving cultural competence

Jean O'Hara

Summary Despite the higher prevalence of intellectual disability among some minority ethnic communities and the greater burden of care, families from these communities with a member who has intellectual disability are doubly disadvantaged as a result of racial discrimination and culturally inappropriate forms of care and service provision. This chapter looks at the issue of discrimination, as well as the generally negative attitudes towards people with intellectual disability, and synthesises these into the concept of 'double jeopardy'. It concludes by proposing ways of developing cultural competence in the delivery of care to this population.

Enormous cultural complexity is found in modern-day families. Spouses may belong to different racial, religious or ethnic groups, and two or more cultures may be represented among the parents and children (Falicov, 1995). Relying on potentially stereotyped and ethnically focused information can be very misleading. Individuals vary considerably in the extent to which they choose to observe religious or cultural customs and conventions; the degree of acculturation may also vary between generations and between men and women. However, there is no doubt that the stigma of intellectual disability (other terms include mental retardation and learning disability) can be shattering and it transcends race, beliefs and culture. It creates profound emotional, practical and psychological experiences for all parents (Shah, 1992).

The 'minority experience'

Ethnicity is a complex concept which includes religious and cultural background, shared histories and common descent. Ultimately, it is the individual's psychological sense of belonging. Although not unique to families from ethnic minorities, there are distinguishing life events that

Box 12.1 The minority experience

Ethnic minority reality – often racism and poverty dominate lives.

Conflicting value systems – almost all minority ethnic groups place greater value on families, historical lineage and the submergence of self for the good of the family.

Biculturalism – many families inherit two cultural traditions. It is important to understand how biculturalism influences family structure, communication and dynamics. There is a need to understand the acculturation process.

Minority status – memories of colonialism, imperialism, slavery and the Holocaust, refugee and immigration status, skin colour and obvious physical differences are important factors that may determine the treatment of individuals and their families.

Migration – whether forced or voluntary

Language – many minority families may not possess vocabulary equivalent to standard English and may appear 'flat', 'non-verbal', 'uncommunicative' or 'lacking in insight'.

Social class – aspects of wealth, name, occupation and status.

(adapted from Sue & Sue, 1999)

differentiate the 'minority experience' from that of White middle-class families (Sue & Sue, 1999; Box 12.1).

The notion of 'White supremacy' has dominated the social and political landscape in much of the world since the 19th century and it has fuelled exploitation and racism. At the same time, its 'scientific' justification in terms of skin colour, skull size and level of 'intelligence' began to emerge.

Fernando (1989) describes racism as much more than just prejudice with social consequences. Once racism is embedded within the structures of society, the prejudice of individuals is no longer the main problem: more damaging is the issue of 'institutionally generated inequality'. Direct racial attack is less common than are perceived discrimination in interpersonal communication and inequity in the receipt of services and justice (Chakraborty & McKenzie, 2002). Studies of Asian families that include someone with a intellectual disability reveal a deprived, isolated group who suffer racial abuse, encounter language barriers and experience significant levels of stress but have little knowledge or understanding of intellectual disability (Nadirshaw, 1997). Although there is little information on the needs of other minority ethnic groups, the literature suggests that, despite formal health policy statements, families from minority ethnic communities with a member who has intellectual disability are doubly disadvantaged as a result of racial discrimination and culturally inappropriate forms of care and service provision. Ethnic identity does not in itself affect health; what does affect it is the daily experience of racism, perceived racism and a discriminatory society (Karlsen & Nazroo, 2002).

Another significant minority experience is that of migration. Whether voluntary or forced, it is a traumatic life event. It is the uprooting of meaning, with disruption of life-long attachments and external stability (Falicov, 1995). Family disruption continues through separations and reunions, and parents who raise their children in a culture that differs from their own often feel disempowered.

Anthropological perspectives

Intellectual disability is a complex label involving interactions between biogenetic and sociocultural factors. The diagnostic criteria are the significant and enduring impairment in social and intellectual functioning evident before adulthood. Deciding on the presence or absence of intellectual disability requires an arbitrary line to be drawn on a continuum of ability. One measure is the IQ test, yet this was once used to prove the innate inferiority of immigrant populations. Eminent psychologists such as Arthur Jensen and Hans Eysenck supported claims that differences in IQ ratings between 'White people' and 'coloured, primitive people' were due to race, although this view is now strongly opposed by many (Fernando, 1989).

The cultural bias of IQ tests is well recognised but they are still administered in a culture-blind fashion. Cultural bias in verbal tests is obvious, but there is no guarantee that non-verbal tests are free from bias (Fernando, 1989). How well children with mild intellectual disability do in school or in adult life and, indeed, how they come to be diagnosed in the first place, largely depends on social and cultural conditions. This type of intellectual disability has been called 'sociocultural' or 'reversible' to emphasise the importance of social and cultural factors. Ramey *et al* (1978) showed in the USA that it was possible to identify children who would need special education before or during their school years, solely on information given on their birth certificate. The children most at risk were male, Black and had been born illegitimately to mothers with little formal education.

Society's views

'In our country, we would not be allowed to treat cattle like that. Perhaps you cannot treat cattle this way in your country either – cattle, after all, are useful, while the retarded are not' (N. E. Bank-Mikkelson, on visiting a state hospital in the USA; quoted in Edgerton, 1984: p. 28).

The neglect and ill-treatment of people with intellectual disability probably exhibits one of the worst histories for any group in society (Sperlinger, 1997; O'Hara & Bouras, 2007). Western reactions have often been brutal. Those with intellectual disability have been killed, kept to entertain guests (a Roman practice that subsequently became common in the courts of European royalty), exhibited as freaks for profit, threatened with eradication and put at risk for the good of others (as in early trials of the measles vaccine). More compassionate views, tempered with pity, horror and contempt, prevailed through the 19th century, with Western attempts to provide institutional treatment and training.

There is little in the literature on the views of non-Western societies of the past. It was assumed that life in such societies was so simple that people with mild intellectual disability would be unexceptional members of their community, whereas the more severely disabled would be killed early in life. However, cross-cultural evidence indicates that even those with very mild intellectual disability were recognised throughout the world. There was a great variation in the treatment they received (Edgerton, 1984): although some societies inflicted casual cruelties, others, including many in Central Asia, India and the Middle East, offered such persons protected and favoured roles.

Cultural and religious attitudes

Cultural and religious attitudes, understanding and beliefs all play their part in how care is ultimately sought, planned, accepted and delivered. Early research interest focused on the attitude of White middle-class parents within a Judaeo–Christian faith. The birth of a child with intellectual disability either stimulated a greater faith or resulted in a complete loss of faith. Some believed that they were being punished for their sins. Fatimilehin & Nadirshaw (1994) found the variations in attitude between Asian and White British families to be related to cultural and religious differences rather than to any descriptive characteristics of the parent or their child (Box 12.2). Some would argue that South Asian cultures are more accommodating of people with disabilities (McGrother et al, 2002).

Many non-Western medical systems do not differentiate between physical and mental states, and the spiritual and supernatural elements are intertwined. The Hindu belief in the concept of karma – the cycle of reward and punishment for all deeds and thoughts as the immortal spirit is reborn into another body – may provide an understanding for what has happened and lead to a sense of resignation or acceptance. Middle Eastern cultures regard disability as a punishment from heaven, emanating from the spirits or caused by an evil eye (Aminidav & Weller, 1995). Many Chinese people believe in fate and use a coping strategy of forbearance, seeking supernatural power and praying to ancestors (Cheng & Tang, 1995). Clinicians have often cited fatalism and the search for a cure as reasons why families from some minority ethnic communities are not interested in educational or habilitative programmes for intellectual disability. It is frequently assumed that Asian parents do not have a positive or encouraging attitude towards disability, precisely because of their religious or superstitious beliefs (Shah, 1992).

An important misconception about intellectual disability held by Asian parents is the notion of curability and that the marriage of someone with intellectual disability may alleviate the condition. Channabasavanna

---

Box 12.2 Differences in attitudes and beliefs of Asian and White British families regarding intellectual disability

Fatimilehin & Nadirshaw (1994) reported the following differences in a cross-cultural study of Asian and White British families

Asian British families

- Had more contact with a 'holy' person ($P<0.05$)
- Were less aware of what their child's problem is called ($P<0.01$)
- Believed in a spiritual explanation/cause for their child's disability ($P<0.05$)
- Fifty per cent said that they did not know the cause of their child's disability
- Believed that religion had something particular to say about intellectual disability ($P<0.005$)
- Their faith helped them to cope but offered little social or practical support
- Wanted care to be provided by a relative when they were no longer able to provide it themselves ($P<0.01$)

White British families

- Most received a medical explanation for their child's disability
- None offered a spiritual explanation for their child's disability
- Only one family felt that it did not know the cause of the child's disability
- Religion/faith offered social support
- Most wanted their child to be cared for in a community home provided by statutory/voluntary services ($P<0.05$)

---

et al (1985) found that neither the severity of disability nor the socio-economic status of the parents had any effect on this attitude. Rather, it was knowledge of the concept of intellectual disability, gained through counselling, that was most influential. An example of good practice in this area is provided by Davis & Rushton (1991).

Gender and social roles

'A woman's Heaven is at her husband's feet' (traditional Asian saying).

Social and gender roles and, in particular, traditional female roles, are interpreted differently in different communities, across generations and within individual families. In 19th-century English literature, men with intellectual disability were portrayed as lacking an essential component of masculine identity, usually because of their inability to handle money (McDonagh, 2000). Women with intellectual disability embodied a paradox, being seen as threatening because of their 'undisciplined sexuality', yet also sexually innocent and in need of protection. This view resulted in mandatory sterilisation and prohibition from marriage. Both practices were still in force in 24 states in the USA as recently as 1971.

Bengali parents' desire to see their intellectually disabled children married is at the heart of their parental responsibility, and services struggle with the ethical issues this situation may pose (O'Hara & Martin, 2003). However, securing a marriage partner also serves to reassure and provide comfort to parents that their child will be cared for after their own death.

Marriage between close biological relatives is generally regarded with suspicion and distaste in Western society (Bittles, 2001). By comparison, other populations perceive marriage outside the family as risky and disruptive. In some communities, consanguineous (first-cousin) marriages continue to account for 33–53% of the total (Jaber *et al*, 2000). Professionals often relate disability explicitly to consanguineous marriage and they may be unsympathetic because they consider the condition to be self-inflicted. An Asian mother of a child with an intellectual disability said: 'the first thing he [the general practitioner] asks is "Is it a first-cousin marriage? You've had one disabled child, then another." He's a good doctor, but, because of his attitude, I only go when I really have to' (Katbamna *et al*, 2002).

Asian women are seen as isolated because of their traditional customs; the failure by Asians to take up services provided by statutory bodies is attributed to their lack of skills relating to Western lifestyles (Fernando, 1989). Women with intellectual disability face 'triple jeopardy' in relation to race, disability/impairment and gender (Mir *et al*, 2001). They may experience simultaneous discrimination and disadvantage and have additional support needs in terms of their sexuality and motherhood. However, there is a growing interest in the health and welfare of women with intellectual disability (e.g. Walsh & Heller, 2002; O'Hara, 2008).

Intellectual disability in minority ethnic communities

The prevalence of intellectual disability among South Asians is three times that in majority communities. Of these families, 19% have more than one member with intellectual disability (Mir *et al*, 2001; Emerson & Hatton, 2004). Unfortunately, prevalence within other minority ethnic communities, and even for different subgroups within the South Asian community, is not well documented. This higher prevalence has been linked to high levels of maternal and social deprivation combined with factors such as inequality in healthcare (Emerson, 1997). The healthcare that is offered may be culturally inappropriate, unwelcoming and discriminatory, with a culture-blaming attitude. It may also have poor standards of communication and offer poor quality of care (Mir *et al*, 2001; Raghavan & Waseem, 2007). For example, prenatal diagnosis is sometimes withheld from Muslim families on the assumption that they will not consider a termination of pregnancy. This denies them information and choice.

There are reports of ethnic differences in the rate of detection of trisomy-21 (Down syndrome) using biochemical markers (e.g. Gilbert *et al*, 1996), with more false positives in ethnic minorities, which lead to unnecessary anxiety and invasive investigations.

The method used to break news of impairment/disability to a family from a minority ethnic community may be particularly poor, with the use of a non-professional interpreter adding to the stress and initiating or perpetuating a cycle of bad health experiences and expectations (e.g. Butt & Mirza, 1996). An information vacuum exists, in terms of culturally appropriate leaflets and audiovisual material, and the type of information that historically has been made available, for example about hygiene and fertility control, may be translated in a way that implies inferior cultural practices (Mir *et al*, 2001).

Carers in minority ethnic communities

In the UK, the burden of care, both socially and financially, is greater for carers from minority ethnic communities than for their White peers (Butt & Mirza, 1996). This is due to a number of contributory factors, including poverty, poor housing, racism, higher levels of unemployment, low pay, minimum pension rights, reduced benefits because of residence status and inadequate education. For example, spouses of adults with intellectual disability from minority ethnic communities are allowed into the UK on the proviso that they do not claim on the welfare state for the first 5 years. There is evidence that general practitioner (GP) consultation rates in minority ethnic communities are significantly higher than in the majority community, but that these patients are less aware of the existence of specialist services (e.g. Katbamna *et al*, 2002; McGrother *et al*, 2002; Raghavan & Waseem, 2007). Psychological and emotional distress may not be recognised, as patients from ethnic minorities tend to present to their GP with somatic symptoms (Nadirshaw, 1997). A discriminatory view is that this is an unsophisticated form of communication (Fernando, 1989). There is also a danger of emphasising people's needs in terms of religion, customs and traditions and overlooking their basic needs for decent housing, access to healthcare and assistance to claim benefits. Factors such as immigration and the quality of housing available, particularly in inner-city areas, often militate against the supportive network traditionally offered by extended families.

A family's failure to spend time with a member with disabilities might be due to insufficient financial and practical support, but it can be perceived by professionals as a lack of interest or engagement with services.

It is a commonly held view that the hierarchical family structure in many non-Western cultures produces 'stress-ridden relationships', and the very strengths of this organisation are seen as a source of actual and potential weakness (Fernando, 1989). Research often pays little attention to the strengths of such a support network. Understanding of and respect for different family organisations are vital to service delivery. Parents may not have sole primary responsibility for looking after their children, as care is shared by a number of adults within the extended family. Extended families may involve grandparents, uncles and aunts, cousins and second cousins and even non-blood 'relatives'. It is important to understand how decisions are made and who has the ultimate authority for making them. In some cultures, out-patient appointments may be seen as a social responsibility, with a large group of family members attending. Likewise, a consultation in the home can often involve the presence of a number of family members. The level of individuals' contacts outside their own ethnic group varies, and this can have profound effects on the perceptions and lifestyles of different generations. Second and third generations may have very different attitudes from their predecessors and this can lead to tension and cultural conflicts within a family. When providing services to families that have a range of different structures and priorities, skills are needed to avoid giving primacy to a particular cultural or ethnic approach (Mir *et al*, 2001).

Ethnic and racial identity

Racism and stigma are pervasive in the lives of people with intellectual disability who are from the South Asian community. Azmi *et al* (1997) found this double discrimination to be a painful reality. However, in their study of such a population, all participants had a strong sense of their ethnic and racial identities and viewed these identities positively. There was a wide variation in the extent to which the 'younger' generation, mostly born in the UK, maintained traditional practices such as arranged marriages, gender roles, family obligations and religious observances. Almost all participants named a religious affiliation matching that of their family, and over 50% reported active observance of their religion. Sixty-three per cent felt that they were treated badly because of their ethnic group (27% did not respond clearly on this issue) and 57% also felt that they were treated badly because of their disability (33% did not respond clearly). Frequently, participants reported abusive behaviour from other people which combined racism and stigma.

An essential part of personal identity is personal appearance, and for some communities it is particularly important to pay attention to cultural factors associated with dress, hair and skin care and personal hygiene. Food is another aspect of basic care where cultural and religious needs might be ignored or inadequately catered for. Behavioural programmes and skills training might be based on White culture, for example teaching someone to use a knife, fork and spoon. Provision of physiotherapy activities such as massage, limb manipulation, dancing and swimming needs to be sensitive to the wishes of the family, especially with regard to modesty and appropriate behaviour. Unless such issues are addressed, people from minority ethnic communities are unlikely to use services that they perceive to be insensitive to their cultural needs.

Knowledge about religious beliefs and cultural practices can enable service providers to ensure that people with intellectual disability from minority ethnic communities experience a range of relevant cultural events and influences. Recurrent themes reported by carers include the need to meet dietary requirements; provide culturally appropriate activities and same-gender centres; increase the number of staff from minority cultures and the number of bilingual workers throughout mainstream services; and adapt materials in a culturally sensitive way. However, the assumption that a family wants support only from someone of their own culture is often misplaced, as workers from other cultures may be perceived as less intrusive (Mir *et al*, 2001). The preference for same-gender staff to carry out intimate personal care and support is curiously portrayed as a requirement specific only to certain religions and cultures, when, in fact, it exists to a large extent in all communities. This belief is unhelpful as it suggests that the preference is 'different' or 'special' and it gives the impression of an additional burden on resources (Baxter, 1996).

Importance of language

> 'Ethnicity patterns our way of thinking, feeling and behaving. Language is one factor in the elaboration of ethnicity' (de Zulueta, 1990).

Communicating with people in a language other than their first language can affect our sensitivity to their attitudes and values (Shah, 1992). Language structures the meaning of communication and contributes to a sense of belonging (Sue & Sue, 1999). We think and feel in our first language, and using a second language can block thoughts and emotions (Bhugra, 2002). Psychosis can appear to be less prominent when bilingual patients are interviewed in their second rather than their first language, and in using their second language they can remain protected from anxiety and hidden meanings and feelings (de Zulueta, 1990). In some cases, health practitioners are themselves using a second language in clinical practice and not enough attention has been paid to the resulting implications, especially in the context of psychotherapeutic approaches. The choice of language used in the delivery of health services to bilingual families may not appear neutral to them. It can be perceived as collusion between the clinician and the most fluent family member; it may allow the child to speak freely in front of the parent; and it may be used to track transgenerational alliances. Complexity increases with family size and the degree of bilingualism of each family member (Raval, 1996).

Interpreters: help or hindrance?

It is unethical and unprofessional to use children to interpret. Interpreting by family members should be avoided because of the possible biases and power relationships within the family (Shah, 1992; Farooq & Fear, 2003). A very high level of interpreting skills is required, with the interpreter at the apex of a triad: 'the interpreter is the person who makes the link between two different languages and cultures… [who] makes sense of unusual questioning, helps contain feelings' (Raval, 1996).

However, interpreters do not have a professional status and their role within services may be ambiguous. They can be seen solely as interpreters of language or as community workers, link workers, advocates, cultural brokers or cultural consultants. Working effectively with interpreters requires training and is a necessary component of providing a high-quality service (Box 12.3). It is not a luxury. Clinicians who have to use interpreters may feel disempowered and culturally ignorant in front of patients and their families, leading to a sense of therapeutic detachment and a mechanical or stilted interview. They may begin to feel deskilled, excluded or resentful and hold a lower opinion of the efficacy of their involvement. They may become dependent on the interpreter in order to carry out their role. Patients or carers, however, can feel more reassured about their ability to communicate freely through a trained interpreter when describing religious beliefs (such as ghost possessions), unsatisfactory environmental conditions, mental illness and even abuse, without fear of being ridiculed (Raval, 1996). Interpreters may feel it culturally inappropriate to translate particular language (e.g. verbal abuse or that related to sexual behaviour). Discussion

---

Box 12.3 Working with interpreters

Skills of a good interpreter

- Fluent communication
- Ability to engage with the patient while speaking as directed by someone else
- Sensitivity and interpersonal skills
- Calm and non-threatening personality
- Capacity to offer comfort in discussing personal and emotional issues

Negotiating the interpreter–clinician relationship

- Insist on mutual briefing and debriefing
- Ensure interpreter is well versed in the information needed and in any specific concepts that may be used
- Agree a model of joint working, e.g. literal translation or translation reflecting cultural context
- Ensure interpreter understands the importance of confidentiality
- Check for compatibility, e.g. in linguistic and religious backgrounds
- Respect the professionalism of the interpreter – do not be suspicious of the relationship between patient/carer and interpreter
- Be patient and open-minded. Ask questions without being intentionally offensive
- Observe gender issues, religious and cultural events
- Be sensitive to the discrimination that patients and families experience in their everyday lives

(Adapted from Shah, 1992 and Nadirshaw, 1997)

of sexuality is surrounded by taboos, more so in some communities than others. Sometimes questions cannot be translated directly and have to be rephrased to make sense in another language. This can result in a translation that is semantically very different from the question originally asked. It is important, therefore, that a method of joint working with the interpreter is agreed prior to the interview.

Developing cultural competence

Services must develop a sense of belonging in people from all cultures, so that everyone feels comfortable using them. Falicov (1995) urges applying a cultural lens to everything we do and taking culture into mainstream thinking, teaching, learning and research (e.g, McCarthy *et al*, 2008). Cultural knowledge is important, but care must be taken not to apply it in a stereotyped manner (Box 12.4).

Ethnic matching of the clinician/doctor and patient is neither necessary nor always desirable, but it is essential that clinicians are aware of the interactions between the parties (Bhugra, 2002). These are often influenced by training, experience, social class, world views and knowledge of one another's culture and ethnicity (Table 12.1). For example, there may be an assumption that the absence of toys scattered around the living room during a home visit indicates that parents do not think that toys are important

---

Box 12.4   The continuum of cultural competence

Cross *et al* (1989) identified the following culturally appropriate or inappropriate behaviour in a healthcare organisation.

- *Cultural destructiveness* – cultural/racial oppression, forced assimilation
- *Cultural incapacity* – discriminatory practices, unchallenged stereotypical beliefs
- *Cultural blindness* – 'we treat everyone the same': this approach ignores cultural strengths. The belief that methods used by the dominant culture are universally applicable can lead to implicit or explicit exclusion of minority ethnic communities
- *Cultural pre-competence* – a false sense of accomplishment; inconsistent policies and practices; practitioners are sensitive to minority issues but these are not an organisational priority
- *Cultural competence* – a vision that reflects multiculturalism, values diversity and views it as an asset: evidence of continuing attempts to accommodate cultural change; careful attention to the dynamics of difference, realising that equal access is not equal treatment
- *Cultural proficiency* – adding to knowledge-base by conducting research; developing new therapeutic approaches based on cultural considerations; follow-through social responsibility to fight social discrimination and advocate social diversity.

Table 12 .1   Value and belief models of world views

	Component values and beliefs	
	Within White culture	**Within BME cultures**
The individual v. the group	Individualism: independence and autonomy highly valued and rewarded	Collectivism: submergence of self for good of family. Interdependence: allegiance to family is of primary importance and takes precedence
Communication	Direct eye contact. Verbal, emotional and behavioural expressiveness. Openness and intimacy. Standard English 'horizontal' pattern of communication	Silence indicates respect. Non-verbal communication important. Strong feelings restrained (i.e. anger, love, affection, frustration). 'Vertical' pattern of communication
Time	Viewed as a commodity. Adherence to time-keeping	Punctuality may be unimportant; things done according to a rational order and not to deadlines
Thinking	Reliance on physical or psychological healing methods. Dismissive/sceptical of supernatural explanations. Emphasis on objective, rational and linear thinking	Reliance on spiritual plane for model of healing. Belief in the spirit world affects circumstances of the living. Relates to nature ('Mother Earth')
Status	Measured by economic possessions, credentials	Honour and respect gained by sharing and giving; refusing to accept a gift/invitation can be taken as an insult
Family structure	Nuclear family as ideal social unit	Hierarchical relationships. Extended family – through to second cousins and non-blood 'relatives'

BME, Black and minority ethnic.
Adapted from Sue & Sue, 1999.

or, more worrying, it may be taken as a sign of neglect or environmental deprivation. The sharing of a parental bed is another culture-bound practice, which may lead to judgemental reactions from practitioners concerned with issues of child protection or adult vulnerability. Criticism, especially in front of others, may be a culture-bound expression of parental concern and the encouragement to better oneself. There is a risk, however, that it may be misconstrued as dysfunctional family dynamics. The diagnosis therefore of 'family conflict' may be no more than a racist assumption about family life (Fernando, 1989).

A strategic approach is required to ensure that the needs of people from minority ethnic communities are not forgotten. These needs are complicated by issues of power, race and gender politics, but they must not be overlooked just because they affect only 'small numbers' in a given population (Cole, 2002; Box 12.5).

'Special-needs' initiatives can provide a much needed focus on the issues to be addressed, but they are often structurally disadvantaged, with inadequate funding. They may appear to meet a need but in fact act as a surrogate form of racism while absolving mainstream services of responsibility. Specialist services do not eliminate the need to remove discriminatory practices and attitudes from mainstream services. This situation is reflected in the wider debates and philosophies underpinning the provision of healthcare in general, and mental healthcare in particular, for people with intellectual disability. Cultural sensitivity is only one element of quality in service provision (Healthcare Commission, 2007). The notion of 'cultural diversity' is intended to move us away from a focus on 'difference' and the consequent perception of additional burden. Managing diversity means offering a level of respect to all. It also leads to recognition that the 'majority' is not a homogeneous population but comprises a number of cultural and social communities with their own needs and aspirations.

Box 12.5 Service principles and action plan for service development

The requirements of service development include:

- a strategic approach
- meaningful consultation with families, carers and community workers
- going beyond consultation to real empowerment
- developing advocacy and self-advocacy, recognising family structures that differ from those of the majority ethnic community
- appropriate publicity for and full access to all service provision
- recruitment of ethnic minority and bilingual staff at all levels and ensuring their adequate support and training
- training for all staff, to increase competence in cultural awareness, sensitivity and flexibility
- person-centred planning, acknowledging discrimination and racism and its impact on the person; drawing up support plans to empower people from different ethnic communities
- accurate information about need – effective monitoring processes, patterns of use, identifying unmet need
- targeting housing and placement opportunities within minority ethnic communities
- commissioning single-culture treatment options, including in-patient and residential facilities, self-help groups, social and psychological therapies
- working with provider agencies that specify 'cultural competence'
- integrated services: the ideal is quality mainstream services sensitive to the needs of all users

(adapted from Mir *et al*, 2001 and Cole, 2002)

References

Aminidav, C. & Weller, L. (1995) Effects of country of origin, sex, religiosity and social class on breadth of knowledge of mental retardation. *British Journal of Developmental Disabilities*, **XLI**, 48–56.

Azmi, S., Hatton, C., Emerson, E., *et al* (1997) Listening to adolescents and adults with intellectual disability in South Asian communities. *Journal of Applied Research in Intellectual Disability*, **10**, 250–263.

Baxter, C. (1996) Sex education: ethnically sensitive services to people with learning disabilities. *Tizard Learning Disability Review*, **1**, 1–6.

Bhugra, D. (2002) Assessing psychiatric problems in ethnic minority patients. *Practitioner*, **246**, 147–163.

Bittles, A. H. (2001) Consanguinity and its relevance to clinical genetics. *Clinical Genetics*, **60**, 89–98.

Butt, J. & Mirza, K. (1996) *Social Care and Black Communities*. TSO (The Stationery Office).

Chakraborty, A. & McKenzie, K. (2002) Does racial discrimination cause mental illness? *British Journal of Psychiatry*, **180**, 475–477.

Channabasavanna, S. M., Bhatti, R. S. & Prabhu, L. R. (1985) A study of attitudes of parents towards the management of mentally retarded children. *Child Psychiatry Quarterly*, **18**, 85–92.

Cheng, P. & Tang, C. S. (1995) Coping and psychological distress of Chinese parents of children with Down's Syndrome. *Mental Retardation*, **33**, 10–20.

Cole, A. (2002) *Developing and Improving Services to Meet the Mental Health Needs of People with Learning Disabilities: A Workbook for Commissioners and Managers in Mental Health and Learning Disability Services*. Institute for Applied Health and Social Policy, King's College.

Cross, T. L., Bazron, B. J., Dennis, K. W., *et al* (1989) *Towards a Culturally Competent System of Care*. Child and Adolescent Service System Program Technical Assistance Center.

Davis, H. & Rushton, R. (1991) Counselling and supporting parents of children with developmental delay: a research evaluation. *Journal of Mental Deficiency Research*, **35**, 89–113.

de Zulueta, F. (1990) Bilingualism and family therapy. *Journal of Family Therapy*, **12**, 255–265.

Edgerton, R. B. (1984) Anthropology and mental retardation: research approaches and opportunities. *Culture, Medicine and Psychiatry*, **8**, 25–48.

Emerson, E. (1997) Is there an increased prevalence of severe learning disabilities among British Asians? *Ethnicity and Health*, **2**, 317–321.

Emerson, E. & Hatton, C. (2004) The prevalence of intellectual disability among South Asian communities in the UK. *Journal of Intellectual Disability Research*, **48**, 201–202.

Falicov, C. J. (1995) Training to think culturally: a multidimensional comparative framework. *Family Process*, **34**, 373–387.

Farooq, S. & Fear, C. (2003) Working through interpreters. *Advances in Psychiatric Treatment*, **9**, 104–109.

Fatimilehin, I. A. & Nadirshaw, Z. (1994) A cross-cultural study of parental attitudes and beliefs about learning disability (mental handicap). *Mental Handicap Research*, **7**, 202–227.

Fernando, S. (1989) *Race and Culture in Psychiatry*. Routledge.

Gilbert, L., Nicholl, J., Alex, S., *et al* (1996) Ethnic differences in the outcome of serum screening for Down's syndrome. *BMJ*, **3**, 94–95.

Healthcare Commission (2007) *Count Me In 2007: Results of the 2007 National Census of Inpatients in Mental Health and Learning Disability Services in England and Wales*. Commission for Healthcare Audit and Inspection.

Jaber, L., Halpem, G. J. & Shohat, T. (2000) Trends in the frequencies of consanguineous marriages in the Israeli Arab community. *Clinical Genetics*, **58**, 106–110.

Karlsen, S. & Nazroo, J. Y. (2002) Agency and structure: the impact of ethnic identity and racism on the health of ethnic minority people. *Sociology of Health and Illness*, **24**, 1–20.

Katbamna, S., Bhakta, P., Ahmad, W., *et al* (2002) Supporting South Asian carers and those they care for: the role of the primary care team. *British Journal of General Practice*, **52**, 300–305.

McCarthy, J., Mir, G. & Wright, S. (2008) People with learning disabilities and mental health problems: the impact of ethnicity. *Advances in Mental Health and Learning Disabilities*, **2** (2), 31–36.

McDonagh, P. (2000) Diminished men and dangerous women: representations of gender and learning disability in early- and mid-nineteenth-century Britain. *British Journal of Learning Disabilities*, **28**, 49–53.

McGrother, W., Bhaumik, S., Thorpe, C. F., *et al* (2002) Prevalence, morbidity and service need among South Asian and White adults with intellectual disability in Leicestershire, UK. *Journal of Intellectual Disability Research*, **46**, 299–309.

Mir, G., Nocon, A., Ahmad, W., *et al* (2001) *Learning Difficulties and Ethnicity*. Department of Health.

Nadirshaw, Z. (1997) Cultural issues. In *Adults with Learning Disabilities: A Practical Approach for Health Professionals* (eds J. O'Hara & A. Sperlinger), pp. 139–153. John Wiley & Sons.

O'Hara, J. (2008) Why should I care about gender? *Advances in Mental Health and Learning Disabilities*, **2**, 463–468.

O'Hara, J. & Bouras, N. (2007) Intellectual disabilities across cultures. In *Textbook of Cultural Psychiatry* (eds D. Bhugra & K. Bhui), pp. 461–470. Cambridge University Press.

O'Hara, J. & Martin, H. (2003) Parents with learning disabilities: a study of gender and cultural perspectives from East London. *British Journal of Learning Disabilities*, **31**, 18–24.

Raghavan, R. & Waseem, F. (2007) Services for young people with learning disabilities and mental health need for South Asian communities. *Advances in Mental Health and Learning Disabilities*, **1** (3), 27–31.

Ramey, C. T., Stedman, D. J., Borders-Petterson, A., *et al* (1978) Predicting school failure from information available at birth. *American Journal of Mental Deficiency*, **82**, 525–534.

Raval, H. (1996) A systemic perspective on working with interpreters. *Clinical Child Psychology and Psychiatry*, **1**, 29–43.

Shah, R. (1992) *The Silent Minority: Children with Disabilities in Asian Families*. National Children's Bureau.

Sperlinger, A. (1997) Introduction. In *Adults with Learning Disabilities: A Practical Approach for Health Professionals* (eds J. O'Hara & A. Sperlinger). John Wiley & Sons.

Sue, D. W. & Sue, D. (1999) *Counseling the Culturally Different: Theory and Practice* (3rd edn). John Wiley & Sons.

Walsh, P. N. & Heller, T. (2002) *Health of Women with Intellectual Disabilities*. Blackwell Science.

CHAPTER 13

Culture and liaison psychiatry

Gopinath Ranjith

Summary   Liaison psychiatry, the branch of psychiatry that operates at the interface of general medicine and psychiatry, faces challenges related both to the different cultures of the two disciplines and to the care of patients who belong to minority cultural backgrounds. In this chapter, cultural issues that are likely to come up in encounters between liaison psychiatrists trained in the West and patients from non-Western cultures are explored. Emotional disorders in the medically ill, medically unexplained symptoms and self-harm are used to illustrate these. Other topics discussed include cultural aspects of ethical problems in the general hospital and cultural sensitivity in psychiatric assessments and treatment. The chapter ends with a model of a culturally capable liaison service.

Liaison psychiatry, also known as consultation-liaison psychiatry, is the subspecialty of psychiatry that provides psychiatric care to patients presenting in medical settings. Services have traditionally been based in general hospitals, where they provide psychiatric consultations on medical and surgical wards, in emergency departments and in out-patient clinics. In spite of recognition as a subspecialty with the achievement of faculty status within the Royal College of Psychiatrists, liaison services remain patchy. Thus, in the UK it is still a growing specialty.

Cultural challenges in liaison psychiatry

In these globalised times hospitals in Western countries, particularly in large cities, see patients from all over the world. The term 'hyperdiversity' has been used to refer to the mix of ethnicities, cultures and identities seen in conurbations (Kirmayer, 2007). Many of them include refugees or asylum seekers with traumatic histories and poor skills in communicating in the dominant language. These patients often do not do well in general hospitals as they are unable to express themselves. It is known that patients with mental illnesses in general hospitals experience stigmatising attitudes (Liggins & Hatcher, 2005) and experience more adverse events during their hospital stay (Daumit et al, 2006). The culturally different patient with a mental illness may thus be the victim of double jeopardy. The liaison psychiatrist, whose role goes beyond psychiatry to psychosocial advocacy

(Smith, 1998), needs to have advanced skills in assessing and treating a patient from a different culture.

When discussing culture and liaison psychiatry another cultural interface must also be considered, as liaison psychiatrists operate in the grey area between medicine and psychiatry. Medicine can be considered a healing culture with its own rituals and codes of conduct. Historically, psychiatry has diverged from medicine and formed its own subculture. A general hospital is, for many psychiatrists, an alien cultural milieu to which they need to adapt. Liaison psychiatrists often finds themselves in a cultural no man's land needing to travel frequently between the two but not quite belonging to either. This dilemma was elegantly expressed by the Australian liaison psychiatrist Graeme Smith, who wrote 'consultation-liaison psychiatrists are doctors who first alienated themselves from the rest of medicine in becoming psychiatrists and then alienated themselves from the rest of psychiatry by moving towards medicine' (Smith, 1998).

In this chapter I describe some common psychiatric presentations in the medically ill that might be strongly influenced by culture. It is not my contention that cultural factors are only relevant in the assessment and treatment of patients belonging to ethnic minorities; indeed, cultural differences are found within communities as much as between communities. But given issues of space, this chapter will concentrate on issues confronting psychiatrists with 'Western' training dealing with patients from a culture different either from their own or from the dominant culture.

Cultural influences in psychiatric presentations in medical settings

Referrals to liaison psychiatrists span the entire range of psychiatric and behavioural disorders, from consequences of brain disorder such as delirium and dementia to consequences of severe life stressors such as adjustment disorders and post-traumatic stress disorder. Tseng (2001) has described different influences of culture on psychiatric disorders: pathogenic (culture directly responsible for causation); pathoselective (culture influences the selection of a particular reaction pattern); pathoplastic (culture influences the manifestation of psychopathology); pathoelaborative (culture reinforces the exaggerated presentation of universal behavioural reactions); patho-facilitative (culture influences the frequency of occurrence of certain disorders in a given society); and pathoreactive (culture moulds reactions towards a particular disorder). For example, in an episode of delirium, culture may have a pathoplastic effect reflected in the content of visual hallucinations. However, it may have a pathogenic role in some episodes of self-harm or a pathoreactive or pathofacilitative effect in certain other disorders such as medically unexplained physical symptoms, adjustment disorders and post-traumatic stress disorder. I discuss next some common clinical problems that are referred to psychiatrists in the general hospital.

Emotional disorders in the medically ill

Low mood is the most common reason for referral to most liaison services. The assessment and classification of depression are difficult at the best of times. When depression occurs in the context of medical illness it raises additional questions (O'Keeffe & Ranjith, 2007). Is the depression related to the pathology that caused the medical illness, as in a post-stroke depression? Is the depression an adverse effect of the treatment for a medical illness, as in interferon-related depression? Is the depression a relapse of an underlying mood disorder triggered by the medical illness? Is the depression an understandable but excessive reaction to the stress of the illness or its consequence, as in an adjustment disorder? Or is it just a normal reaction to an unusually stressful life situation, as in demoralisation?

In patients from cultures where a rigid mind–body dichotomy is not practised, emotional distress may be presented in a somatic way (Parker et al, 2001). The interviewer, to circumvent this initial presentation with somatic symptoms, would need to use the techniques described under the rubric of the reattribution model (Goldberg et al, 1989). The other option when psychological symptoms are not easily elicited is to give more importance to objective signs such as psychomotor retardation and biological symptoms such as insomnia and weight loss rather than expressed low mood or anhedonia. Since many biological symptoms of depression may be signs of the coexisting medical illness rather than of depression, liaison psychiatrists often base their diagnosis on depressive cognitions rather than on biological symptoms. As will be clear in light of the above discussion, this approach requires modification in cross-cultural settings.

The process of adjusting to a medical illness is a complex biopsychosocial one in which cultural factors play a major role. Prior knowledge about the illness, coping resources and societal responses, including stigma, play a role in shaping an individual's reaction. Thus, when assessing disordered adjustment to an illness a cultural framework is essential. Without a good understanding of the perceptions regarding a particular illness in a particular culture and the attendant stigma, normal reactions may be pathologised or vice versa. The fictitious vignette below shows how the stigma of HIV led a patient with a maladaptive illness behaviour to be diagnosed with depression and referred to a liaison psychiatry service.

Vignette 1

Mr A, a 25-year-old Malawian student, was diagnosed with HIV infection after being investigated for weight loss. After hearing the diagnosis he stopped interacting with doctors and nurses and hardly got out of bed. He also did not accept the antiretroviral medications prescribed by his doctors. He was referred to a liaison psychiatrist for assessment and treatment for 'depression'. On talking to a friend who was visiting the ward, the trainee liaison psychiatrist found that Mr A's cousin and another close friend had died in the past year in Malawi after an HIV-related illness.

His friend also explained that in the village Mr A came from there was no access to treatment for HIV. The liaison psychiatrist spoke to Mr A in a joint consultation with the ward doctor, with the close friend present, and explained that the prognosis was good with antiretroviral treatment. Mr A soon started interacting and adhering to the treatment. The team had underestimated the meaning of the diagnosis of HIV – to him it was equal to a death sentence.

Medically unexplained symptoms

Medically unexplained symptoms are common in medical settings, in both primary and secondary care. The currently accepted aetiological model considers increased attention to bodily sensation, aberrant experience through somatosensory amplification and attribution of these to a disease prompting help-seeking. Cultural factors influence these processes, from the choice of the symptom or body part to the attribution based on folk views. Broader sociocultural influences such as familial and community factors, reinforcement by doctors or other healers and the availability of disability benefits and societal attitudes to disability may be important in perpetuating the disorder (Kirmayer & Sartorius, 2007). When formulating the link between culture and physical symptoms, the model provided by Mumford (1989) is useful: language and idiom as determinants of symptom expression, concepts of health and disease as influences on symptom interpretation and culturally sanctioned illness behaviour as predictive of symptom presentation.

Functional somatic syndromes are constellations of symptoms, including fatigue and multiple physical symptoms, often attributed to a medical causative factor. These syndromes enjoy some amount of medical legitimacy and are endorsed by different medical specialties such as gastroenterology (irritable bowel syndrome), rheumatology (fibromyalgia) and infectious diseases (chronic fatigue syndrome). Researchers who have looked at the symptoms of these various syndromes have identified more similarities than differences among them and suggested that rather than consider these as separate syndromes they may be considered presentations of a single functional somatic syndrome (Wessely *et al*, 1999). Most of the functional somatic syndromes described so far have been diagnoses popular in Western medicine. We have proposed, citing the example of *dhat* syndrome, in which men complain of loss of semen through urine, that some 'culture-bound syndromes' may actually be considered functional somatic syndromes (Ranjith & Mohan, 2006). According to this model, young men with anxiety about sex and masturbation and a predisposition to amplification of somatic symptoms may focus attention on physiological changes such as turbidity of urine and tiredness, and misattribute them to loss of semen in the light of widely prevalent health beliefs. This attribution may then be confirmed by traditional views as well as by local practitioners subscribing to similar beliefs. Taboos regarding the open discussion of sexual matters prevent disconfirmation of these beliefs.

Vignette 2

A 19-year-old Bangladeshi man had been in the UK only for 6 months, working as a kitchen assistant in a restaurant. His supervisor advised him to see his general practitioner as he was constantly complaining of tiredness. He ended up being referred to the genitourinary medicine (GUM) clinic as he talked of a whitish discharge in the urine. The GUM clinic referred him to the liaison psychiatrist to rule out a somatic delusion. The liaison psychiatrist, familiar with semen loss as an idiom of distress, spent some time on psychosocial enquiry. He elicited a history of poor adjustment in the young man's new workplace, homesickness and guilt about masturbation. After simple reassurance about the normality of masturbation and supportive sessions taking a problem-solving approach, the young man was doing well and no longer had any symptoms.

Self-harm

Self-harm results in around 140 000 presentations a year to accident and emergency departments in England and Wales (Hawton *et al*, 1997). This may still be an underestimate, as mild episodes of self-harm often do not come to the attention of medical services. Many studies have identified increased rates of self-harm in certain ethnic and cultural groups. There are methodological problems with these studies, such as lumping together heterogeneous groups as 'South Asian' or 'Black' and investigation of cultural conflict between groups using questionnaires that are relevant to one group but not the other. Nevertheless, the findings offer pointers to broad trends and I will discuss some key studies here.

Among the main minority ethnic groups within the UK most research on self-harm has been done in South Asian communities. In a series of studies conducted in west London, Bhugra and colleagues looked at self-harm presentations to four hospitals in a particular catchment area (Bhugra *et al*, 1999*a,b*). They found that the rate of self-harm among Asian women was 1.6 times that for White women and 2.5 times that for Asian men. When the analysis was restricted to those below the age of 30, the rate for Asian women was 2.5 times that for White women and 7 times that for Asian men. Comparing the Asian women with the White women, they also found that the former had experienced more adverse life events, whereas the latter more often had a psychiatric disorder, and that the Asian women expressed more regret at being alive despite taking fewer tablets (in overdose). In this study, rates of self-harm in the Black group were lower than expected.

A more recent study from Manchester also found higher rates of self-harm among South Asian women than among South Asian men and White men and women (Cooper *et al*, 2006). The South Asian women reported more intrafamilial conflicts and endorsed depressive symptoms less frequently. They also found that South Asians of both genders were less likely to be offered psychiatric follow-up. A recent systematic review (Bhui *et al*, 2007) confirmed the findings of higher rates among South Asian women compared with their White counterparts. It also noted the dearth of high-quality studies with African–Caribbean participants.

Ethical problems in the general hospital

Although there are significant differences in perspective between a psychiatric consultation and an ethics consultation, psychiatric consultations in general hospitals often involve ethical issues. A not uncommon reason for referral to liaison psychiatrists is the patient's refusal of treatment (Ranjith & Hotopf, 2004). There are legal frameworks in place in different jurisdictions within the UK to deal with the assessment of mental capacity and to assist in decision-making in incapacitated patients. A seemingly unwise or irrational decision in itself does not equate with lack of mental capacity but often triggers an assessment of capacity. In such cases it is important to determine the cultural context in which the decision was made.

For patients lacking capacity, the clinician has to make a 'best interests' decision-taking into consideration the values, wishes and world view of the patient, having consulted widely with people close to the patient. Some of the views expressed regarding continuation or discontinuation of treatment may appear baffling to clinicians. But rather than dismiss the views of carers and relatives and make a decision solely on medical best interests it behoves a clinician to consider cultural and religious factors as much as clinical ones. There is little research into the impact of cultural differences on decision-making in healthcare settings. The following four are considered pillars of Western biomedical ethics: autonomy, beneficence, non-maleficence and justice (Beauchamp & Childress, 2001). Among these, autonomy is often given the status of first among equals. One of the questions confronting a clinician working with a patient from a different culture is whether this prominence given to autonomy is an imposition of a Euro-centric ethical view on people from collectivist cultures. The counter-argument is that autonomy is a non-negotiable principle that needs to be upheld regardless of the cultural milieu. There may not be a clear answer to such dilemmas in clinical practice but this highlights the importance of debating these issues and consulting with one's colleagues as well as those well versed in a particular culture before making a final decision.

Other ethical issues also often confront the liaison psychiatrist working with medically ill patients. Some issues recently discussed with reference to palliative care psychiatry may be directly relevant to liaison psychiatrists working with a diverse group of medically ill patients (Chaturvedi, 2008). One of the issues is about disclosing the diagnosis, as in many cultures it is common for the patient to be spared hearing the diagnosis of a potentially life-threatening illness such as cancer. The clinicians involved in the patient's care, including the physician and the liaison psychiatrist, may have to play a delicate balancing act between the pressure of the well-meaning family and the obligation to be truthful and honest with the patient. In patriarchal societies with large extended families, treatment choices are often made by family or clan elders. In such situations, the clinician often is caught between the need to consider the cultural context and respect the family versus the need to make sure that the patient's voice is heard and his or her needs are not ignored. Other situations in which cultural and/or religious factors might be relevant include end-of-life care, the concept of a good death and use of complementary and alternative medications.

Cultural sensitivity in assessments in the general hospital

Cultural competence has become a buzzword in recent years and training in cultural competence is now mandatory for health professionals. Although there is no widely accepted definition of cultural competence, it is generally considered to constitute a set of skills or processes that enable health professionals to provide services that are culturally appropriate for the diverse populations they serve (Bhui *et al*, 2007). It includes concepts such as cultural sensitivity, cultural knowledge and cultural skills and can be considered at the level of the individual clinician and the level of the organisation. At a practical level, the clinician may need to move beyond a checklist approach to cultural competence as it risks pigeonholing patients into groups such as 'Chinese' or Caribbean'. The alternative is to use an idiographic cultural formulation approach such as that described by the Committee on Cultural Psychiatry of the Group for the Advancement of Psychiatry (Group for the Advancement of Psychiatry, 2002); this lends itself well to use in liaison psychiatry training.

A practical example of using a cultural formulation approach is given by Ahmed *et al* (2007), who offer a guide to the assessment of self-harm in women hailing from the Indian subcontinent. In addition to the questions routinely asked in determining the risk after an episode of self-harm, they suggest concentrating on personal factors such as low self-esteem and social isolation, family factors such as arranged and forced marriages, problems with inter-racial or inter-caste relationships, cultural factors such as poor acculturation, gender-role expectations and misuse of religion to control women, and socioeconomic factors such as racism and sexism.

The following fictitious vignette shows the difficulties faced by a psychiatry trainee treating a South Asian woman who was assessed in the accident and emergency department following an overdose of amitriptyline.

Vignette 3

A 20-year-old Indian woman was seen by the liaison psychiatrist in the intensive care unit after she had taken an overdose of her mother's amitriptyline tablets. She informed the assessing psychiatrist that her family had been planning to send her to India to marry her off, as they objected to her relationship with a fellow White student. She did not report any depressive symptoms prior to the overdose and did not have any ongoing suicidal ideas. The psychiatrist recommended discharge from hospital with a referral to the team psychologist for problem-solving therapy. Two weeks later, the psychiatrist received a letter from the psychologist saying that when she had called the home number she had been informed that the young woman was in India. The psychiatrist was left wondering whether she had totally ignored the cultural stressor and whether she could have done something different.

Culturally aware treatments in liaison psychiatry

There is a limited evidence base for psychological therapies in liaison psychiatry (Guthrie, 2006). However, one area in which the evidence is robust is cognitive–behavioural therapy (CBT) for medically unexplained symptoms and syndromes. It is also the recommended therapy for common mental disorders, such as anxiety and depression, that often affect medically ill patients (Pilling et al, 2009). Since most trials have been carried out in the West, with poor representation of patients from other cultures, there is scepticism about whether their results can be extrapolated to other contexts. Sumathipala et al (2000) found that psychiatrist-administered CBT for medically unexplained symptoms among out-patients in a clinic in Sri Lanka was efficacious. However, in a subsequent larger trial involving primary care physicians who had received a brief training in CBT, the intervention was no more efficacious than structured care (Sumathipala et al, 2008).

Drawing on 15 years of experience working with patients with medically unexplained symptoms in Sri Lanka, Sumathipala and colleagues produced a manual to help practitioners (Sumathipala et al, 2006). One of the most interesting aspects of their manual is that they describe the modifications they made to the standard technique. They emphasise the need to explain the treatment to patients using appropriate language and they give many examples of using culturally apt metaphors and analogies. For example, they use the 'Why an elephant is called an elephant' analogy to explain how medically unexplained symptoms are diagnosed on the basis of positive, inclusive features ('an elephant is an elephant because it has a trunk and tusks') rather than solely on that of negative, excluding factors ('because it is not a rat or a cat') such as normal investigations. This example and others throughout the manual show how treatments need to be adapted to the cultural context. Rather than dismiss patients from other cultures as 'not psychologically minded' it is incumbent on therapists to make adaptations.

Appropriate and safe use of psychopharmacology with medically ill patients is one of the core skills of a liaison psychiatrist. The field of ethnopharmacology deals with differences between different ethnic and racial groups in response to psychotropic medications (Ng & Klimidis, 2008). These differences are influenced by many biological and non-biological factors that may influence acceptance of psychotropic medications and adherence to them. Among the non-biological factors are psychological and sociocultural factors such as illness explanatory models and beliefs about treatments, personal meaning related to accepting psychiatric treatments, stigma of psychiatric illness and treatments, attitudes of the family and the community, and preference for traditional medicines.

In addition to an awareness of the psychosociocultural factors, the liaison psychiatrist also needs a good grounding in aspects of the absorption and metabolism of psychotropic medications and their pharmacodynamics. To give an example, there are wide variations in drug metabolism owing to genetic variations in the drug-metabolising enzymes (Chaudhury *et al*, 2008; Lambert & Norman, 2008). From the perspective of the psycho-pharmacologist the most important are the cytochrome P450 (CYP) group of enzymes, particularly CYP1, CYP2 and CYP3. The enzyme CYP2D6 is involved in the metabolism of many psychotropic medications. A larger proportion of patients of Asian or African ancestries are poor metabolisers with regard to CYP2D6 compared with those of Caucasian ancestry. As 'normal' doses are based on studies involving Caucasian participants, this may translate in clinical practice as lower required doses and an excess of adverse effects. Given the likelihood that many patients seen by liaison psychiatrists will be on other medications that also inhibit the metabolism of psychotropic medications, such adverse effects may be more marked. A more detailed discussion of ethnopsychopharmacology is beyond the scope of this chapter, and readers are advised to consult specialist books or journal articles such as Ng *et al* (2008) and Chaudhury *et al* (2008).

Culturally capable liaison psychiatry services

The principles of developing effective and equitable mental health services for multicultural societies has been described elsewhere (Minas, 2007). Like any other mental health service, psychiatric services in general hospitals need to be culturally capable. This needs to go beyond mandatory courses in cultural competence and increasing knowledge about different cultures, although they are undoubtedly important. Cultural capability also does not mean matching clinicians and patients according to ethnicity and cultural background or developing separate services for different cultural groups, although either of these may be relevant in some situations. What is needed is a structural change in the organisation of services so that cultural factors are given the same weight as others in assessment, and a willingness among practitioners to reflect on the cultural assumptions they bring to the clinical setting. At the level of service organisation, attention to issues of diversity would have to be central. Provision of ready access to interpreters and availability of information in different languages are essential. Quality indicators and outcome measures should include items relating to cultural needs in addition to clinical and psychosocial ones.

A culturally capable service, organised using the above principles, would adopt a stepped-care approach to issues of culture in a general hospital. A cultural formulation would be used to enrich the understanding of problems in all cases. In instances when cultural issues are found to be central either in precipitating a psychiatric disorder or in maintaining it, the liaison psychiatrist would have access to a cultural consultant – the cultural consultation model (Kirmayer *et al*, 2003). This may involve advice on further exploration of cultural issues or on managing the disorder. In the most complex cases, the cultural consultant would directly assess the patient and work closely with the liaison team in managing their illness.

References

Ahmed K., Mohan, R. & Bhugra, D. (2007) Self-harm in South Asian women: a literature review informed approach to assessment and formulation. *American Journal of Psychotherapy*, **61**, 71–81.

Beauchamp, T. L. & Childress, J. F. (2001) *Principles of Biomedical Ethics* (5th edn). Oxford University Press.

Bhugra, D., Desai, M. & Baldwin D. S. (1999*a*) Attempted suicide in West London. I. Rates across ethnic communities. *Psychological Medicine*, **29**, 1125–1130.

Bhugra D., Baldwin D. S., Desai, M., *et al* (1999*b*) Attempted suicide in West London. II. Inter-group comparisons. *Psychological Medicine*, **29**, 1131–1139.

Bhui, K., McKenzie, K. & Rasul, F. (2007) Rates, risk factors and methods of self-harm among minority ethnic groups in the UK: a systematic review. *BMC Public Health*, **7**, 336.

Chaturvedi, S. K. (2008) Ethical dilemmas in palliative care in traditional developing societies, with special reference to the Indian setting. *Journal of Medical Ethics*, **34**, 611–615.

Chaudhury, I. B., Neelam, K., Duddu, V., *et al* (2008) Ethnicity and psychopharmacology. *Journal of Psychopharmacology*, **22**, 673–680.

Cooper, J., Husain, N., Webb, R., *et al* (2006) Self-harm in the UK: differences between South Asians and Whites in rates, characteristics, provision of services and repetition. *Social Psychiatry and Psychiatric Epidemiology*, **41**, 782–788.

Daumit, G. L., Pronovost, P. J., Anthony, C. B., *et al* (2006) Adverse events during medical and surgical hospitalizations for persons with schizophrenia. *Archives of General Psychiatry*, **63**, 267–272.

Goldberg, D., Gask, L. & O'Dowd, T. (1989) The treatment of somatization: teaching of reattribution. *Journal of Psychosomatic Research*, **33**, 689–695.

Group for the Advancement of Psychiatry (2002) *Cultural Assessment in Clinical Psychiatry*. American Psychiatric Publishing.

Guthrie, E. (2006) Psychological treatments in liaison psychiatry: the evidence base. *Clinical Medicine*, **6**, 544–547.

Hawton, K., Fagg, J., Simkin, S., *et al* (1997) Trends in deliberate self-harm in Oxford, 1985–1995. Implications for clinical services and the prevention of suicide. *British Journal of Psychiatry*, **171**, 556–560.

Kirmayer L. J. (2007) Cultural psychiatry in historical perspective. In *Textbook of Cultural Psychiatry* (eds D. Bhugra & K. Bhui). Cambridge University Press.

Kirmayer L. J. & Sartorius, N. (2007) Cultural models and somatic syndromes. *Psychosomatic Medicine*, **69**, 832–840.

Kirmayer, L. J., Groleau, D., Guzder, J., *et al* (2003) Cultural consultation: a model of mental health service for multicultural societies. *Canadian Journal of Psychiatry*, **48**, 145–153.

Lambert, T. & Norman, T. R. (2008) Ethnic differences in psychotropic drug response and pharmacokinetics. In *Ethno-psychopharmacology: Advances in Current Practice* (eds C. H. Ng, K.-M. Lim, B. S. Singh, *et al*). Cambridge University Press.

Liggins, J. & Hatcher, S. (2005) Stigma towards the mentally ill in the general hospital: a qualitative study. *General Hospital Psychiatry*, **27**, 359–364.

Minas, H. (2007) Developing mental health services for multicultural societies. In *Textbook of Cultural Psychiatry* (eds D. Bhugra & K. Bhui). Cambridge University Press.

Mumford, D. B. (1989) Somatic sensations and psychological distress among students in Britain and Pakistan. *Social Psychiatry and Psychiatric Epidemiology*, **24**, 321–326.

Ng, C. H. & Klimidis, S. (2008) Cultural factors and the use of psychotropic medications. In *Ethno-psychopharmacology: Advances in Current Practice* (eds C. H. Ng, K.-M. Lim, B. S. Singh, et al). Cambridge University Press.

Ng, C. H., Lin, K.-M., Singh, B. S., *et al* (2008) *Ethno-psychopharmacology: Advances in Current Practice*. Cambridge University Press.

O'Keeffe, N. & Ranjith, G. (2007) Depression, demoralisation, or adjustment disorder? Understanding emotional distress in the severely medically ill. *Clinical Medicine*, **7**, 478–481.

Parker, G., Cheah, Y. C. & Roy, K. (2001) Do the Chinese somatize depression? A cross-cultural study. *Social Psychiatry and Psychiatric Epidemiology*, **36**, 287–293.

Pilling, S., Anderson, I., Goldberg, D., *et al* (2009) Depression in adults, including those with a chronic physical health problem: summary of NICE guidance. *BMJ*, **339**, 1025–1027.

Ranjith, G. & Hotopf, M. (2004) 'Refusing treatment – please see': an analysis of capacity assessments carried out by a liaison psychiatry service. *Journal of the Royal Society of Medicine*, **97**, 480–482.

Ranjith, G. & Mohan, R. (2006) Dhat syndrome as a functional somatic syndrome: identifying a sociosomatic model. *Psychiatry*, **69**, 142–150.

Smith, G. C. (1998) From consultation-liaison psychiatry to psychosocial advocacy; maintaining psychiatry's scope. *Australian and New Zealand Journal of Psychiatry*, **32**, 753–761.

Sumathipala, A., Hewege, S., Hawella, R., *et al* (2000) Randomized controlled trial for repeated consultations for medically unexplained complaints: a feasibility study in Sri Lanka. *Psychological Medicine*, **30**, 747–757.

Sumathipala, A., Siribaddana, S., Mangwana, S., *et al* (2006) *Management of Patients with Medically Unexplained Symptoms: A Practical Guide*. Battaramulla: Forum for Research and Development (http://www.irdsrilanka.org/Upload/book.pdf).

Sumathipala, A., Siribaddana, S., Abeyasingha, M. R. N., *et al* (2008) Cognitive–behavioural therapy v. structured care for medically unexplained symptoms: randomised controlled trial. *British Journal of Psychiatry*, **193**, 51–59.

Tseng, W.-S. (2001) *Handbook of Cultural Psychiatry*. Academic Press.

Wessely S., Nimnuan, C. & Sharpe, M. (1999) Functional somatic symptoms: one or many? *Lancet*, **354**, 936–939.

CHAPTER 14

Addiction in ethnic minorities

Bhaskar Punukollu, Zarrar A. Chowdary and Gideon Felton

Summary This chapter describes the challenges that drug and alcohol addiction services face when providing care for service users from Black and minority ethnic groups. Initially, little was known about the pattern of substance misuse within each ethnic minority, as Black and minority ethnic service users appear to be underrepresented in these services, resulting in a paucity of data. Underreporting of addictions among this group of patients may account for this underrepresentation, and reasons for a lower level of engagement with addiction services need to be explored. Over the past decade there have been more studies that demonstrate the extent of substance misuse within specific minority ethnic groups as well as some biological and social factors that influence this. Drug and alcohol treatment services now face the challenge of responding to this new information so that they can provide a more accessible and improved service for these individuals.

There has been increasing concern that current addiction services have not been effective in meeting the needs of patients from ethnic minorities. The Home Office Briefing *Delivering Drug Services to Black and Ethnic-Minority Communities* (Sangster *et al*, 2002) highlighted this problem, stating that existing services appear more equipped to cater for the needs of the White population, citing strong evidence that Black and minority ethnic groups are underrepresented in addiction services. These problems were also acknowledged by the National Treatment Agency for Substance Misuse (2002), an organisation set up by the government in 2001 to improve drug treatments in the UK. This agency, having identified diversity as a key objective, recognised that significant sections of the population seemed to be excluded from treatment.

Before 2001, few high-impact peer-reviewed publications addressed the relationship between ethnicity and illicit drug use. Notably, as recently as 1995, the government strategy document *Tackling Drugs Together* (Department of Health, 1995) made no mention of ethnicity at all. A review of drug treatment services in England published in the following year did discuss ethnicity, but it concluded that there was insufficient evidence to judge whether patients from Black and minority ethnic backgrounds find drug treatment agencies less accessible than the rest of the drug-using population (Task Force to Review Services for Drug Misusers, 1996).

In 1998, the government's ten-year strategy for tackling drug misuse reported evidence of reduced accessibility, noting that drug users from Black and minority ethnic groups viewed drug treatment services as 'run by White people for White people' (Department of Health, 1998). As a result of these findings, service commissioners were encouraged to consider issues such as cultural diversity in the delivery of addiction services.

The problem of under-utilisation of treatment agencies by drug users from ethnic minorities was reiterated in government's updated drug strategy in 2002, in which 'significant shortcomings in ... service provision for ethnic minority women' were described (Home Office, 2002). The need for training staff on equality and diversity and designing services to attract substance misusing clients from ethnic minorities was recognised.

The most recent drug strategy *Drugs: Protecting Families and Communities* (Home Office, 2008) also addresses the need to remove barriers to treatment for underrepresented groups, including ethnic minorities. However, to date it is not clear how effective drug services have been in addressing the needs of the Black and minority ethnic population and only a few comprehensive needs assessments have taken place.

To address identifiable shortcomings in service provision to drug users from ethnic minorities, it is important to develop further understanding in the following areas:

- prevalence and factors influencing drug and alcohol misuse in different ethnic groups
- patterns and types of drugs most commonly used by each ethnic group
- how drug and alcohol services can respond to the challenge of addressing substance misuse in ethnic minorities.

Prevalence of drug use in ethnic minorities

Data on the prevalence of drug misuse among ethnic minorities remains poor. There is a paucity of high-quality information to establish the extent and nature of substance misuse among different groups. The lack of research evidence may reflect a colour-blind attitude towards the subject. Available evidence does not adequately tell us whether substance misuse is lower in ethnic minorities compared with the majority population or simply underreported and not known to public agencies.

Black and Black British

Home Office surveys conducted in four major cities in the UK showed comparable rates of self-reported drug use among White and African–Caribbean respondents (Leitner *et al*, 1993). The 1992 British Crime Survey showed identical levels of drug use among 16- to 29-year-old White and African–Caribbean people (30%) (Home Office, 1993). The 1996 survey, however, showed inconclusive results, with the proportion of respondents

183

among Black and other ethnic minorities being too small to draw any meaningful conclusions about the prevalence of substance misuse in the group (Home Office, 1998). Individuals from Black and minority ethnic groups usually present to services at a late stage of drug use, so it is difficult to estimate the number of people from these groups using substances but not accessing services (Sangster et al, 2002).

Asian and Asian British

There have been difficulties in accurately estimating the prevalence of drug use within Asian populations. Evidence suggests that the observed lower levels of substance misuse may be influenced by underreporting and under-diagnosing of such problems in this ethnic group, and that heroin and crack misuse is in fact on the rise in this population (Fountain et al, 2003).

In the 1992 British Crime Survey, Asians were found to have a lower rate of lifetime drug use (10%) than any other ethnic group (Home Office, 1993). However, Gilman (1993) highlighted the need to increase awareness of changing patterns of drug use among Asians, especially women. A 1966 survey of substance misuse among 15- to 25-year-old Asian women in Bradford, in the north of England, found that nearly half of respondents had used an illicit substance at sometime in their lives but it could not draw reliable conclusions on the current prevalence of such use (Bridge Project, 1996). Bentley & Hanton (1997) discovered high levels of drug use among young Asians interviewed in Nottingham, another northern English city. An analysis of a regional drug misuse database in Anglia and Oxford (Sheikh et al, 2001) found that 30% of new presentations to drug treatment services were from Black and minority ethnic groups, with a significant number of Asians enrolled in services.

The problem of the growing use of illicit substances among Asians was highlighted by White (2001), who found that heroin misuse among Bangladeshi men living in London had increased from negligible levels in the early 1990s to levels proportionally higher than those for equivalent White populations. However, despite further studies describing increasing drug use among Chinese and South Asian populations, the prevalence of problem drug use in this group is still reported to be lower than in the general population (Ross et al, 2004).

Among Asian heroin users attending a substance misuse service in north London, heroin and crack cocaine were usually ingested by smoking; none had a history of injecting. Among the White heroin users, however, almost all clients injected the drug and they were also more likely to have used other drugs in the past (Fernandez, 2004). A higher proportion of Asian clients relapsed soon after detoxification compared with White clients. Asians were more likely to see drug treatment from a medical perspective, hoping that detoxification would provide the solution for their dependence. They had less focus on psychosocial aspects of treatment and their desire for an early detoxification was influenced strongly by their family.

White minority ethnic groups

Kalunta-Crumpton (2003) described forms of social exclusion that compound problem drug use in Portuguese and Italian communities living in the UK. People from White minority ethnic groups may be as disadvantaged as those from Black and Asian groups. At present there is little research on substance misuse in White immigrants to the UK and more needs to be done in this area.

Ethnic minorities in prisons

There is evidence that substance misuse and dependence are prevalent among male prisoners from minority ethnic groups. Compared with the White British prison population, among whom the drug of choice was heroin, crack cocaine was the most common drug used by a small sample of male prisoners from minority ethnic groups (80% were Black and 20% Asian/mixed race) interviewed in 2001: 85% reported using it in the year before prison, 65% of whom were dependent on it (Home Office, 2003). Only 35% had used heroin during that period. There was a high comorbidity of crack and alcohol misuse in this group.

Prisoners from minority ethnic groups tend not to present to prison detoxification or rehabilitation services, which may be partly explained by a lack of minority ethnic staff and/or a perceived or actual lack of cultural understanding in prison services. Treatment programmes for crack cocaine should be a focus for minority ethnic men, paying particular attention to the relationship between crack cocaine and alcohol use. The development of culturally sensitive anxiety management strategies in prison and on release will be important for this group (Home Office, 2003).

Factors influencing addiction in minority ethnic communities

People's perception of existing drug treatment services

There is evidence to indicate that ethnic minorities have perceived services as being for the majority White population only (Awiah et al, 1990, 1992). As mentioned above, this has been acknowledged in the government's 1998 drug strategy (Department of Health, 1998).

Considerable stigma surrounds alcohol misuse in minority ethnic groups. This is particularly so for Asian communities in the UK, where people from an older generation are unwilling to recognise alcohol misuse within their communities. Younger generations may share this view and perceive their actions as reflecting the behaviour of the whole family. As a result people with alcohol problems may try to cope on their own rather than use local alcohol services (of which they may even be unaware). A different set of influences may operate in Irish immigrant communities, where perceived negative stereotyping by health professionals might explain the low rates of primary care consultation for alcohol-related problems (Rao, 2006).

Norms and attitudes

Patterns of alcohol and drug use can be influenced by an ethnic group's norms and attitudes. The norms refer to how one should behave in relation to alcohol and drugs – for example, how much alcohol it is appropriate for a parent to drink in the presence of small children, for a man at a bar with friends, or for someone at a party at another person's home. The attitudes refer to general beliefs about drinking and drugs, such as whether drinkers have more friends, whether a party is not really a party unless alcoholic beverages are served, and whether 'getting drunk' occasionally is acceptable (Caetano & Clark, 1999).

People belonging to minority ethnic groups in England have less knowledge about the harmful effects of smoking on their health (Health Development Agency, 2000). The proportions of African–Caribbean, Bangladeshi and Pakistani men who say that their smoking has 'no effect' on their current health are 12%, 22% and 20% respectively, and all of these are above the general population. Religion may have an influence on attitudes to smoking in some ethnic groups: some religious leaders view sale of tobacco and smoking as prohibited by Islam (Khayat, 2000).

Acculturation

In addition to an ethnic group's norms and attitudes, the degree of its acculturation to the broader society may also play a role in determining drug misuse among its members. Acculturation is the extent to which minority ethnic groups adopt the culture of the country to which they have moved. In a study conducted in the USA, Japanese Americans reported drinking patterns that were closer to those of Whites than to those of Japanese living in Japan (Higuchi et al, 1994). The association between acculturation and drinking patterns has been seen among other minority ethnic groups in the USA. For example, using an assessment of acculturation based on 12 survey items (measuring areas such as the daily use of and ability to speak, read and write English; a preference for media in English; the ethnicity of the people with whom one interacts; and values thought to be characteristic of the way of life of the group), Caetano (1987) revealed that Hispanics who had acculturated to life in the USA had adopted US patterns of drinking.

Acculturation to drinking patterns may not be the same across different ethnic groups or even for all subcategories of nationalities within the same ethnic group (e.g. there may be differences between Bangladeshi, Pakistani and Indian communities among Asians/British Asians). One factor that contributes to how the association between acculturation and drinking patterns develops for a particular ethnic group or subgroup is the drinking patterns of that group's country of origin. Many factors influence the role that acculturation plays in the development of drinking patterns among minority ethnic groups (Caetano, 1987). Research needs to be done to examine the effect of acculturation on drug use in minority ethnic groups in the UK population.

Social class, poverty and unemployment

Alcohol misuse and ethnicity are both independently associated with social disadvantage. In the UK, the clustering of first-generation Irish people in areas of socioeconomic deprivation may explain their higher prevalence of alcohol use (Acheson, 1998). A similar observation has been noted in Mexican Indians in the USA, who have higher rates of alcohol dependence and misuse than other Mexicans in the country, but these differences disappear when adjustment is made for socioeconomic factors (Alderete *et al*, 2000).

Genetic influences

There are lower rates of alcohol misuse and dependence among people of East Asian origin in the USA than in any other ethnic group. This may be related to a genetic variation that exists in this population (Makimoto, 1998). People of Chinese, Korean and Vietnamese background are more likely to have a variant of the aldehyde dehydrogenase gene (*ALDH2*). If a person with the *ALDH2* allele drinks alcohol they experience headaches, facial flushing, dizziness, nausea and palpitations. The presence of this allele may mean that people of East Asian background are less likely to drink alcohol and therefore have a lower prevalence of alcohol dependence compared with other ethnic groups. This allele may therefore provide East Asians some protection against heavy drinking and alcohol dependence (Yin *et al*, 1988; Makimoto, 1998). However, the prevalence of the *ALDH2* allele varies among Asian groups. In a study of college students in the USA, 48% of participants of Chinese background had this allele, compared with 35% of those of Korean background (Luczak *et al*, 2001). The Chinese students also had a lower rate of binge drinking (7%) compared with the Korean students (30%). An increase in triplet repeat of the *CNR1* gene in African–Caribbean men was found to be associated with cocaine dependence with or without schizophrenia in one study (Ballon *et al*, 2006). It is possible that other gene loci are implicated in differences in drug use between ethnic groups, but more research in this area is needed to verify this.

Patterns of addiction among ethnic groups

Alcohol

In the UK population, a number of ethnic groups have higher levels of alcohol use than the general population (Rao, 2006). Thirty-four per cent of Irish men drink above the weekly recommended limit of 21 units of alcohol, compared with 29% of the general Irish population and 27% of the general British population (Department of Health, 2001). Among South Asian Sikh male immigrants to the UK, problem drinking is higher than in the Sikh population in South Asia and similar to that of the UK general population (Cochrane & Bal, 1990). Irish and Sikh groups in the UK also have higher rates of alcohol-related morbidity and mortality than the general population (Douds *et al*, 2003). In the USA, similar patterns have been observed in Hispanic men, among whom the prevalence of alcohol misuse has remained static while it has fallen among White (non-Irish) men (Galvan & Caetano, 2003).

Cannabis

According to the British Crime Survey 2001/02, cannabis is the most commonly used drug in all ethnic groups (Austin & Smith, 2003). The survey reports that although there are no differences in lifetime rates of cannabis use between people of White and African–Caribbean origin, cannabis use in the previous year was reported more often by African–Caribbean people than Whites. Important generational differences were pointed out in the report; people in the 36–59 years age group from a Black ethnic background were more likely to have used cannabis than White British, but this difference was absent in the 16–24 and 25–35 years groups. Rodham *et al* (2005) reported that cannabis use among Black (49.3%) and Other (44.3%) males was significantly higher than in the White group (33.5%). There were also gender differences, as Black females had a slightly higher use of cannabis than White females whereas Asian females reported a much lower use. Jayakody *et al* (2006) reported that lifetime cannabis use was significantly higher among Black Caribbean and mixed ethnicity young people, but was lower among Bangladeshi, Indian and Pakistani adolescents.

Crack cocaine

Sangster *et al* (2002) reported that Black Caribbean people are more likely than other ethnic groups to present to UK drug services for crack cocaine use. Cocaine was reported as the main drug of use among Black Caribbean drug users, who used reported higher use than people of South Asian or White British background (Daniel, 1993; Perera *et al*, 1993). Sheikh *et al* (2001) reported evidence of crack cocaine use among young Bangladeshis and Kashmiris in the UK.

Heroin

Heroin is the drug of choice among South Asians, particularly Pakistanis and Bangladeshis, in England and is often the first drug used by this group (Gilman, 1993; Perera, 1996, 1998; Chaudry *et al*, 1997; Patel *et al*, 2001; Sheikh *et al*, 2001). This is in contrast to the prison population described earlier, in which it appears that Asian prisoners had higher levels of crack cocaine than heroin use (Home Office, 2003). Heroin use has also been reported among people of Chinese, Iranian and Vietnamese origin (Patel *et al*, 1998). The 'holiday habit' among Pakistanis is the one way in which the Asian heroin experience differs from that of the wider community: young men become dependent on heroin after using the drug while visiting Pakistan. Several young Asians interviewed in Bradford said that they had friends whose heroin habits had started in this way (Butt, 1992: p. 17).

The Black and minority ethnic population is under-represented in data for injected heroin use, as fewer users from Black and minority ethnic groups present to needle exchange programmes compared with White British users (Sangster *et al*, 2002). However, a survey of drug users known to a number of agencies in south London indicated that Black heroin users (largely of African–Caribbean descent) were much less likely to inject than their White counterparts (Mirza *et al*, 1991). Although South Asian users seem to prefer to smoke opiates, injecting does occur in these communities (Siddique, 1992; Sangster *et al*, 2002). Participation in needle exchange programmes is low among South Asian drug injectors, but they are known to access injecting equipment though White British friends or partners (Patel *et al*, 1998; Sheikh *et al*, 2001). Dangerous injecting practices have been recorded among South Asian female street workers (Hall, 1999).

Khat

Khat use is largely confined to minority ethnic communities in England, notably the Somali and Yemeni population (Kennedy *et al*, 1983). The vast majority who use khat do so by chewing; a small number ingest it by making a drink from dried leaves and even fewer smoke dried leaves. Possession and use of khat is not illegal in the UK, although its active ingredients cathinone and cathine are class C drugs. Khat has stimulant properties and it is used to enhance performance and alertness (Kalix, 1984). There is a belief among Yemeni users that khat is beneficial for minor ailments such as headaches and colds, and also for depression (Kennedy *et al*, 1983). A survey among Somalis living in England revealed that two-thirds of both males and females had used khat at some time and 6% were still using it (Griffith, 1998). For Somali men, khat houses have been described as equivalent to pubs for British men (Nabuzoka & Badhade, 2000).

Cigarettes and tobacco

Among men from minority ethnic groups in England, smoking rates are particularly high in Bangladeshi (40%), Irish (30%) and Pakistani (29%) populations (compared with the national average for men of 24%). Among women, rates are low (at 8% or below), except in Black (24%) and Irish (26%) groups, compared with the national average for women of 20% (Action on Smoking and Health, 2006; Department of Health, 2006). By 2007, the number of smokers (men and women combined) in the general population had fallen to 21% (Office for National Statistics, 2009), but 2007 data on smoking among ethnic minorities are not available.

Chewing tobacco is used by some minority ethnic groups, especially people of South Asian origin. Tobacco chewing is most common among Bangladeshis, with 9% of men and 16% of women reporting use (Department of Health, 2006). This is a reduction from 1999 levels, when 19% of men and 26% of women from the Bangladeshi community reported tobacco chewing (Department of Health, 2006). There may be underreporting of tobacco use in this group, however.

Smoking in the home in the UK is as common in Black Caribbean, Indian, Pakistani and Bangladeshi households as in the general population. Children from minority ethnic groups may be attracted by the marketing of gutka (a combination of betel leaf, areca nut, slaked lime and tobacco), which is sold in brightly coloured foil parcels and is subject to no marketing regulations. They may also be at risk of smoking bidis (a thin, often flavoured cigarette made of tobacco wrapped in a tendu leaf), which are cheaper and more easily available than ordinary cigarettes (Action on Smoking and Health, 2006). Individuals from minority ethnic groups have a higher risk of diabetes and heart disease than the general UK population. For example, in 1999, Bangladeshi men and women living in England were nearly six times more likely (after standardising for age) than the general population to report having diabetes. Risk ratios among Pakistani men and women were almost as high as those for the Bangladeshi group. Indian men and women were almost three times as likely as the general population to report having diabetes (National Statistics, 2002). Thus, increasing people's awareness of the effects of smoking on these diseases could reduce morbidity associated with these conditions, with consequent cost savings for health services.

'Club drugs'

There is high usage of ecstasy and LSD (lysergic acid diethylamide) among young people attending night-time Bhangra scenes in England. The clientele are mostly Asian, although increasing numbers of young people of African–Caribbean origin are joining them (Patel et al, 1998; Perera, 1998). There is also evidence of heroin use within this group. The alcoholic drinks consumed are similar to those generally preferred by young people in Britain today: 'designer' beers and ciders with a high alcohol content (Patel & Pearson, 2007). In African–Caribbean communities, ecstasy and LSD use is limited: in the northern city of Bradford these substances, together with cocaine, were considered 'drugs for White people' (Gilman, 1993).

Behavioural addiction

'Behavioural addiction' encompasses a range of addictive behaviours, including problem and pathological gambling, compulsive buying, hyper-sexuality, compulsive overeating, excessive exercise, and technological addictions, for example to video games or the internet. Pathological gambling has been well researched, whereas the other area behaviours are emerging areas of research in addiction psychiatry. In a report prepared for the Responsibility in Gambling Trust, Abbott *et al* (2004) predict that the expansion of the gambling industry in the UK with the more liberal gambling laws might be expected to disproportionately affect young people, women and ethnic and new immigrant minorities. They note that funding will be needed for culturally appropriate treatment services to help problem gamblers from ethnic minorities and that it would be beneficial to provide information in various languages. The report recommends that counsellors working in agencies involved with ethnic minorities be trained in diagnosis and appropriate referral pathways for problem gamblers among their clients.

How can services address addiction in ethnic minorities?

Overcoming barriers to uptake of services

Fountain *et al* (2003) commented that commissioners of drug services may be reluctant to develop specific services for people from ethnic minorities owing to a fear of appearing racist by placing particular emphasis on the needs of service users from minority ethnic groups. However, there is no evidence to indicate that this observation is valid. The Race Relations Amendment Act (2000) places a requirement on all public bodies to promote racial equality, and the Commission for Racial Equality has produced codes of practice on the implementation of quality frameworks. In particular, the Act attempts to address institutional racism, which has been defined by Sir William Macpherson as: 'the collective failure of an organisation to provide an appropriate and professional service to people because of their colour, culture, or ethnic origin. It can be seen or detected in processes, attitudes and behaviour which amount to discrimination through unwitting prejudice, ignorance, thoughtlessness and racist stereotyping which disadvantage minority ethnic people' (Macpherson, 1999: p. 9).

In its *Models of Care for the Treatment of Drug Misusers*, the National Treatment Agency for Substance Misuse set out a common framework for the commissioning and delivery of drug services in England (National Treatment Agency for Substance Misuse, 2002). The document highlights the fact that women from Black and minority ethnic groups may miss out on harm minimisation interventions as a result of late entry to treatment. One of the most significant recommendations of Models of Care is that drug and alcohol action teams (DAATs) and local drug agencies give detailed consideration to ethnic and racial equality, and that commissioning be 'needs led' according to the requirements of the local community.

Community involvement is essential in the planning of services, and service user feedback is necessary for continuing improvement of existing services. Community engagement and outreach work can help in improving contact between drug services and ethnic minorities. Providing education on drug misuse and dependence and advertising drug services through Asian and African–Caribbean radio stations, newspapers and local organisations would be helpful in increasing uptake of treatment by people from these groups. Recruiting ethnically diverse staff who have knowledge of the locality and who can speak the language of the local population would encourage uptake as well. Liaison with local counselling and voluntary support agencies and use of interpreters during meetings with substance misusers from minority ethnic groups might also be beneficial. Further information on voluntary organisations in the UK that support people from ethnic minorities who have drug or alcohol problems and provide materials in minority languages is available from the charity DrugScope.

Responding to the challenges that lie ahead

Both generic general adult psychiatric services and specialised addiction services face many of the same challenges in terms of effective, culturally sensitive service delivery to patients from ethnic minorities. Historically, the cultural needs of these patients were overlooked for a considerable length of time before a problem was even identified. The potential suffering caused by 'culturally insensitive' service provision has resulted in hostility towards services among some of these patients. Service providers have often been slow to react in the face of this hostility and the need for change has been driven by external factors.

In the past 10 years, efforts have been made to identify the needs of minority ethnic patients. Despite procedural difficulties of accurate data collection and analysis in this field, progress has been made, particularly in generic psychiatric services. This improvement is manifested by the development of both statutory and voluntary organisations in the UK (DrugScope, 2006) with specialised knowledge of problems specific to particular ethnic groups. These ancillary organisations often work in partnership with the National Health Service addiction services.

Another driver of change is the increasing involvement of patients in decisions regarding service delivery. Like other healthcare services, addiction services have to work more closely with their patients than previously. Clinicians are now actively encouraged to participate in service user forums, which may increase their awareness of cultural sensitivity, particularly if they practice in an area with a high density of patients from minority ethnic backgrounds.

Both measures run the risk of producing geographical variations in quality of care. Ancillary organisations are more likely to be established in areas with a higher density of patients from minority ethnic groups. Consequently, patients in these areas may have more resources than patients from less ethnically diverse areas and may therefore have better outcomes.

The increasing accountability of the National Health Service has brought with it some improvements for patients from minority ethnic backgrounds. More importantly, it has generated constructive debate.

References

Abbott, M. W., Volberg, R. A., Bellringer, M., *et al* (2004) *A Review of Research on Aspects of Problem Gambling*. Responsibility in Gambling Trust.

Acheson, D. (1998) *Report of the Independent Inquiry into Inequalities in Health*. TSO (The Stationery Office).

Action on Smoking and Health (2006) *Tobacco and Ethnic Minorities (Essential Information 26)*. ASH.

Alderete, E., Vega, W. A., Kolody, B., *et al* (2000) Effects of time in the United States and Indian ethnicity on DSM–III–R psychiatric disorders among Mexican Americans in California. *Journal of Nervous and Mental Disease*, **188**, 90–100.

Austin, R. & Smith, N. (2003) *Ethnicity and drug use: key findings from the 2001/2002 British Crime Survey (Home Office Research Findings No. 209)*. Home Office.

Awiah, J., Butt, S. & Dorn, N. (1990) The last place I would go: Black people and drug services in Britain. *Druglink*, **5** (5), 14–15.

Awiah, J., Butt, S. & Dorn, N. (1992) *Race, Gender and Drug Services (ISDD Research Monograph 6)*. Institute for the Study of Drug Dependence.

Ballon, N., Leroy, S., Roy, C., *et al* (2006) (AAT)n repeat in the cannabinoid receptor gene (CNR1): association with cocaine addiction in an African–Caribbean population. *Pharmacogenomics Journal*, **6** (2), 126–130.

Bentley, C. & Hanton, A. (1997) *A Study to Investigate the Extent to Which There is a Drug Problem among Young Asian People in Nottingham. How Effective are Drug Services in Providing Assistance for Such Minority Ethnic Groups?* Nottingham ADAPT.

Bridge Project (1996) *A Report of a Survey of Asian Women Aged 14–25*. Bridge.

Butt, S. (1992) Asian males and access to drug services in Bradford. In *Race, Gender and Drug Services (ISDD Research Monograph 6)* (eds J. Awiah, S. Butt & N. Dorn), Institute for the Study of Drug Dependence.

Caetano, R. (1987) Acculturation and drinking patterns among U.S. Hispanics. *British Journal of Addiction*, **82**, 789–799.

Caetano, R. & Clark, D. (1999) Trends in situational norms and attitudes toward drinking among whites, blacks, and Hispanics: 1984–1995. *Drug and Alcohol Dependence*, **54**, 45–56.

Chaudry, M. A., Sherlock, K. & Patel, K. (1997) *Drugs and Ethnics Health Project: Oldham and Tameside 1997. A Report to North Pennine DAT*. Manchester Lifeline/University of Central Lancashire.

Cochrane, R. & Bal, S. (1990) The drinking habits of Hindu, Muslim and white men in the West Midlands: a community survey. *British Journal of Addiction*, **85**, 759–769.

Daniel, T. (1993) Ethnic minorities' use of drug services. *Druglink*, **8** (1), 16–17.

Department of Health (1995) *Tackling Drugs Together: A Strategy for England 1995–1998*. TSO (The Stationery Office).

Department of Health (1998) *Tackling Drugs to Build a Better Britain: The Government's Ten-Year Strategy for Tackling Drugs Misuse*. TSO (The Stationery Office).

Department of Health (2001) *Health Survey for England: The Health of Minority Ethnic Groups '99*. Department of Health.

Department of Health (2006) *Health Survey for England 2004: The Health of Minority Ethnic Groups*. The Information Centre.

Douds, A. C., Cox, M. A., Iqbal, T. H., *et al* (2003) Ethnic differences in cirrhosis of the liver in a British city: alcoholic cirrhosis in South Asian men. *Alcohol and Alcoholism*, **38**, 148–150.

DrugScope (2006) *Black and Minority Ethnic Groups (Pathfinders series no.7)*. DrugScope (http://www.drugscope.org.uk/Resources/Drugscope/Documents/PDF/Info/pathethnic.pdf).

Fernandez, J. (2004) Cultural considerations – improving community involvement. *Substance Misuse Management in General Practice*, Network No. 9, September.

Fountain, J., Bashford, J., Winters, M., et al (2003) *Black and Minority Ethnic Communities in England: A Review of the Literature on Drug Use and Related Service Provision*. National Treatment Agency for Substance Misuse.

Galvan, F. H. & Caetano, R. (2003) *Alcohol Use and Related Problems among Ethnic Minorities in the United States*. National Institute on Alcohol Abuse and Alcoholism.

Gilman, M. (1993) *An Overview of the Main Findings and Implications of Seven Action Studies into the Nature of Drug Use in Bradford*. Bradford Drugs Prevention Team.

Griffith, P. (1998) *Qat Use in London: A Study of Khat Use among a Sample of Somalis Living in London (Home Office Paper 26)*. TSO (The Stationery Office).

Hall, C. (1999) *Drug use and HIV infection in South Asian and Middle Eastern Communities in the UK: A Literature Review*. Naz Project London.

Health Development Agency (2000) *Tobacco and England's Ethnic Minorities: A Research Report*. Health Development Agency.

Higuchi, S. (1994) Relationship between age and drinking patterns and drinking problems among Japanese, Japanese-Americans, and Caucasians. *Alcoholism, Clinical and Experimental Research*, **18**, 305–310.

Home Office (1993) *British Crime Survey, 1992*. TSO (The Stationery Office).

Home Office (1998) *British Crime Survey, 1996*. TSO (The Stationery Office).

Home Office (2002) *Updated Drugs Strategy 2002*. TSO (The Stationery Office).

Home Office (2003) *The Substance Misuse Treatment Needs of Minority Prisoner Groups: Women, Young Offenders and Ethnic Minorities (Home Office Development and Practice Report 8)*. TSO (The Stationery Office).

Home Office (2008) *Drugs: Protecting Families and Communities. The 2008 Drug Strategy*. TSO (The Stationery Office).

Jayakody, A. A., Viner, R. M. & Haines, M. M. (2006) Illicit and traditional drug use among ethnic minority adolescents in East London. *Public Health*, **120**, 329–338.

Kalix, P. (1984) The pharmacology of khat. *General Pharmacology*, **15**, 179–187.

Kalunta-Crumpton, A. (2003) Problematic drug use among 'invisible' ethnic minorities. *Journal of Substance Use*, **8**, 170–175.

Kennedy, J. G., Teague, J. & Rokaw, W. (1983) A medical evaluation of use of qat in North Yemen. *Social Science and Medicine*, **17**, 783–793.

Khayat, M. H. (2000) *Islamic Ruling on Smoking*. World Health Organization, Regional Office for Eastern Mediterranean.

Leitner, M., Shapland, J. & Wiles, P. (1993) *Drug Usage and Drugs Prevention: The Views and Habits of the General Public*. TSO (The Stationery Office).

Luczak, S. E., Wall, T. L., Shea, S. H., et al (2001) Binge drinking in Chinese, Korean, and White college students: genetic and ethnic group differences. *Psychology of Addictive Behaviors*, **15**, 306–309.

Macpherson, W. (1999) *The Stephen Lawrence Inquiry. Report of an Inquiry by Sir William Macpherson of Cluny*. TSO (The Stationery Office).

Makimoto, K. (1998) Drinking patterns and drinking problems among Asian Americans and Pacific Islanders. *Alcohol Health and Research World*, **22**, 270–275.

Mirza, H. S., Pearson, G. & Phillips, S. (1991) *Drugs, People and Services in Lewisham: Final Report of the Drug Information Project*. Goldsmiths College, University of London.

Nabuzoka, D. & Badhade, F. A. (2000) Use and perception of Khat among young Somalis in a UK city. *Addiction Research*, **8**, 5–26.

National Statistics (2002) News Release: minority ethnic groups in the UK. National Statistics (http://www.statistics.gov.uk/pdfdir/meg1202.pdf).

National Treatment Agency for Substance Misuse (2002) *Models of Care for the Treatment of Drug Misusers: Promoting Quality, Efficiency and Effectiveness in Drug Misuse Treatment Services in England. Part 2: Full Reference Report*. National Treatment Agency for Substance Misuse.

Office for National Statistics (2009) Smoking: smoking habits in Great Britain. ONS (http://www.statistics.gov.uk/cci/nugget.asp?id=313).

Patel, K. & Pearson, G. (2007) *Outreach among Asian Drug Injectors in Bradford. A Report Prepared for the Home Office and the Mental Health Foundation*. Bridge Project & Goldsmiths College, University of London.

Patel, K., Sherlock, K., Chaudry, M., *et al* (1998) *Drug Use among Asian Communities in Cheetham Hill*. Manchester Lifeline & University of Central Lancashire.

Patel, K., Wardle, J., Bashford, J., *et al* (2001) *The Evaluation of Nafas: A Bangladeshi Drug Service*. Ethnicity and Health Unit, University of Central Lancashire.

Perera, J. (1996) *Drug Misuse in Bedfordshire: Preliminary Report to Inform Further Assessment Research. Report to Public Health Specialist and DAT Coordinator*. Action Research Consultancies.

Perera, J. (1998) *Assessing the Drug Information Needs of Asian Parents in North Hertfordshire: A Brief Report to Inform the Planning of a Drugs Education Programme*. Action Research Consultancies.

Perera, J., Power, R. & Gibson, N. (1993) *Assessing the Needs of Black Drug Users in North Westminster*. Hungerford Drug Project & Centre for Research on Drugs and Health Behaviour.

Rao, R. (2006) Alcohol misuse and ethnicity. *BMJ*, **332**, 682.

Rodham, K., Hawton, K., Evans, E., *et al* (2005) Ethnic and gender differences in drinking, smoking and drug taking among adolescents in England: a self-report school-based survey of 15 and 16 year olds. *Journal of Adolescence*, **28**, 63–73.

Ross, A. J., Heim, D., Bakshi, N., *et al* (2004) Drug issues affecting Chinese, Indian and Pakistani people living in Greater Glasgow. *Drugs: Education, Prevention and Policy*, **11**, 49–65.

Sangster, D., Shiner, M., Patel, K., *et al* (2002) *Delivering Drug Services to Black and Minority-Ethnic Communities (DPAS Briefing P16)*. Home Office Drug Prevention and Advisory Service.

Sheikh, N., Fountain, J., Bashford, J., *et al* (2001) *A review of current drug service provision for Black and minority ethnic communities in Bedfordshire. Final report to Bedfordshire Drug Action Team, August 2001*. Centre for Ethnicity and Health, University of Lancashire.

Siddique, M. (1992) *Action Studies on the Misuse of Drugs in Manningham, Bradford*. Bradford Drug Prevention Team.

Task Force to Review Services for Drug Misusers (1996) *Report of an Independent Review of Drug Treatment Services in England*. TSO (The Stationery Office).

White, R. (2001) Heroin use, ethnicity and the environment: the case of the London Bangladeshi community. *Addiction*, **96**, 1815–1824.

Yin, S.J., Cheng, T. C., Chang, C. P., *et al* (1988) Human stomach alcohol and aldehyde dehydrogenases (ALDH): a genetic model proposed for ALDH III isozymes. *Biochemical Genetics*, **26**, 343–360.

CHAPTER 15

Sex and culture

Sheraz Ahmad and Dinesh Bhugra

Summary   Culture has a profound influence over sex, relationships and sexuality. This chapter highlights similarities and differences in sexual behaviour, sexual dysfunction and attitudes across cultures. Themes include how 'sex-positive' or 'sex-negative' a culture is, epidemiology of sexual dysfunction and sexual diversity. Clinical approaches to management of sexual problems are offered, with an emphasis on tailoring to the needs of individuals and couples. Observations are set in the context of increasing globalisation and an appreciation of levels of acculturation in people who present with sexual dysfunction and relationship difficulties.

To any practising clinician it will be apparent that taking into account an individual's cultural identity is an important aspect of assessment. It allows a mutual understanding of cultural factors that may be causing or contributing to the patient's problem and that can be used in planning and delivering appropriate and acceptable treatment. This is even more important in the arena of sexuality and psychosexual therapy, where cultures dictate models of explanation and help-seeking. Sexual expectations, practices and preferences are strongly shaped by culture, as well as by gender, class and ethnicity (Mahay et al, 2000). In our increasingly multicultural and globalised society, understanding the way in which our sexuality and relationships with one another develop is vital for the clinician.

Sex is one of the basic human instincts: over the centuries its function has vacillated between procreation and pleasure, and societies have fluctuated between sex-positive and sex-negative cultures. Sex and sexual behaviour have been viewed in different tones and shades, perhaps with fear or respect or as magico-religious experiences. Although historical data may be inaccurate (Bullough, 1972), it seems that attitudes to sex and sexual behaviour fluctuate and are strongly influenced by prevalent social norms (Gregersen, 1986; Segall et al, 1986). Inevitably, religion, state control and economic factors have at different times also profoundly shaped the way sex, sexuality and sexual practices are seen in a given culture.

Sexual function across cultures

Early literature was based on religious texts, which are a rich source of information on sexual behaviour (Bhugra & De Silva, 1995). The assumptions they contain about sex and its purpose have been greatly influential (Bullough, 1976); reinforced by centuries of religious observation, some remain deeply ingrained in many cultures.

Male and female patterns of sexual behaviour and sexual orientation are socially learnt alongside genetic encoding. Heterosexual coitus is the most prevalent sexual behaviour for the majority of individuals in any given society, although society defines what is 'deviant' and what is 'normal' (Ford & Beach, 1951; Segall *et al*, 1986; Bhugra, 1997). It has been suggested that societies accept or tolerate non-heterosexual behaviour at times when they have a sufficiently stabilised population and perhaps do not face a threat of annihilation (Bullough, 1972).

In most societies, a patriarchal structure ensures that males possess the greater power, via control of social institutions, thereby shaping gender roles in ways that accord themselves greater sexual privilege (Reiss, 1986). With feminism came the most significant sea change in this imbalance, particularly in the West; although few would argue that there is 'equality', feminism has had a profound effect on sex and sexuality. It led the way for increasing openness about sexual abuse, sexual assault and domestic abuse, altering the way marriages and relationships are perceived. This process also made it possible for society to have more open discussion of homosexuality, transsexualism and sexual preference.

Sex-positive and sex-negative cultures

Cultures may be described as being sex-positive or sex-negative (Bullough, 1976). It has been argued persuasively that sex-positive cultures consider sex to be life-affirming and pleasurable, whereas sex-negative cultures view the sexual act as purely procreative. The pleasure involved is strongly influenced by gender roles and in some sex-positive cultures sexual pleasure is meant to be experienced only by males. This in turn dictates how the society defines and understands it.

A commonly cited example is ancient India, with its erotic literature and sex manuals. Describing at great length various sexual acts and sex aids for pleasure these indicate a culture less fearful and more approving of sex than contemporary Western counterparts (Bullough, 1976). There is evidence of this in other ancient cultures – the early Greeks and Romans also wrote sex manuals (King, 1994).

Early Christians and Christianity influenced attitudes towards sex in the West and the Church still continues to do so. It can be hypothesised that this may have reflected the need for the newly formed 'Christian tribe' to survive and thrive in its infancy. Subjugation of the body along with the

197

potential to attain perfection through renunciation may have contributed to negative attitudes towards sex. Early Christianity saw justification of sexual intercourse only between a male and female in marriage and for procreation. Celibacy was the highest good and goal; sex was simply animal lust allowed within specific boundaries. Most Christian cultures, and particularly Irish (Roman) Catholicism, have viewed marriage as 'permission to sin' (McGoldrick *et al*, 2005). It has been suggested that Islamic cultures, on the other hand, are sex-positive (Al-Sawaf & Al-Issa, 2000), seeing sex as a necessary and healthy part of marriage. This attitude to sex is also held in Jewish culture. For Jews, the element of obligation is prominent and denial of sex by either partner is considered grounds for annulment of a marriage (Blech, 2003; Ribner & Rosenbaum, 2005).

The celebration of sex as sacred and positive in Eastern cultures is, however, limited to heterosexual activity. Muslim culture views monogamy as the ideal, polygamy as 'a concession to human nature' (Pickthall, 1953) and celibacy as the least acceptable state – anything outside of heterosexual activity is not acceptable at all.

Sexual dysfunction

The literature on psychosexual problems and culture is sparse (Bhugra & De Silva, 1993) and definitions vary widely. This makes it difficult to interpret and compare data. This is particularly relevant in countries such as the UK, where the major ethnic minorities – South Asian and African–Caribbean communities – are approaching second and third generations. Many difficulties that arise may be the product of the conflict of cultures for this group rather than any one prevailing ideology.

Similarly, although the USA has a growing proportion of non-Caucasians, estimated at about 27% in 2000, the vast majority of research on sexual functioning has been conducted among Whites. An examination of 1123 papers published in two major sexuality journals between 1971 and 1995 showed that the ethnicity of the study population was reported in only 26% of studies; only 4% included interethnic comparisons, mainly between Caucasian and African Americans (Wiederman *et al*, 1996). Studies that do examine racial/ethnic differences tend to compare only two groups, thus making it difficult to generalise more widely. Although Laumann *et al* (1994) included Caucasians, African Americans, Hispanics and Asians in their sample, the number of non-Caucasians was quite small, especially of older people.

There is a growing body of work looking not only at how cultural backgrounds influence sexuality but also at the role of acculturation in immigrant populations (Richardson & Goldmeier, 2005; Meston & Ahrold, 2008). Interestingly, a distinction in the literature between exploring immigrant and native populations is emerging. In the USA the larger minority groups of Black American, Latino and East Asian are being studied, while in the UK researchers are focusing on South Asian and Black British communities.

It is very difficult to reach conclusions from the literature on these disparate subject areas. Both sexual and cultural identity change radically with time and depending on context. With globalisation, the internet, immigration and greater mobility comes clash of culture, bringing integration and evolution, as well as conflict and confusion.

Epidemiology of sexual dysfunction between cultural groups

A UK study surveyed in detail sexual attitudes and lifestyles of 18 876 individuals (Johnson et al, 1994). One finding was a trend towards earlier first sexual intercourse: for 16- to 19-year old men the mean age of first sexual intercourse was 17, whereas for men aged 55–59 it was 20. A similar drop in age was recorded for women. Racial and ethnic differences were also found. Compared with White British individuals, people of South Asian origin were much less likely to report having had sexual intercourse before the age of 16, whereas this was more likely among Black British men and women. The median age for first sexual intercourse for men was higher for Asian participants and lower for Black participants in comparison with White. Religion also played a role in this interaction, with those belonging to the Church of England or other Christian churches (excluding the Roman Catholic Church) were less likely to report underage sexual intercourse.

Comparing cultural and biological factors regarding the sexual health and marital satisfaction of men in Germany and the USA, Mazur et al (2002) found that sexuality declined with age in both populations and neither testosterone levels nor psychological depression could explain this. Sexual health and marital satisfaction were related to sexuality among the Americans but not the Germans. They concluded that in both cultural settings, the wife's desire and the man's ability to maintain an erection and his imagination/fantasy may play a role.

Studies show both similarities and differences in the prevalence and associations of erectile dysfunction across different nations and cultures. Of 799 men aged 40–70 interviewed in a Belgian study, over 60% complained of erectile dysfunction (Mak et al, 2002). Participants reported a significant increase in dysfunction with age, in wide agreement with the literature, including a large racially diverse US study (Saigal et al, 2006), which noted an elevated risk of erectile dysfunction among Hispanics compared with other ethnic groups in the study.

A study involving 1250 men recruited from four sites in the Thai city of Bangkok found that age was not a significant factor in the prevalence of erectile dysfunction, but that diabetes and hypertension were (Kongkanand, 2000).

In a three-nation study of men aged 35–70 attending primary care clinics, erectile dysfunction was reported by 57.4% of the men interviewed in Nigeria, 63.6% of those in Egypt and 80.8% of those in Pakistan (Shaeer

199

et al, 2003). Older age, diabetes, peptic ulcer, prostate disease, depression-related symptoms and caffeine intake appeared to be independently associated with increased prevalence of erectile dysfunction.

In a UK population, significantly higher rates of rapid (premature) ejaculation were noted among Muslim men or men of South Asian origin (Richardson & Goldmeier, 2005). When this was explored in a subsequent qualitative study, anxiety regarding first sexual experience, particularly before or outside of marriage, resulting in cognitions involving fear of discovery and wanting to finish quickly, were prominent themes (Richardson *et al*, 2006). In a Canadian sample, similarly high rates of sexual dysfunction were found among East Asians compared with their White Canadian counterparts (Brotto *et al*, 2007); degree of acculturation rather than length of residency was a more reliable predictor of sexual problems.

Data gathered from 97 infertile Nigerian women who completed questionnaires regarding their sexual history revealed that 78% reported 'frigidity' and 58% dyspareunia (painful coitus) (Audu, 2002). A fifth had difficulties with sexual arousal and the same proportion had problems with reaching orgasm. This study reflects how sexual dysfunction is related to infertility: in many cultures sexual problems are framed as inability to conceive, so that the first point of contact for help is with obstetric and gynaecological services.

Bancroft *et al* (2003) surveyed 987 White and African American women aged 20–85 to measure 'distress' about heterosexual sex. In total, 22% of this sample reported marked distress about the sexual relationship and/or their own sexuality. Physical aspects of the women's sexual response, including arousal, vaginal lubrication and orgasm, were reported as poor predictors. Although the study is weakened by its use of conceptual terms such as 'distress', which do not map onto diagnostic criteria, it does include African American women.

A population-based study involving 728 women in Casablanca (Morocco) aged 20 and over found that 27% had a lifetime or 6-month prevalence of DSM–IV sexual dysfunction (Kadri *et al*, 2002). Hypoactive sexual desire disorder was the most common finding; age, financial dependency, number of children and sexual harassment were positively associated with symptoms of sexual dysfunction. Only 17% had sought help for symptoms.

In 2005, *Ebony* magazine in the USA sent out a questionnaire to its readers with the aim of exploring the sex lives and sexuality of African American women (Ashby, 2005). Of the 7800 respondents, 37% self-reported sexual abuse at the hands of immediate and/or extended family; 33% had experienced inability to reach orgasm in the past year and 47% had not sought medical help for any symptoms of sexual dysfunction.

Of 242 Nigerian women of child-bearing age recruited from out-patient clinics at a teaching hospital, 63% reported sexual dysfunction (Fajewonyomi *et al*, 2007) such as disorder of desire ($n = 20$; 8.3%), disorder of arousal ($n = 13$; 5.4%), disorder of orgasm ($n = 154$; 63.6%) and dyspareunia ($n = 55$; 22.7%). Dysfunction was most common in the 26–30 age group and among women of higher educational status. Unsatisfactory sexual life was mainly attributed to medical illness and psychosexual factors (uncaring partners, excessive domestic duties, lack of adequate foreplay, competition between wives in polygamous marriages, previous sexual abuse and guilt about a termination of pregnancy). The authors regarded the male-dominated culture, in which women were afraid of rejection and divorce if they complained about sexual matters, as a perpetuating factor in sexual dysfunction. They called for urgent attention to this social and psychological problem.

Among South Asian couples in Leicester, male partners often spoke on behalf of their female partners regarding sexual dysfunction, and sex therapy referrals were more likely to come from secondary care (Bhugra & Cordle, 1986, 1988).

Homosexuality across cultures

His studies in the USA, Guatemala, Brazil and the Philippines led Whitam (1983) to suggest that male homosexuality is a fundamental form of human sexuality acted out in different cultural settings. He offered six tentative conclusions about the cultural invariability of homosexuality (Box 15.1).

Same-sex behaviours have been described across all societies and cultures at different times (Bullough, 1979) with varying societal responses. However, legal proscription of such behaviour in some countries forces individuals to conceal their sexuality, clouding evidence of prevalence.

Ancient Hindu texts and literature contain detailed descriptions of same-sex attraction in both men and women (Bullough, 1979; Vanita, 2005). As mentioned above, sex was at that time seen as an activity in which both genders took pleasure. Hinsch (1990) noted that during certain periods in China 'homosexuality was widely accepted and even respected, had its

---

Box 15.1 Observations on the cultural invariability of homosexuality

- All societies include homosexuals
- All societies include similar (and stable) percentages of homosexuals
- The emergence of homosexual orientation is not hindered or encouraged by social norms
- All societies of sufficient size have homosexual subcultures
- Homosexuals in different societies tend to share certain behavioural interests and occupational choices
- The continuum from overtly masculine to overtly feminine homosexuals is similar in all societies

(Whitam, 1983)

own formal history and had a role in shaping Chinese political conventions and spurring artistic creations'. In ancient China, as in ancient Rome and Greece, kings were allowed to keep male sexual partners. The role of same-sex relationships has been well noted and described in ancient Greece (Bullough, 1979), where such behaviour was accepted not as a phase but as part of the bisexual nature of humans.

A study of the coming-out of 145 lesbian, gay and bisexual youths in the USA reported no significant ethnic/racial differences in the milestones of sexual development, or in sexual orientation, sexual behaviour and sexual identity (Rosario et al, 2004). The Black participants participated in fewer social activities in the gay and lesbian community and felt less comfortable with others knowing their sexual identity than the White participants. Over time, though, their positive attitudes towards homosexuality and certainty in their sexual identity increased more than those of their White counterparts. Both the Black and Latino participants disclosed their sexual identity to fewer people than did White participants. The authors concluded that these findings 'support [their] hypothesis that cultural factors do not impede the formation of identity but may delay identity integration'. Indeed, it has been suggested that the conflict of cultural identity with anti-homosexual attitudes in the Black community and of sexuality with racism in the homosexual community may result in poor self-concept and coping techniques (Icard, 1986).

Approaching cultural aspects of sexual dysfunction

An important issue to highlight is the individual's cultural context. In this respect, identity must be considered in all its multifaceted aspects. Specifically, historical cultural ideas, current attitudes in countries of origination and differing levels of cultural integration of immigrant populations at different stages need to be explored. Relationships between individuals of differing cultural origin may present particular issues.

Although many cultures attempt to maintain endogamy, globalisation has influenced the proportion of individuals who choose partners from their own background. An exploration of the process of assimilation of immigrant cultures using marriage data (Rosenfeld, 2002) found a drop in the proportion of endogamous marriages in the USA from 77% in 1970 to 66% in 1990. However, problems with generalising these data were noted, including the limitations of using data only on marriages and not on relationships in general, and different rates of assimilation between different ethnic groups.

The role of the clinician lies not only in asking the right questions about cultural differences but also in helping people to understand the influence of these differences on their sexuality. For example, for mixed-race couples the clinician might explore the stereotypes and prejudices that may have affected their partner choice: 'white men or women may be sought out for their access to white privilege, Asian women for their compliance, African Americans for their sexual prowess, Latinos as passionate lovers, etc.' (McGoldrick *et al*, 2006). The very factors that may have sparked initial sexual attraction can later undermine relationships. Consideration must also be given to the acculturation of the couple: a significant proportion of South Asian couples in Britain are formed of a second- or third-generation individual and a partner from the originating country.

Interestingly, presentations previously regarded as 'culturally bound syndromes' have been revisited. Typical symptoms associated with the value of semen and its loss (*dhat* syndrome) have been noted in several cultures, including the USA, UK and Australia. Thus, although originally thought to be a solely Asian phenomenon, the syndrome cannot be attributed as clearly to culture but may well be a manifestation of more general psychological disturbance (Bhui, 1998; Sumathipala *et al*, 2004).

A further consideration is the relationship between the couple and their therapist, particularly when there are obvious internal or external differences such as culture, ethnicity, language, religion, class and/or education. The therapist may be from the majority culture and the couple from a minority culture, or vice versa; both therapist and couple may be from the same minority culture or different minority cultures; and the partners in the couple might both be from minority cultures, or one might be from the majority and one from a minority culture (Bhugra & de Silva, 2007). These different permutations can result in various problems for psychosexual therapy. A majority-culture therapist may be 'colour blind', assuming that a minority-culture couple are the same; conversely, too much may be made of racism and cultural issues, over-identifying differences. However, matching of patients to therapists on the basis of ethnicity or culture is not a straightforward solution, as some people prefer therapists from a different background (Bhui, 1998). The usual power imbalance in the patient–therapist relationship can become intensified by cultural differences (D'Ardenne, 1991).

Box 15.2 summarises the key issues that the therapist should consider during assessment and the formulation.

Management of sexual problems

There is a paucity of literature available on how to manage sexual problems in people from minority ethnic groups. Although there is an emphasis on making services more accessible, there is the question of how appropriate it is to use therapeutic methods that reflect Western definitions of sexuality. Clinicians must remain mindful that culture is not homogeneous: different attitudes and beliefs proliferate in any ethnic group, and studies pertaining to a particular group may not always apply to everyone belonging to it (Petrak & Keane, 1998). The mainstream of sex therapy remains closely based on the work of Masters & Johnson (1970), which emphasises teaching the giving and receiving of pleasure. Given the differing perspectives on

---

Box 15.2 Key issues to consider during assessment and formulation

- The level of acculturation of the couple
- Any disparity in acculturation between the two
- Gender roles in relationships
- Gender roles of the couple and of their family
- The influence of the family on their relationship
- The role of the family in the initiation of their relationship
- Whether the relationship was arranged in any way
- The pressure/expectation (on the part of the individuals and others) to have children
- If married, whether there was pressure to marry
- Any normative age for marriage
- Whether certain achievements are expected before marriage

---

sex in different cultures, techniques focusing on a pleasuring framework developed in a largely White, heterosexual, well-educated, middle-class group may be unacceptable or inaccessible to the wider population.

Factors such as high drop-out rates and the missing of sessions are also pertinent. In one survey, 83% of Asian couples dropped out of therapy, compared with 29% of White couples (Bhui, 1998). Patients' pursuit of organic explanations, along with educational and language barriers, may explain some of the low uptake and success rates (Bhui *et al*, 1994). There may be cultural bias against help-seeking or individuals may not know where to go for help. Only 17% of women with sexual dysfunction in Casablanca asked for help, although they were aware of their disorder and its negative impact on their lives (Kadri *et al*, 2002). Only 2% of men and women in Korea had talked to a medical doctor about their sexual problems. Many individuals did not seek help because they did not think that the problem was important, they could not access or afford medical care and/or they were not aware that treatment was available (Moreira *et al*, 2006). A cross-national survey of the attitudes of men with erectile dysfunction in six countries reported that all of the men interviewed described their dysfunction as a source of great sadness for themselves and their partners, and that half of them said they would do 'nearly anything' to cure it. Participants in the USA and the UK were less willing to accept the problem, more motivated to find a cure and less likely to consider erectile dysfunction to be result of psychological problems (Perelman *et al*, 2005).

Clinical practice

Once an individual with a sexual problem has presented, the real work of the clinician can begin. As a starting point it is worth bearing in mind the basic sex therapy framework of the PLISSIT model: permission, limited information, specific suggestions and intensive therapy (Annon, 1976). Although as old as the Masters & Johnson (1970) models, PLISSIT is relevant and useful, especially with culturally diverse groups where permission-giving, limited information and specific suggestions may be as far as the clinician gets. This may well be enough to help resolve the problem, but it also provides a staged approach leading to more intensive therapy if appropriate. Masturbation or self-pleasure is frowned on in some cultures – many religions forbid it and this can be a major block in management of problems such as premature ejaculation. For some Muslim and Jewish patients, for example, gaining permission to masturbate from a religious figure may facilitate its use in a 'medical' context (Gupta *et al*, 1989; Ribner, 2004). Artificial penetration and sex toys may also be prohibited, as they are regarded as being for pleasure rather than for procreation. This might be a problem in the treatment of vaginismus. It is inevitable that such cultures approve only heteronormative penetrative intercourse. In some communities, sexual dysfunction is framed as physical or spiritual failure or weakness. This will undoubtedly undermine psychological approaches. Therefore, pursuit of physical aetiologies and lack of psychological mindedness may undo attempts to explore problems and so patients' expectations of treatment must be established early.

In addition to the difficulties described in Box 15.3, special consideration must be given to working with couples from differing cultural backgrounds. In light of the increasing numbers of such couples and also increasingly complex family structures, it has been suggested that family genograms be used to explore these issues (McGoldrick *et al*, 2006). Treatment must

---

Box 15.3 Difficulties with psychosexual therapy for people from minority ethnic groups

- Disapproval of masturbation
- Prohibition of artificial penetration and sex toys
- Concepts such as foreplay, sensual touch and oral sex may seem alien and unwelcome
- Lack of privacy or time alone, making homework/exercises difficult
- The framing of sexual dysfunction as physical or spiritual failure or weakness
- The pursuit of physical causes for sexual problems and lack of psychological mindedness
- It may be unacceptable for women to have sex therapy, especially with a male therapist
- Treatment approaches that require the female to take an active initiatory role may fail
- Men may find it difficult to speak to a female therapist, particularly when asked to carry out tasks and give feedback

be carefully tailored to the situation. One of the few published examples of this approach concerns the treatment of members of the Bangladeshi community in east London. Diagrams and drawings, the involvement of senior family figures and an 'authoritative' approach were found to facilitate therapy (D'Ardenne & Crown, 1986).

Mapping out family trees can prompt questions about different attitudes between backgrounds towards sex, relationships, gender roles and coping with difficulties. Identifying role models in the family, features of their culture that the individual values and aspects they wish to leave behind, examples in the family of marrying outside the culture, and aspects of one partner that are congruent with and contradictory to the other partner can all help the clinician's understanding.

Conclusion

Although there is little evidence of how sex therapy can be effectively adapted to a multicultural community, the shift to a more multifaceted model of intervention (Daines & Hallam-Jones, 2007) is helpful. Clinicians may not be able to attend to the details of every cultural permutation, but a body of work is accumulating on key cultural groups. In the USA, these are the African–Caribbean, East Asian and Hispanic populations and in the UK, the South Asian and African–Caribbean communities. Of course, newer immigrant groups and globalisation continue to alter the mix of patients presenting, but themes are emerging that can help clinicians to both encourage attendance and provide appropriate intervention when patients do attend.

References

Al-Sawaf, M. & Al-Issa, I. (2000) Sex and sexual dysfunction in an Arab-Islamic society. In *Al-Junun: Mental Illness in the Islamic World* (ed. I. Al-Issa). International Universities Press.

Annon, J. S. (1976) The PLISSIT model: a proposed conceptual scheme for the behavioral treatment of sexual problems. *Journal of Sex Education and Therapy*, **2**, 1–15.

Ashby, H. E. (2005) The Ebony Sex Survey and the sex lives of African–American women: a call to healthcare providers. *Ethnicity and Disease*, **15**, S40–4.

Audu, B. M. (2002) Sexual dysfunction among infertile Nigerian women. *Journal of Obstetrics and Gynaecology*, **22**, 655–7.

Bancroft, J., Loftus, J. & Long, J. S. (2003) Distress about sex: a national survey of women in heterosexual relationships. *Archives of Sexual Behavior*, **32**, 193–208.

Bhugra, D. (1997) Experiences of being a gay man in urban India. *A descriptive study. Sexual and Relationship Therapy*, **12**, 371–375.

Bhugra, D. & Cordle, C. (1986) Sexual dysfunction in Asian couples. *BMJ (Clinical Research Edition)*, **292**, 111–2.

Bhugra, D. & Cordle, C. (1988) A case–control study of sexual dysfunction in Asian and non-Asian couples 1981–1985. *Sexual and Marital Therapy*, **3**, 71–76.

Bhugra, D. & De Silva, P. (1993) Sexual dysfunction across cultures. *International Review of Psychiatry*, **5**, 243–252.

Bhugra, D. & De Silva, P. (1995) Sexual dysfunction and sex therapy. An historical perspective. *International Review of Psychiatry*, **7**, 159–166.

Bhugra, D. & De Silva, P. (2007) Management of sexual dysfunction across cultures. In *Textbook of Cultural Psychiatry* (eds D. Bhugra & K. Bhui). Cambridge University Press.

Bhui, K. (1998) Psychosexual care in a multi-ethnic society. *Journal of the Royal Society of Medicine*, **91**, 141–143.

Bhui, K., Herriot, P., Dein, S., *et al* (1994) Asians presenting to a sex and marital therapy clinic. *International Journal of Social Psychiatry*, **40**, 194.

Blech, B. (2003) *The Complete Idiot's Guide to Understanding Judaism*. Alpha Books.

Brotto, L. A., Woo, J. S. & Ryder, A. G. (2007) Acculturation and sexual function in Canadian East Asian men. *Journal of Sexual Medicine*, **4**, 72–82.

Bullough, V. L. (1972) Sex in history: a virgin field. *Journal of Sex Research*, **8**, 101–116.

Bullough, V. L. (1976) *Sexual Variance in Society and History*. John Wiley & Sons.

Bullough, V. L. (1979) *Homosexuality: A History*. Plume Books.

D'Ardenne, P. (1991) Transcultural issues in couple therapy. In *Couple Therapy: A Handbook* (eds D. Hooper & W. Dryden). Open University Press.

D'Ardenne, P. & Crown, S. (1986) Sexual dysfunction in Asian couples. *BMJ (Clinical Research Edition)*, **292**, 1078–1079.

Daines, B. & Hallam-Jones, R. (2007) Multifaceted intervention sex therapy (MIST). *Sexual and Relationship Therapy*, **22**, 339–350.

Fajewonyomi, B. A., Orji, E. O. & Adeyemo, A. O. (2007) Sexual dysfunction among female patients of reproductive age in a hospital setting in Nigeria. *Journal of Health, Population and Nutrition*, **25**, 101–106.

Ford, C. S. & Beach, F. A. (1951) *Patterns of Sexual Behavior*. Harper.

Gregersen, E. (1986) Human sexuality in cross-cultural perspective. In *Alternative Approaches to the Study of Sexual Behavior* (eds D. Byrne & K. Kelly). Lawrence Erlbaum Associates.

Gupta, P., Banerjee, G. & Nandi, D. (1989) Modified Masters–Johnson technique in the treatment of sexual inadequacy in males. *Indian Journal of Psychiatry*, **31**, 63.

Hinsch, B. (1990) *Passions of the Cut Sleeve: The Male Homosexual Tradition in China*. University of California Press.

Icard, L. (1986) Black gay men and conflicting social identities. Sexual orientation versus racial identity. *Journal of Social Work and Human Sexuality*, **4**, 83–93.

Johnson, A. M., Wadsworth, J., Wellings, K., *et al* (1994) *Sexual Attitudes and Lifestyles*. Blackwell Scientific.

Kadri, N., Mchichi Alami, K. H. & Mchakra Tahiri, S. (2002) Sexual dysfunction in women: population based epidemiological study. *Archives of Women's Mental Health*, **5**, 59–63.

King, H. (1994) Sowing the field: Greek and Roman sexology. In *Sexual Knowledge, Sexual Science: The History of Attitudes to Sexuality* (eds R. Porter & M. Teich). Cambridge University Press.

Kongkanand, A. (2000) Prevalence of erectile dysfunction in Thailand. *International Journal of Andrology*, **23** (suppl. 2), 77–80.

Laumann, E. O., Michael, R. T. & Gagnon, J. H. (1994) A political history of the national sex survey of adults. *Family Planning Perspectives*, **26**, 34–38.

Mahay, J., Laumann, E. O. & Michaels, S. (2000) Race, gender, and class in sexual scripts. In *Sex, Love and Health in America: Private Choices and Public Policies* (eds E. O. Laumann & R. T. Michael). University of Chicago Press.

Mak, R., De Backer, G., Kornitzer, M., *et al* (2002) Prevalence and correlates of erectile dysfunction in a population-based study in Belgium. *European Urology*, **41**, 132–138.

Masters, W. H. & Johnson, V. E. (1970) *Human Sexual Inadequacy*. Little, Brown.

Mazur, A., Mueller, U., Krause, W., *et al* (2002) Causes of sexual decline in aging married men: Germany and America. *International Journal of Impotence Research*, **14**, 101–106.

McGoldrick, M., Giordano, J. & Garcia-Preto, N. (2005) *Ethnicity and Family Therapy*. Guilford Press.

McGoldrick, M., Loonan, R. & Wohlsifer, D. (2006) Sexuality and Culture. In *Principles and Practice of Sex Therapy* (ed. S. R. Leiblum). Guilford Press.

Meston, C. M. & Ahrold, T. (2008) Ethnic, gender, and acculturation influences on sexual behaviors. *Archives of Sexual Behavior*, Epub, doi: 10.1007/s10508-008-9415-0.

Moreira, E. D. Jr., Kim, S. C., Glasser, D., *et al* (2006) Sexual activity, prevalence of sexual problems, and associated help-seeking patterns in men and women aged 40–80 years in Korea: data from the Global Study of Sexual Attitudes and Behaviors (GSSAB). *Journal of Sexual Medicine*, **3**, 201–211.

Perelman, M., Shabsigh, R., Seftel, A., *et al* (2005) Attitudes of men with erectile dysfunction: a cross-national survey. *Journal of Sexual Medicine*, **2**, 397–406.

Petrak, J. & Keane, F. (1998) Cultural beliefs and the treatment of sexual dysfunction: an overview. *Sexual Dysfunction*, **1**, 13–17.

Pickthall, M. (1953) *Glorious Meaning of the Koran*. New American Library.

Reiss, I. L. (1986) *Journey into Sexuality: An Exploratory Voyage*. Prentice Hall.

Ribner, D. S. (2004) Ejaculatory restrictions as a factor in the treatment of Haredi (ultraorthodox) Jewish couples. *Archives of Sexual Behavior*, **33**, 303–308.

Ribner, D. S. & Rosenbaum, T. Y. (2005) Evaluation and treatment of unconsummated marriages among Orthodox Jewish couples. *Journal of Sex and Marital Therapy*, **31**, 341–353.

Richardson, D. & Goldmeier, D. (2005) Premature ejaculation – does country of origin tell us anything about etiology? *Journal of Sexual Medicine*, **2**, 508–512.

Richardson, D., Wood, K. & Goldmeier, D. (2006) A qualitative pilot study of Islamic men with lifelong premature (rapid) ejaculation. *Journal of Sexual Medicine*, **3**, 337–343.

Rosario, M., Schrimshaw, E. W. & Hunter, J. (2004) Ethnic/racial differences in the coming-out process of lesbian, gay, and bisexual youths: a comparison of sexual identity development over time. *Cultural Diversity and Ethnic Minority Psychology*, **10**, 215–228.

Rosenfeld, M. J. (2002) Measures of assimilation in the marriage market: Mexican Americans 1970–1990. *Journal of Marriage and the Family*, **64**, 152–162.

Saigal, C. S., Wessells, H., Pace, J., *et al* (2006) Predictors and prevalence of erectile dysfunction in a racially diverse population. *Archives of Internal Medicine*, **166**, 207–212.

Segall, M. H., Dasen, P. R., Berry, J. W., *et al* (1986) *Human Behavior in Global Perspective*. Pergamon Press.

Shaeer, K. Z., Osegbe, D. N., Siddiqui, S. H., *et al* (2003) Prevalence of erectile dysfunction and its correlates among men attending primary care clinics in three countries: Pakistan, Egypt, and Nigeria. *International Journal of Impotence Research*, **15** (suppl. 1), S8–14.

Sumathipala, A., Siribaddana, S. H. & Bhugra, D. (2004) Culture-bound syndromes: the story of *dhat* syndrome. *British Journal of Psychiatry*, **184**, 200–209.

Vanita, R. (2005) *Love's Rite: Same Sex Marriage in India and the West*. Palgrave Macmillan.

Whitam, F. L. (1983) Culturally invariable properties of male homosexuality: tentative conclusions from cross-cultural research. *Archives of Sexual Behavior*, **12**, 207–226.

Wiederman, M. W., Maynard, C. & Fretz, A. (1996) Ethnicity in 25 years of published sexuality research: 1971–1995. *Journal of Sex Research*, **33**, 339–342.

CHAPTER 16

Culture in child and adolescent psychiatry

Nisha Dogra

Summary Almost everyone continues to develop throughout life, but at no time is development more marked than in childhood and adolescence. Culture can influence this process in many ways and mental health clinicians and researchers need to be aware of this. Everyone has some sort of family, and definitions and compositions of families are changing all the time. Children are dependent on families in many ways so the family structure needs to be taken very much into account. A third area, apart from culture and family, that must be considered is the potential cultural mismatch between young people and their carers, which may affect presentations to mental health services. The relationship between culture and mental illness has been discussed elsewhere in this volume, so here I focus on the impact of culture on the practice of child and adolescent psychiatry and the context in which this psychiatric specialty is practised.

There are many definitions of culture, but for reasons discussed in chapter 27 and elsewhere (Dogra *et al*, 2007*a*) I use here that of the Association of American Medical Colleges (AAMC):

> Culture is defined by each person in relationship to the group or groups with whom he or she identifies. An individual's cultural identity may be based on heritage as well as individual circumstances and personal choice. Cultural identity may be affected by such factors as race, ethnicity, age, language, country of origin, acculturation, sexual orientation, gender, socioeconomic status, religious/spiritual beliefs, physical abilities, occupation, among others. These factors may impact behaviours such as communication styles, diet preferences, health beliefs, family roles, lifestyle, rituals and decision-making processes. All of these beliefs and practices, in turn can influence how patients and heath care professionals perceive health and illness, and how they interact with one another. (Task Force on Spirituality, Cultural Issues, and End of Life Care, 1999: p. 25.)

A key advantage of this definition for psychiatry is its patient-centred nature: it allows patients to define which aspects of their whole are important to them and when. Although children can and do make choices about some of the aspects outlined above, they often find that choices are made for them without their involvement. There can be great pressure on children to behave in accordance with the most obvious aspect of themselves such as their 'ethnic' or 'cultural' background even if that is not how they feel about themselves. This pressure, unintended or intended, may come from the family and peers. Children of mixed racial heritage are often forced to identify more with one part of their heritage than with another (Lincoln, 2009).

The concept of childhood is itself culturally influenced, as are expectations of children's behaviour and protection. In 'Western' cultures, for example, as a more autonomous sense of self has developed, the rights of children have been increasingly recognised – a process that started in British society in Victorian times (Heywood, 2001).

Culture and child development

There is no doubt that culture influences child rearing, the way in which children are encouraged to grow up and how they are swayed by their peers and siblings. It also affects the roles and responsibilities that accompany their development in the physical, emotional, social, cognitive and moral domains. The influences of culture on social and emotional development are most evident, but it can be difficult to identify its specific effects on any particular child as there will be other complex dynamic features at work.

In seminal research, Baumrind (1966) identified three parenting (child-rearing) styles: authoritative, authoritarian and permissive. Macoby & Martin (1983) subsequently divided permissive parenting into two subtypes – neglectful and indulgent. From a 'Western' clinical perspective, authoritative parenting is the 'preferred norm' in that parents demonstrate high control but are also responsive to the child's needs. Authoritative parents value compliance and set behavioural standards, while respecting the child's developing autonomy and independence. They expect developmentally and age-appropriate behaviour. Children brought up by authoritative parents are the most competent, being more self-reliant, content, socially responsible, self-controlled and cooperative (Baumrind, 1966). This style of parenting is less likely in 'Eastern' cultures, where authoritarian parenting may more often be considered the norm as it fits the notion of a collectivist agenda that emphasises responsibility to others, obedience and dutifulness.

McLoyd et al (2000) argue that variations in child-rearing practices identified in different ethnic groups may demonstrate diversity within groups and/or the lack of rigorous research rather than real differences. Furthermore, interactions between parenting style and other factors may affect outcome. For example, the child's perception of discipline and that of the parent may influence the way a particular style plays out. It is difficult to separate culture from social context and gender issues. In a Palestinian sample, parents varied their parenting styles depending on the issues they felt they were faced with (Dwairy, 2004). A study with an Egyptian sample found that in rural communities parents used authoritarian styles with boys and authoritative styles with girls whereas in urban areas the authoritarian style was used for girls (Dwairy & Menshar, 2006).

Such external factors strongly influence emotional and social development and the sense of self. The interplay between a child's sense of self and the expectations of its parents, family and wider society are of great relevance in the practice of child psychiatry.

The family

Although parenting styles may be influenced by culture, individual families remain unique entities. It is often difficult to define what a family is: for example, the 'nuclear' family on which so many Western ideas of child development are based is increasingly changing in shape and content.

Child and adolescent mental health services in the UK have been influenced by the family life-cycle model of Carter & McGoldrick (1989). However, mental health professionals in India openly acknowledged that this model is not immediately transferable to the Indian context and that even in the West the model has been criticised (Dogra et al, 2005). Nevertheless, the family life-cycle model does highlight that life and development inherently bring with them change in social contexts and practices. The way that families as a whole or individuals within them manage that change has implications for all involved. Although the stages of the family life cycle may vary between and within cultures, the concept of different stages of development is likely to hold true. Practitioners can therefore use the model as a template of stages, the features of which can be altered to fit with their own experiences and those of the families with whom they have worked. It is then unnecessary to debate whether the model is right or wrong, as its structure offers families and practitioners a framework that can be adapted to the specific context. Table 16.1 shows the Carter & McGoldrick model used as a template for family life-cycle issues identified by mental health professionals in India. This clearly shows that Indian families are influenced by more than just culture; social class can significantly alter expectations and roles, as can rural or urban dwelling.

An additional complication in child and adolescent psychiatry is family members are also stakeholders in the young person's treatment. The clinician may have to contend with different viewpoints within the family, all of which will affect the assessment and the treatment that can be agreed. Garland et al (2004) interviewed 170 adolescents, their caregivers and their therapists to identify three desired treatment outcomes for each stakeholder. The most commonly reported desired outcome across all three stakeholder groups was to reduce anger and aggression. However, when individual cases were compared, almost two-thirds of the triads did not agree on even one desired outcome of the adolescent's treatment. The adolescents

Table 16.1 Family life-cycle models

Stage	The Carter–McGoldrick (1989) model	Traditional Indian society (Dogra et al, 2005)
1 Family-of-origin experiences	Maintaining relationships with parents, siblings and peers Completing school	Relationships are not only with parents but also with extended family. Social and emotional attachment to mother very strong and socially expected. Differential attachment with fathers, whose role is authoritative. Specific gender hierarchy and gender roles. Many children never attend school; those that do may not be able to complete their education. Girls are directed towards domestic skills and boys towards education. Difference between classes strong.
2 Leaving home	Differentiation of self from family of origin and development of adult-to-adult relationship with parents Development of intimate peer relationships Beginning a career	Leaving home is not a stage for most Indian families: it is not expected or socially sanctioned. No attempt to differentiate the self, as individual stays with family. Adult-to-adult relationship with parents develops later. Religion has an important impact on lives. Intimate peer relationships are fewer, but more common with same gender. Beginning a career is likely to mean participating in family business. Gender roles and social class affect career: the lower the social class, the greater the economic input of women to the family. If both parents are working, domestic issues remain the women's responsibility. There will be differences between rural and urban families, for example rural families may adhere to more traditional roles than urban families. Individuals from rural backgrounds may also be less well educated. Before marriage, women may move into the home of their future spouse.
3 Premarriage stage	Selecting partners Developing a relationship Deciding to marry	Parents often decide on their children's marriage and select the partner. Social class is important: lower classes – parents do not ask a daughter's views; middle classes – consent from the both partners is sought; higher classes – individuals choose their own partner. The need to raise a dowry may influence how this life stage is addressed.

Continued opposite

212

Table 16.1 continued

Stage	The Carter–McGoldrick (1989) model	Traditional Indian society
4 Childless couple stage	Developing a way to live together based on reality rather than mutual projection Realigning relationships with families of origin and peers to include spouses	Childless couples often live with extended family. The welcome of girls into their spouse's home depends on the attitudes of his parents. There is an expectation to have children. Issues relating to new relationships.
5 Family with young children	Adjusting marriage to make space for children Adopting parenting roles Realigning relationships with families of origin to include parenting and grandparenting roles Children developing peer relationships	Family with young children or adolescents are not discrete stages. Life is based on experiences of others, e.g. extended families, religion, books. Children are not allowed to experience things for themselves. 'Guilt-producing' culture: depression common in childless marriage. Strictly defined roles based on religious expectations.
6 Family with adolescents	Adjusting parent–child relationships to allow adolescents more autonomy Adjusting marital relationships to focus on midlife marital and career issues Taking on responsibility of caring for families of origin	
7 Launching children	Adjusting to living as a couple again Adjusting to including in-laws and grandchildren within the family circle Dealing with disability and death in the family of origin	Negotiating adult relationship with children is not necessary as it is perceived to have been done already. Disability is not discussed or addressed. Senior family members make decisions. Adaptation to extended family. Social roles/regulations of society.
8 Later life	Coping with physiological decline Adjusting to the children taking a more central role in family maintenance Experience of and making room for the elderly Dealing with loss of spouse and peers Preparation for death, life review and integration	Coping with decline. Elderly people continue to make decisions but, given social roles, there may be conflict over who has the power. Later life more involved with grandchildren and spiritual matters. Preparation for death. Sharing of experiences and problem-solving.

and therapists were each more likely than the parents to report desired outcomes that related to the family environment; adolescents were the least likely to report desired outcomes that were related to their own symptom reduction. The study revealed lack of agreement on the desired outcome among key stakeholders and on desired outcome priorities for adolescent services. This lack of consensus may limit engagement in treatment and the effectiveness of care. This highlights a fundamental problem for child and adolescent mental health services: deciding who is the client.

Culture and mental health problems

Not all mental health problems are culture-related and not all will be responsive to change. However, an understanding of the cultural context of a young person's problems may help clinicians present the issues in ways that are acceptable to the family and thereby amenable to intervention. There are very few culturally specific problems, but some disorders are more likely to occur in some contexts than in others (Dogra *et al*, 2007*b*). For example, the eating disorder anorexia nervosa is more common in Western contexts than elsewhere. Rousseau *et al* (2008) surveyed the literature on culture and DSM–IV diagnoses in child psychiatry. They concluded that although the DSM–IV diagnostic categories may be found cross-culturally, clinicians need to be aware of how culture may influence the diagnostic process.

The Office for National Statistics Survey (Green *et al*, 2005) highlights that children living in the UK had different prevalence rates of psychiatric disorders, with rates for Indian girls being considerably lower than for other ethnic groups. However, the small numbers of children from minority ethnic groups represented makes it difficult to be conclusive. Goodman *et al* (2008), in a systematic review which included the Office for National Statistics data, concluded that there is evidence to suggest that there are inter-ethnic differences in the prevalence of mental health problems among children in the UK but that the differences are largely unexplained. Klineberg *et al* (2006) found that differences in social support did not explain ethnic differences in psychological distress in an ethnically diverse adolescent group. In common with other studies, they found that low social support was associated with poor mental health, but this relationship did not vary with ethnicity.

Culture may influence the development of mental health problems by the influence it has on how gender roles, parenting styles and so on are enacted. Culture and religion may also influence how mental health problems and the interventions used to address them are viewed (Yeh *et al*, 2004). In a study of children's fears, Meltzer *et al* (2009) found that the most marked associations were fears of the dark, loud noises and imagined supernatural beings in younger children; fear of animals was more common among girls than among boys and among children from Black and minority ethnic groups than among White boys. They concluded that children's fears differ in nature across different ethnic groups. Culturally mediated beliefs, values and traditions may play a role in their expression. Not only is culture a relevant factor in the development of mental health problems, it can be relevant in whether children are presented to psychiatric services or not. Hackett & Hackett (1993) found differences between Gujarati and White English parents in how they viewed normal and deviant behaviours with respect to conduct and bedwetting but not self-care. Pumariega et al (2005) speculated that Latinos and African Americans were perhaps more accepting of hyperactivity than 'Caucasian' and Asian Americans. This in turn could affect prevalence rates.

Professional perspectives may also influence whether children are referred or not. When referral patterns were analysed for different agencies and professional groups, Daryanani et al (2001) found that general practitioners were more likely to refer proportionally more White children, whereas paediatricians referred more Black and South Asian children, education services more Black children, and social workers more mixed-race children. This may say more about the professional's bias than the child's problems or presentation. Thus, clinicians must be aware of their own perspectives and how these influence their interactions with culturally diverse groups.

Clients from minority ethnic groups often have a higher level of unmet health need, which may reflect differential access, referral pathways and service utilisation (Dogra, 2004; Pumariega et al, 2005). It may also reflect different patterns of care if services are accessed. Culture influences not only the presentation of problems but also the interpretation of symptoms, to whom people first turn (for example, for some ethnic groups religious leaders may be the first point of access when there are concerns about children's behaviour) and which treatment options a family accepts (some of the principles of family therapy may be unacceptable to authoritarian parents).

Implications for practice

Cultural sensibility

A 'cultural sensibility' approach based on the definition of culture at the start of this chapter enables the practitioner to find out about the unique cultural situation of child and family and to use the assessment process to gain information that will ensure that any treatment plan incorporates the cultural perspective of the family and is thereby acceptable to them (Dogra et al, 2007a; chapter 27, this volume). Additional information about the life of the child can be gained by understanding its everyday aspects such as toys and the nature of play that the child engages with, the way they dress and how their lives are structured (Mukherji, 1997). Nevertheless, much of this will be influenced by parental, cultural and economic choices.

It is essential that clinicians identify their own biases and prejudices about children and families, as this is the baggage taken into the clinical encounter or consultation. Understanding of one's personal perspectives is important not only because they may lead to a poorer quality of care for those towards whom there is prejudice, but also because they may cause overcompensation – for example, a clinician who is uncomfortable dealing with a particular group but does not acknowledge this might be sympathetic and supportive when the more appropriate response may have been to expect the young person to take some responsibility. In training, this is often glossed over as 'awareness'. It needs to be more critical and clinicians' assumptions need to be challenged as a matter of routine.

Garland *et al*'s (2004) findings that adolescents, caregivers and therapists have different expectations of outcomes of the consultation also reveal how culture might influence who is allowed to express themselves at meetings. Family expectations may mean that the therapist is not supposed to give as much weight to the young person's perspective as to that of adults, or that the father's view should override the maternal perspective. Such assumptions require careful negotiation and sensitivity but cannot be ignored. I have discussed elsewhere, using vulnerable children as an example, how to ensure that those working in child psychiatry make sure that the care they provide is 'culturally appropriate' (Dogra, 2007).

The 'cultural sensibility' framework is adaptable. It has not yet been formally tested, but at face value it is an approach that focuses on the needs of the child and acknowledges that the clinician is not a neutral being but a real person who is flawed.

Patient-centred interviewing

The key areas of exploration in patient-centred interviewing, as discussed by Platt *et al* (2001), are outlined in Box 16.1. It may be argued that this is nothing more than good psychiatric interviewing and is all part of a comprehensive assessment, but it is useful to state them here. To ensure that care is culturally appropriate, one needs to consider how the

---

Box 16.1 The key questions in patient-centred interviewing

- Who is this person, what constitutes their life? What are their interests, work, important relationships and main concerns?
- What does the patient want from the physician? What are their values and fears? What do they hope to accomplish today or over the longer term?
- How does the patient experience their illness or problems?
- What are the patient's ideas about the illness or problem
- What are the patient's main feelings about the illness?

(Platt *et al*, 2001)

responses to the questions posed fit in with the wider world and also with the provider's own perspective. In working with young people, the perspectives of the adults involved in their lives might also have to be taken into account.

As with adults, children's experiences may have made them suspicious of mental health services. They may also have been given misinformation about who they are going to see. After introductions have been made, a useful opening question is to ask the young person (and anyone else present) what they anticipate will happen. It is important to explore where they have obtained these ideas from as their sources may be unreliable. Young people need to know that they are valued and are not being negatively judged.

Respect

Respect means different things to different people. Rather than falling back on stereotypes, it is probably best negotiated with each individual. Children who come from families in which parents are authoritarian (and this can be from any cultural background) or in which children are 'seen but not heard' may be less forthcoming. Clinicians need to be open to the idea that children may need different levels of coaxing. If a child does not say much it cannot be assumed that they have nothing to say. It is worth paying attention to contexts. Exploring the meaning of mental health to the child and the family will reveal much about their understanding and the work that lies ahead for everyone. It is important to avoid making assumptions or trying to explain things in a way that supports one's own world view.

Clinical case example

At a workshop, a clinician asked how he should best manage a situation in which a Pakistani Muslim father always spoke for his female child. The clinician was unsure whether it would be appropriate for him as a male to ask to see the child alone.

There are, of course, different ways to approach this potential dilemma. One way forward is to consider for whom the clinician has primary responsibility. Although child psychiatrists have a responsibility to ensure that parents' perspectives are heard, the overriding responsibility is to the young person. Children and adolescents should be offered an opportunity to meet alone with the clinician. If both the child and the parent feel that this is inappropriate, this should be accepted unless there are other concerns such as abuse. However, it does not mean there is no need to explore what worries the parent about the child being seen alone. If the parent does not wish for the child to be seen alone but the child indicates that they would like to take this option, weight has to be given to the child's view, especially if they are older. Some clinicians fear that this will set up tensions in the family, but it is likely that the situation only illustrates what is already happening or what underlies the presentation. Furthermore, there are legislative frameworks within which clinicians are obliged to work. The Convention on the Rights of the Child 1989 covers all children in the UK irrespective of race, ethnicity or religion. Whether authoritarian parents want their children to have a viewpoint or not is not the point: children have a right to be heard.

Developing attitudes

Younger children will often accept their families values and what their family tells them, although wider societal or cultural expectations can sometimes override the family even at this stage. As children move into adolescence, cultural expectations are more likely to influence their developing sense of identity and they may challenge and question the values that they have grown up with. It is often assumed that there are more likely to be 'cultural differences' between parents and young people in minority ethnic families, especially when the children experience one culture at home and another outside the home. The explanation given is that the parents may hold views consistent with their ethnic origin, whereas adolescents face the task of integrating the wider culture in which they are growing up with their family's culture. It is often described in terms of the collective sense of identity of 'Eastern cultures' versus the focus on the individual of 'Western cultures'. In practice, most families have their own unique culture. Furthermore, cultural practices often vary between the private (usually the home) and public domains (school or work). Different families and young people manage in different ways. Some integrate the culture of origin and the culture of the new country, some switch between cultures depending on the context, and some fuse elements of both cultures (Dogra, 2009).

Box 16.2 lists some of the problems that commonly arise as children approach adolescence and adulthood. The young person may respond by challenging their parents, rebelling and becoming non-compliant, self-harming and/or becoming moody and withdrawn. They may become depressed, especially if they feel there is no possibility of resolution.

Bhui et al (2005) investigated cultural identity as a factor for mental health problems among adolescents. Integrated friendships (that is, friendships across groups) conferred advantages in all cultural groups. Girls with integrated (non-traditional) clothing choices and boys with integrated friendship choices had fewer mental health problems. This highlights how young people have to negotiate their way round a public world and their private lives. Referring back to the AAMC definition, it enables us to see that young people have a myriad of options and depending on the context will express different parts of themselves.

Kirmayer et al (2003) reported on a cultural consultation service designed to improve the delivery of mental healthcare in mainstream settings for a culturally diverse population. Their evaluation of the first 100 cases referred to the service demonstrated the impact of previous cultural misunderstandings: incomplete assessments, incorrect diagnosis,

Box 16.2 Issues that may give rise to problems during late childhood and adolescence

- Pressures to conform to the family's religious or other practices that the young person cannot reconcile with their own beliefs
- Pressures to conform to expected gender roles (e.g. boys wanting to pursue careers generally considered to be in the female domain, such as nursing or child care, and vice versa)
- Pressures to conform to the family's social norms (e.g. an expectation that a young person will go on to further education even if they do not want to)
- Pressures to conform to family expectations that differ from what the young person wants (e.g. an expectation that the young person will work in the family business)
- Sexual orientation
- Impending forced marriages
- Difficulty in reconciling the culture in the private and public domains

inadequate or inappropriate treatment and failed treatment alliances. Clinicians reported satisfaction with the new service. The authors concluded that such an approach can improve existing services and that clinicians need training in working with interpreters and culture brokers.

Such problems arise not only where two ethnically different cultures interact. Young people and their parents may have different cultural preferences regarding mental healthcare providers. In a survey of Gujarati families in the UK, a number of adults said that it might be useful to have a mental healthcare provider who spoke Gujarati; this was not something that young people raised (Dogra *et al*, 2007c). For some parents, language was linked to appropriate communication and accessible care. However, it can be difficult to distinguish language from cultural and ethnicity issues, and cultural values are variously interpreted. In our study, the quality of the service overall appeared to be more important than any other factor to both young people and their parents. Ethnicity did not appear to be an overriding factor for the participants. These findings indicate the need for caution, for further evidence and for debate on whether Black and minority ethnic families should be treated as a homogeneous group. Rather than passing on the responsibility to culture brokers, it might be argued that clinicians should be acquiring the appropriate skills to ensure they better meet the needs of their patients.

Conclusion

Cultural influences play a role in child and adolescent mental healthcare that is perhaps more complex than in other areas of psychiatry. First, the child's own the attitudes and behaviour are to a greater or lesser extent culturally influenced. Second, children are dependent on their families, and the culture and beliefs of those families – the meaning of family and how families respond to their children – will affect the child and be brought into the consultation room. Third, there may be a complex relationship between the wider culture and the micro-familial culture. And fourth, the challenge of trying to balance the wider culture and the culture of their family might itself have led the young person to mental health services. In practising child psychiatry, the clinician must strike a balance between the concerns and perspectives of the parents and those of the child. Negotiating this with families requires sensitivity but cannot be ignored. To initiate appropriate interventions, clinicians need to ensure that they are mindful of their own perspectives and how these interplay with those of the family and the child. Only if these issues are acknowledged and addressed will it be possible to devise management plans that are clinically sound but also acceptable to the young patient and the family.

References

Baumrind, D. (1966) Effects of authoritative parental control on child behaviour. *Child Development*, **37**, 887–907.

Bhui, K., Stansfield, S., Hood, J., *et al* (2005) Cultural identity, acculturation, and mental health among adolescents in east London's multiethnic community. *Journal of Epidemiology and Community Health*, **59**, 296–302.

Carter, E. A & McGoldrick, M. (1989) *The Changing Family Life Cycle: A Framework for Family Therapy* (2nd edn). Gardner.

Daryanani, R., Hindley, P., Evans, C., *et al* (2001) Ethnicity and the use of a child and adolescent mental health service. *Child Psychology and Psychiatry Review*, **6**, 127–132.

Dogra, N. (2004) Commissioning and delivering culturally diverse child and adolescent mental services. *Current Opinion in Psychiatry*, **17**, 243–247.

Dogra, N. (2007) Cultural diversity issues. In *Mental Health Interventions and Services for Vulnerable Children and Young People* (ed. P Vostanis): pp. 233–243. Jessica Kingsley.

Dogra, N. (2009) Culture and society. In *The Young Mind: An Essential Guide to Mental Health for Young Adults, Parents and Teachers* (eds S. Bailey & M. Shooter): pp. 210–217. Bantam Press.

Dogra, N., Frake, C., Bretherton, K., *et al* (2005) Training CAMHS professionals in developing countries: an Indian case study. *Child and Adolescent Mental Health*, **10**, 74–79.

Dogra, N., Vostanis, P. & Frake, C. (2007a) Child mental health services: cultural diversity training and its impact on practice. *Clinical Child Psychology and Psychiatry*, **12**, 137–142,

Dogra, N., Vostanis, P. & Karnik, N. (2007b) Child and adolescent psychiatric disorders. In *Textbook of Cultural Psychiatry* (eds D. Bhugra & K. Bhui): pp. 301–313. Cambridge University Press.

Dogra, N., Vostanis, P., Abuateya, H., *et al* (2007c) Children's mental health services and ethnic diversity: Gujarati families' perspectives of service provision for mental health problems. *Transcultural Psychiatry*, **44**, 275–291.

Dwairy, M. (2004) Parenting styles and mental health of Palestinian-Arab adolescents in Israel. *Transcultural Psychiatry*, **41**, 233–252.

Dwairy, M. & Menshar, K. E. (2006) Parenting style, individuation and mental health of Egyptian adolescents. *Journal of Adolescence*, **29**, 103–117.

Garland, A. F., Lewczyk-Boxmeyer, C., Gabayan, E. N., *et al* (2004) Multiple stakeholder agreement on desired outcomes for adolescents' mental health services. *Psychiatric Services*, **55**, 671–676.

Goodman, A., Patel, V. & Leon, D. A. (2008) Child mental health differences amongst ethnic groups in Britain: a systematic review. *BMC Public Health*, **8**, 258.

Green, G., McGinnity, A., Meltzer, H., *et al* (2005) *Mental Health of Children and Young People in Great Britain, 2004*. Office for National Statistics (http://www.data-archive.ac.uk/doc/5269%5Cmrdoc%5Cpdf%5C5269technicalreport.pdf).

Hackett, L. & Hackett, R. (1993) Parental ideas of normal and deviant child behaviour. A comparison of two ethnic groups. *British Journal of Psychiatry*, **162**, 353–357.

Heywood, C. (2001) *A History of Childhood: Children and Childhood in the West from Medieval to Modern Times*. Polity Press.

Kirmayer, L. J., Groleau, D., Guzder, J., *et al* (2003) Cultural consultation: a model of mental health services for multicultural societies. *Canadian Journal of Psychiatry*, **48**, 145–153.

Klineberg, E., Clark, C., Bhui, K. S., *et al* (2006) Social support, ethnicity and mental health in adolescents. *Social Psychiatry and Psychiatric Epidemiology*, **41**, 755–760.

Lincoln, B. (2009) A mixed race experience. Intermix (http://www.intermix.org.uk/Events/Bradley%20Lincoln.asp).

Macoby, E. E. & Martin, J. A. (1983) Socialisation in the context of the family: parent–child interaction. In *Handbook of Child Psychology. Vol. 4: Socialisation, Personality and Social Development* (4th edn) (eds P. H. Mussen & E. M. Hetherington): pp. 1–101. John Wiley & Son.

McLoyd, V., Cauce, A., TakeuchI, D., *et al* (2000) Marital processes and parental socialization in families of color: a decade review of research. *Journal of Marriage and the Family*, **62**, 1070.

Meltzer, H., Vostanis, P., Dogra, N., *et al* (2009) Children's specific fears. *Child: Care, Health and Development*, **35**, 781–789.

Mukherji, C. (1997) Monsters and muppets: the history of childhood and techniques of cultural analysis. In *From Sociology to Cultural Studies* (ed. E. Long): pp. 155–184. Blackwell Publishers.

Platt, F. W., Gaspar, D. L., Coulehan, J. L., *et al* (2001) Medical writing. Tell me about: the patient-centered interview. *Annals of Internal Medicine*, **134**, 1079–1085.

Pumariega, A. J., Rogers, K. & Rothe, E. (2005) Culturally competent systems of care for children's mental health: advances and challenges. *Community Mental Health Journal*, **41**, 539–555.

Rousseau, C., Measham, T. & Bathide-Suidan, M. (2008) DSM–IV, culture and child psychiatry. *Journal of the Canadian Academy of Child and Adolescent Psychiatry*, **17**, 69–75.

Task Force on Spirituality, Cultural Issues, and End of Life Care (1999) Task Force report: spirituality, cultural issues and end of life care. In *Report III: Contemporary Issues in Medicine. Communication in Medicine* (eds Association of American Medical Colleges). Association of American Medical Colleges.

Yeh, M., Hough, R., McCabe, K., *et al* (2004) Parental beliefs about the causes of child problems: exploring racial/ethnic patterns. *Journal of the Canadian Academy of Child and Adolescent Psychiatry*, **43**, 605–612.

CHAPTER 17

Black and minority ethnic issues in forensic psychiatry

David Ndegwa

Summary This chapter looks at some of the experiences of patients of Black (African and African–Caribbean) descent in forensic psychiatric hospitals and the likely effects of some aspects of the new mental health legislation in England and Wales. It describes the difficulties in meeting the objectives set out in the government's Delivering Race Equality programme and makes suggestions on the way forward through a focus on reducing length of stay in institutions, implementing preventive strategies to reduce the number of people who move into tertiary psychiatric services and improving the experience of those in hospital through a cultural consultation intervention.

The experience of Black service users within forensic psychiatric services in the UK has remained largely unchanged over the past decade. It is similar to that of Black patients in secondary mental healthcare services, as summarised in a Department of Health publication *Inside Outside* (Sashidharan, 2003). This document brought together evidence from clinical and epidemiological research, clinical observations, anecdotal accounts and testimonies of service users and carers. It summarised the problems of mental healthcare as experienced by Black and minority ethnic groups to be:

- the overemphasis on institutional and coercive models of care
- the prioritising of professional and organisation requirements over individual needs and rights
- institutional racism within mental healthcare services.

Institutional racism

Despite the conclusion reached by Professor Sashidharan in *Inside Outside*, the Department of Health disagrees with the existence of institutional racism (also called structural or systemic racism) in mental healthcare services. Retired judge Sir John Blofield, in the independent report following the death of David Bennett in a medium secure unit, reported that institutional racism was present throughout the National Health Service (NHS) and that greater effort was needed to combat it. He noted that until that problem is addressed, people from Black and minority ethnic communities will not be treated fairly. He described the experiences of patients poignantly: 'the black and minority ethnic community have a very real fear of the Mental Health Service. They fear that if they engage with the mental health services they will be locked up for a long time, if not for life, and treated with medication which may eventually kill them' (Norfolk, Suffolk & Cambridgeshire Strategic Health Authority, 2003: p. 42). In rejecting Judge Blofield's charge of institutional racism, the then Health Minister Rosie Winterton is reported to have said that the term institutional racism was not helpful and that organisations often used it as an excuse for their failure to tackle discrimination (Batty 2005). She did, however, acknowledge that there was clear evidence that Black people and people from ethnic minorities were less likely to access mental health services early enough, more likely to be forcibly treated and detained and more likely to be given medication and electroconvulsive therapy than psychological therapies.

Not surprisingly, the concept and existence of institutional racism have been subject to debate in the field of psychiatry. In October 2007, the *Psychiatric Bulletin* devoted its Opinion & debate section to the subject, led by Professor Swaran P. Singh (Singh, 2007).

Experiences

A number of documents have summarised the general experience of people from the UK's Black and minority ethnic groups in secure care as particularly negative and often not aiding recovery (e.g. Sainsbury Centre for Mental Health, 2002; Sashidharan, 2003; Department of Health, 2005). Compared with the White British population, they are at increased risk of coercive care, of admission or transfer to a secure unit, particularly a medium or high secure facility, on average they spend more time in hospital and they are less likely to have social care and psychological needs met in care planning and treatment processes. Black people also have an increased risk of readmission.

These experiences are reinforced by the Count Me In census reports for 2008 (Healthcare Commission, 2008). This annual census was first conducted in 2005 and will be repeated until 2010. The 2008 census collected information from 31 020 in-patients in mental health hospitals and 4107 in-patients in learning disability (intellectual disability) hospitals in both NHS and independent healthcare in England and Wales. It showed that compulsory admission rates, admissions from the criminal justice system, numbers of people placed on Section 37/41 of the Mental Health Act 1983 (a Section 37 hospital order together with a Section 41 restriction order), control and restraint and seclusion incidents remained higher for

Black people than for any other ethnic group. The recently published 2009 census shows that the situation is broadly similar to that in 2008 (Care Quality Commission, 2010).

Coid *et al* (2001) reported high rates of admission of Black men to secure forensic psychiatric services and high-risk patterns of escalating criminal and dangerous behaviour among this group, associated with repeated admissions to increasing levels of security. They found that these patterns were more prevalent among African–Caribbean men than among all other groups, suggesting that community-based services may be less successful in interventions with this group, and recommended preventive interventions to improve aftercare for high-risk patients. Both Coid *et al* (2001) and Guite (2003) found a linear relationship between admission rates to secure forensic psychiatric services and measures of social economic deprivation in the patients' catchment area of origin. Guite (2003) recommended a review of the provision of services to people with mental health and drug-related problems, and a review of pathways to special hospital care and to mental health and secure mental healthcare for minority ethnic groups. She also recommended a detailed examination of what goes on inside secure units.

I believe that one reason for the pressure to increase numbers of secure beds might be the failure to discharge patients fit for discharge because of a lack of clinical, financial or managerial incentives.

Problems and solutions

Anecdotal evidence and my own observations of practice in medium secure units indicate problems that might explain the long periods of stay for both White and minority ethnic patients. These observations, some of which are listed in Box 17.1, need to be grounded in research of what goes on inside medium secure units.

In addition to understanding what goes on inside medium secure units once patients are admitted, we have a long way to go before understanding the reasons behind the high rates of compulsory admissions to secure services. Research on conduct disorder and personality disorder may help shed some light and lead to preventive interventions in primary or secondary care.

The presence of personality disorder (with or without co-occurring disorders such as substance misuse) might explain the difficulty that primary and secondary services have with patients who later end up offending or showing challenging behaviours that can be only be managed in forensic establishments. Personality disorders in Black patients are rarely diagnosed within the NHS (National Institute for Mental Health in England, 2003) and one can speculate on the reasons for this. Hodgins & Müller-Isberner (2004) identified a group of forensic patients with a history of offending before the age of 18, alcohol misuse or dependence at first admission, antisocial personality disorder and deficient affective experience

---

Box 17.1 Observed problems in medium secure units

- Infrequent or absent formal risk assessments based on appropriate tools such as structured clinical judgement tools
- Infrequent or absent objective assessment of psychopathology, with absence of interventions directed at offending behaviour or delays in providing appropriate interventions
- Use of polypharmacy or high-dose medication
- Inappropriate use of seclusion
- Lack of innovative unit design and practices in managing violence
- Problems in diagnosis for Black and minority ethnic patients
- Slow decision-making or indecisiveness on the part of clinicians
- Lack of assertive delivery of interventions or use of good clinical practice guidelines
- Failure to recognise the heterogeneous nature of presentations (assessed needs, diagnosis) and failure to match this with staff skills and competencies
- Ineffective interventions and treatments
- Fostering of a dependency culture and a culture of low expectations

---

and showed that their pathway in and out of service differed from that of other forensic patients with mental illness.

Black ethnic minorities are over-represented among children and adolescents with conduct disorder (Meltzer *et al*, 2000). McCabe *et al* (2001) found that individual and family factors were more strongly related to childhood-onset conduct disorder, whereas minority ethnic status and exposure to 'deviant' peers were more strongly associated with onset in adolescence. Coid *et al* (2002) reported similar findings, identifying differences between Black and White prisoners in terms of upbringing and the prevalence of risk factors thought to be proxy measures of poor parenting during childhood. These differences appear to be accounted for by adolescent- and late-onset criminality in the Black prisoners. About half of the children with conduct problems develop antisocial personality disorder in adulthood. Studies show that the younger the age at onset of conduct disorder in Black children, the more likely is its persistence and transition to antisocial personality disorder, although this may be different in different ethnic communities (De Brito & Hodgins, 2009). They also hypothesise that among Black children living in socially disadvantaged neighbourhoods of the UK whose conduct problems start in adolescence, for reasons not currently understood there is a high rate of transition to antisocial personality disorder in adulthood and the factors associated with the persistence of their antisocial behaviour into adulthood are specific to this group. Among people who develop schizophrenia in adulthood the prevalence of conduct disorder prior to age 15 is much higher than in the general population. Studies have shown that using large doses of cannabis during adolescence is a trigger for psychosis (Arseneault *et al*,

2004; Konings *et al*, 2008). Hodgins (2008) hypothesises that adolescents with conduct disorder are at very high risk of cannabis misuse. Research on gene–environmental interplay between cannabis and psychosis may identify other risk factors (Henquet *et al*, 2008).

The studies of the association between conduct disorder, development of mental illness and pathways in the psychiatric system indicate an urgent need for examination of the prevalence and impact of personality disorder in Black patients with psychosis and for assessment of the impact of comorbid personality disorder on pathways into and out of care, engagement with community services before and during admission, and risk of harm to others. Studies of the association between conduct disorder and mental illness also strengthen the case for early intervention in childhood and adolescence to disrupt the transition from conduct disorder to antisocial personality disorder (Matthew & Scott, 2005) and to increase resilience and reduce vulnerability to developing psychosis.

Policy

In 2005, the UK government launched a 5-year action plan entitled Delivering Race Equality in Mental Healthcare (Department of Health, 2005), the objectives of which are listed in Box 17.2. The focus of the programme was equality of access, equality of experience and equality of outcomes. Unfortunately, the results of the 2008 and Count Me In censuses suggest that these objectives are unlikely to met soon. Part of this failure is that they are not supported by any performance management frameworks within the NHS, so there are no incentives to meet them. Another major reason is that clinicians who are key decision makers in the admission and discharge process and in what goes on in hospital have not been properly engaged in the programme.

Challenges

There is a paucity of interventions that can reduce compulsory admissions to hospital, improve the experience of those who are detained in hospital, increase the period spent in remission in the community or increase rates of referral back to primary and secondary care services for Black and minority ethnic individuals. The absence of a particular focus on ensuring that clinicians find ways of reducing coercion through service redesign, reorganisation, preventive interventions or new treatments means that the current situation is likely to continue.

Managers and clinicians also need to ask themselves what can be done to early intervention services, home treatment services, partial hospitalisation programmes and assertive outreach services to improve their accessibility and ability to engage people from ethnic minorities, for whom such services

---

Box 17.2   Key objectives of Delivering Race Equality

- To reduce fear of mental health services among Black and minority ethnic communities and service users
- To increase satisfaction with services
- To reduce the rate of admission of people from Black and minority ethnic communities to psychiatric in-patient units
- To reduce the disproportionate rates of compulsory detention of Black and minority ethnic service users in in-patient units
- To reduce the number of violent incidents that are secondary to inadequate treatment of mental illness
- To reduce the use of seclusion of patients from Black and minority ethnic groups
- To prevent deaths in mental health services following physical interventions
- To enable more Black and minority ethnic service users to reach self-reported states of recovery
- To reduce the ethnic disparities found in prison populations
- To achieve a more balanced range of effective therapies such as peer support services and psychotherapeutic and counselling treatments, as well as pharmacological interventions that are culturally appropriate and effective
- To give Black and minority ethnic communities and service users a more active role in the training of professionals, the development of mental health policy and the planning and provision of services
- To achieve a workforce and organisation capable of delivering appropriate and responsive mental health services to Black and minority ethnic communities

(Department of Health, 2005)

---

will be expected to be more acceptable, given their non-institutional nature. The active ingredients of services (mainly focusing on non-psychotic disorders) led by or specifically for the Black and minority ethnic community that have been reported to have particularly good relationships with ethnic minorities need to be identified and incorporated into existing or new services.

Outreach and Support in South London (OASIS), run by a multidisciplinary team within the South London and Maudsley NHS Foundation Trust, focuses on identifying and intervening with people in the prodrome of psychosis or in at-risk mental states. It has been particularly successful at engaging people from ethnic minorities. Moreover, among those managed by OASIS, there are no significant differences between ethnic groups in rates of psychosis, hospital admission and use of the Mental Health Act (P. Byrne, personal communication, 2009).

Community development workers who are the focus of the recruitment and training under the Delivering Race Equality programme may not have the background, knowledge and status to make any long-term impact on the clinical policy and procedures that are relevant in reducing coercion.

Box 17.3 Community treatment orders and restriction orders

Community treatment orders:

- were brought in by the 2007 Amendments to the Mental Health Act 1983
- patients can be treated in the community for their mental disorder without their consent
- apply only to patients who had previously been under Section 3 of the Mental Health Act or to unrestricted Part 3 patients
- patients must have a mental disorder of a nature or degree that makes it appropriate for them to receive medical treatment

Restriction orders:

- are a form of community treatment order – they differ in that they are a Court sentence for persons convicted of an imprisonable offence
- they are added to a hospital order when the Courts feel that they are necessary to protect the public from harm.

In England at least, Black patients are likely to be over-represented among those receiving the new community treatment orders (Box 17.3), just as they are over-represented among those who are in receipt of a Section 37/41 under the Mental Health Act. The history of poor relations with psychiatric services is likely to be repaid by large numbers on these new orders. In my view, the patients who are likely to be vulnerable to be placed on these orders are those with a history of poor adherence with medication in the community, of a revolving-door relationship with services, of hostility to services, of what clinicians describe as insight or attitude problems and of antisocial behaviour (even where these are not related to psychosis). Added to these aspects of the patient's history is the clinician's need to act defensively and the fear that patients from Black and minority ethnic groups generate in services as a result of issues such stereotyping, bias and racism. This is all compounded by any perceptions the clinician might have that responses to previous challenging and difficult behaviours have been inadequate and that new powers to compel patients to comply with treatment are needed.

There is very little literature critical of restriction orders, which suggests that they are generally well accepted by clinicians. In my experience, Black patients, however, see these orders as a type of a life sentence. Despite the concerns of the Black community, it seems likely that more Black patients are going to end up on them. In my view, patients in the community perceive restriction orders to be intrusive and coercive, and their primary effect thus far has been to increase the duration of in-patient stays in secure units. Forensic clinicians need to address these different experiences and perceptions.

Cultural competency

It is possible that increasing the cultural competency of individuals and organisations will improve the relationship between patients from Black and minority ethnic groups and their clinicians. However, as Kleinman & Benson (2006) have warned, there is a danger that the concept of 'cultural competency' may suggest that culture can be reduced to a technical skill in which clinicians can be trained to develop expertise. Thus, cultural competency becomes simply a series of do's and don'ts that define how to treat a patient from a given ethnic background. These authors argue that this problem stems from how culture is defined in medicine, which is at variance with its use in anthropology (where the concept originated). They believe that the optimum way to increase clinicians' sensitivity to cultural difference is to train them in ethnography. Ethnography differs from cultural competency in that it does not use the trait approach and instead emphasises engagement with others and the practices that people undertake in their local worlds. The clinician tries to understand the illness as the patient understands, feels, perceives and responds to it. An approach that has been used to synthesise the products of the ethnographic study of a case is the cultural formulation, the best known of which appears in the Appendix of DSM–IV (American Psychiatric Association, 1994). Kleinman & Benson suggest modifications to this approach and describe six steps of a culturally informed care (Box 17.4). They emphasise that the most important thing is for clinicians to ask the patient what matters most to them in their experience of illness and treatment. The clinician can then use that information in thinking through treatment decisions and negotiating with patients.

Most of Kleinman & Benson's objectives can be delivered within cultural consultancy interventions (Kilshaw *et al*, 2002; Kirmayer *et al*, 2003; Bhui *et al*, 2007). Cultural consultancy involves a process of eliciting cultural narratives through an ethnographic study of the patient, then using the material generated to construct a cultural formulation which

---

Box 17.4   Six steps of culturally informed care

- Determine whether ethnic identity is an important part of the self
- Evaluate what is at stake
- Describe the patient's illness narrative
- Describe psychosocial stressors
- Describe the influence of culture on clinical relationships
- Take into account the question of efficacy, e.g. potential side-effects of a cultural competency approach

(Kleinman & Benson, 2006)

---

is used in assessment and care planning. This approach can lead to an improvement in communication, improved patient experience, fewer cultural misunderstandings, fewer incomplete assessments, fewer incorrect diagnoses and fewer instances of inadequate or inappropriate treatment and failed treatment alliances. There is also increased patient ownership of the product of the intervention, ranging from ownership of the formulation and diagnosis to the treatment plan. There is a reduction in conflict and stigma. Information on cultural narratives that is obtained in the consultation can be used in interventions designed around the needs of ethnic minorities, e.g. forms of narrative therapy. The aim of cultural consultancy is to change the patient experience, thus changing the relationship with the clinician, making services more relevant, changing patients' use of services and in the process reducing patients' vulnerability to coercion.

Conclusion

One of the most important interventions to improve the experience of people from Black and minority ethnic groups in forensic services would be to focus on reducing the length of in-patient stay. This should occur in the context of a culturally sensitive environment. Reduction in length of stay will require better assessments of presenting psychopathology and risk. It will require more assertive treatments using the best available clinical practice guidelines and incorporating cognitive–behavioural interventions for reducing antisocial and offending behaviour. A recovery-based approach will increase patients' involvement in their care and improve their acquisition of self-management skills. It will also challenge current ideologies in forensic services and foster a more collaborative approach to working with patients. In the community, emphasis should be on relapse prevention for both antisocial behaviour and illness, while at the same the reducing dependence and increasing social inclusion.

References

American Psychiatric Association (1994) *Diagnostic and Statistical Manual of Mental Disorders (4th edn) (DSM–IV)*. APA.

Arseneault, L., Cannon, M., Witton, J., *et al* (2004) Causal association between cannabis and psychosis: examination of the evidence. *British Journal of Psychiatry*, **184**, 110–117.

Batty, D. (2005) NHS 'not institutionally racist'. *Society Guardian*, Tuesday 11 January.

Bhui, K., Warfa, N., Edonya, P., *et al* (2007) Cultural competence in mental health care: a review of model evaluations. *Biomed Central Health Services Research*, **7**, 15.

Care Quality Commission (2010) *Count Me In 2009: Results of the 2009 National Census of Inpatients and Patients on Supervised Community Treatment in Mental Health and Learning Disability Services in England and Wales*. Care Quality Commission.

Coid, J., Kahtan, N., Cook, A., *et al* (2001) Predicting admission rates to secure forensic psychiatry services. *Psychological Medicine*, **31**, 531–539.

Coid, J., Petruckevitch, A., Bebbington, P., *et al* (2002) Ethnic differences in prisoners. 2: Risk factors and psychiatric service use. *British Journal of Psychiatry*, **181**, 481–487.

De Brito, S. A. & Hodgins, S. (2009) Antisocial personality disorder. In *Personality, Personality Disorder and Violence: An Evidence Based Approach* (eds M. McMurran & R. Howard): pp. 133–154. John Wiley & Sons.

Department of Health (2005) *Delivering Race Equality in Mental Health Care: An Action Plan for Reform Inside and Outside Services and the Government's Response to the Independent Inquiry into the Death of David Bennett*. TSO (The Stationery Office).

Guite, H. (2003) *South East London Mentally Disordered Offenders Needs Assessment 1 & 2*. Greenwich PCT for the South East London Public Health network.

Healthcare Commission (2008) *Count Me In 2008: Results of the 2008 National Census of Inpatients in Mental Health and Learning Disability Services in England and Wales*. Commission for Healthcare Audit and Inspection.

Henquet, C., Di Forti, M., Morrison, P., *et al* (2008) Gene–environment interplay between cannabis and psychosis. *Schizophrenia Bulletin*, **34**, 1111–1121.

Hodgins, S. (2008) Violent behaviour among people with schizophrenia. A framework for investigations of causes, and effective treatment, and prevention. *Philosophical Transactions of The Royal Society B*, **363**, 2505–2518.

Hodgins, S. & Müller-Isberner, R. (2004) Preventing crime by people with schizophrenic disorders: the role of psychiatric services. *British Journal of Psychiatry*, **185**, 245–250.

Kilshaw, S., Ndegwa, D. & Curran, J. (2002) *Between Worlds – Interpreting Conflict between Black Patients and their Clinicians*. Lambeth, Southwark & Lewisham Health Action Zone (http://www.selphnet.nhs.uk).

Kirmayer, L. J., Groleau, D., Guzder, J., *et al* (2003) Cultural consultation: a model of mental health service for multicultural societies. *Canadian Journal of Psychiatry*, **48**, 145–153.

Kleinman, A. & Benson, P. (2006) Anthropology in the clinic: the problem of cultural competency and how to fix it. *PLoS Medicine*, **3** (10): e294.

Konings, M., Henquet, C., Maharajh, H. D., *et al* (2008) Early exposure to cannabis and risk for psychosis in young adolescents in Trinidad. *Acta Psychiatrica Scandinavica*, **118**, 209–213.

Matthew, W. & Scott, S. (2005) Evidence-based management of conduct disorders. *Current Opinion in Psychiatry*, **18**, 392–396.

McCabe, K. M., Hough, R., Wood, P. A., *et al* (2001) Childhood and adolescent onset conduct disorder: a test of the developmental taxonomy. *Journal of Abnormal Child Psychology*, **29**, 305–316.

Meltzer, H., Gatward, R., Goodman, R., *et al* (2000) *Mental Health of Children and Adolescents in Great Britain*. TSO (The Stationery Office).

National Institute for Mental Health in England (2003) *Personality Disorder: No Longer a Diagnosis of Exclusion. Policy Implementation Guidance for the Development of Services for People with Personality Disorder*. Department of Health.

Norfolk, Suffolk & Cambridgeshire Strategic Health Authority (2003) *Independent Inquiry into the Death of David Bennett*. NSCSHA.

Sainsbury Centre for Mental Health (2002) *Breaking the Circles of Fear: A Review of the Relationship between Mental Health Services and African and Caribbean communities*. Sainsbury Centre for Mental Health.

Sashidharan, S. P. (2003) *Inside Outside: Improving Mental Health Services for Black and Minority Ethnic Communities in England*. Department of Health.

Singh, S. P. (2007) Institutional racism in psychiatry: lessons from inquiries. *Psychiatric Bulletin*, **31**, 363–365.

CHAPTER 18

Cultural perspectives on eating disorders

Rahul Bhattacharya, Anish Unadkat and Frances Connan

Summary Evidence suggests that both the presentation and prevalence of eating disorders has changed across history and cultures. This challenges earlier conceptualisations of these disorders as culture-bound syndromes, and raises important questions about aetiology. Culture may play a role in shaping the presentation as well as possibly affecting the prevalence of eating disorders. Although the evidence base is limited, current evidence of the pathoplastic role of culture in shaping the presentation of eating disorders and the pathofacilitative role of culture in the aetiology of the condition are discussed. The role of gender is similarly explored. Finally, the importance of cultural sensitivity in the development of future diagnostic criteria, treatment and service provision is discussed.

Eating disorders constitute a range of conditions associated with abnormal eating behaviour, with related cognitive, emotional, behavioural and physiological components. Anorexia nervosa and bulimia nervosa are the two most well-described eating disorders. Although a medical conceptualisation of anorexia nervosa goes back to the last quarter of the 19th century, bulimia nervosa was first described as a 'variant' of anorexia nervosa only three decades ago (Russell, 1979). Anorexia nervosa and bulimia nervosa remain the most commonly studied eating disorders, but the majority of people presenting for treatment in the UK do not meet the diagnostic criteria for these disorders and are classified as 'eating disorder not otherwise specified' (EDNOS) (Fairburn & Bohn, 2005). Prevalence of the different forms of eating disorders vary across cultures, e.g. among African–Caribbean and Latino people in the USA binge eating disorder was found to be the most common diagnosis (Hudson et al, 2007).

Eating disorders were once thought to affect only young women in affluent Western societies. This led to the suggestion that anorexia nervosa may be a culture-bound syndrome of the West (Prince, 1983). This notion was later challenged by the demonstration that eating disorders are not confined to one particular culture or socioeconomic class (Hoek et al, 2003). Eating disorders may therefore be culturally reactive rather than culture-bound phenomena (Caradas *et al*, 2001), and their expression may be influenced by gender and culture (Reiger, 2007). Cultural plasticity presents a challenge in understanding and diagnosing eating disorders for the forthcoming fifth revision of the *Diagnostic and Statistical Manual of Mental Disorders* (Striegel-Moore & Wonderlich, 2007).

Cultural psychiatry is concerned with understanding the impact of social and cultural differences on mental illness and aims at minimising misunderstandings resulting from misinterpretations across cultures. The study of mental illnesses in non-Western countries has demonstrated commonalities of certain conditions across the globe, along with awareness of new and unusual syndromes, which have subsequently been described as culture bound. Culture influences psychopathology in many ways (Tseng, 2001). We believe that two of these processes are relevant in understanding how culture affects both the presentation and the prevalence of eating disorders. Culture can shape the manifestations of symptoms in such a way that disorders are recognised as 'atypical' or 'variations' of the recognised Western stereotype of the condition. This is described as a *pathoplastic* impact of culture on a mental illness. This is relevant in the atypical or 'non-fat-phobic' variants of anorexia nervosa. Culture can also make it easier for certain conditions to develop and increase their prevalence in certain populations, without affecting the presentation of individual cases. This is known as the *pathofacilitative* effect. Concern about body shape and association of slimness with female beauty may lead to discontent with one's own body shape, adversely affecting eating behaviours and resulting in an increase in disordered eating and bulimic behaviours with Westernisation. We discuss these phenomena in more detail in the following sections.

The pathoplastic model

The focus on the drive for thinness in the eating disorders literature is often attributed to Hilde Bruch, a German-born American psychoanalyst, through her works in the second half of the 20th century. The universality of this drive for thinness in both anorexia and bulimia nervosa is questionable. Non-fat-phobic or atypical variants of eating disorders have been documented historically in the West and in contemporary non-Western cultures.

From a historical perspective, Vandereycken & van Deth (1994) have suggested that self-starvation is a pervasive phenomenon in human history. In medieval times many women who ultimately became saints engaged in self-starvation, including Hedwig of Silesia (13th century) and Catherine of Siena (14th century). Saint Catherine of Sienna lost a significant amount of weight during her adolescence by fasting and by vomiting after eating. She described her motivation as an expression of her dedication to God. Although advised to pray so that she would be able to eat again, she was unable to give up fasting. There is no mention of a wish to be thin. Anorexia nervosa was first described by Sir William Withey Gull and Dr R. Lasègue, in 1874 and 1873 respectively. Of note is that neither Gull nor Lasègue considered anything resembling a drive for thinness in their description of the condition. At the Mayo Clinic in the USA between 1917 and 1929, 103 out of 107 patients with anorexia nervosa attributed their weight loss to gastrointestinal disturbances, including vomiting (56%), fullness and bloating. Issues of weight and shape were not mentioned (Berkman, 1930). Western society has changed significantly over the past century. Anorexia nervosa is now a well-recognised trans-Atlantic phenomenon. It is possible that as Western culture has changed, the content of beliefs about the illness has evolved, bringing a fear of fatness to the fore.

In a recent study of anorexia nervosa among female secondary school students in Ghana, the body mass index (BMI) of 668 students was measured. The 10 students with a BMI <17.5 kg/m^2 appeared to have self-starvation as the only cause of their low weight. All 10 viewed their food restriction positively and in religious terms. The content of beliefs about the illness included ideas of self-control and denial of hunger, without the typical anorexic concerns about weight or shape (Bennett et al, 2004). These beliefs bear a striking resemblance to those of the fasting saints of medieval Europe. A survey among adolescents in London found that Asian adolescents were more likely than their White British peers to use fasting as a way to control weight, and presented this in a religious context. Fasting as a religious matter is common among the Indian diaspora (Bhugra & Bhui, 2003). A survey looking into the prevalence of abnormal eating attitudes among South African schoolgirls from different ethnic backgrounds reported that mixed-race and Black participants exhibited less concern about body image and lower levels of dissatisfaction with their bodies than White participants (Caradas et al, 2001). A non-fat-phobic variant of anorexia nervosa is not uncommon in non-Western cultures. In a Hong Kong study, 41 out of 70 patients with anorexia nervosa had no fear of fatness. Instead, they reported epigastric fullness, bloating and a lack of appetite (Lee 1993). In the UK, South Asian adolescents with eating disorders in north London presented less frequently with fat phobia or weight preoccupation and more frequently with loss of appetite than White British adolescents (Tareen et al, 2005). Similarly, American Asian adolescents had lower scores on the Eating Disorder Examination questionnaire subscales, particularly the restraint and weight concern subscales, compared with the non-Asian sample (Lee & Lock, 2007). This variance in phenomenology across cultures suggests a pathoplasticity to the expression of the disorder that warrants further study. It is possible that the concepts of control and restraint might not translate well across different cultures, but a myriad of other possibilities may explain this phenomenon.

Although religious sanction for fasting perhaps provided justification for food avoidance in medieval Europe and contemporary African cultures, alternative explanatory models of mental health, such as yin and yang, may be more pertinent in Hong Kong and some Asian American populations. In eating disorders, particularly anorexia nervosa, the motivation associated with food restriction and weight loss appears to be shaped by the person's cultural beliefs and value system. Therefore there is a pathoplastic effect on manifestation of eating disorders, particularly surrounding the symptoms of pursuit of thinness and fear of fatness. These findings raise the question of whether pursuit of thinness and fear of fatness should be considered 'core symptoms' in future editions of diagnostic classifications.

The pathofacilitative model

Westernisation and acculturation

Western society has, for at least the past 50 years, idealised a thin female body shape. For example, 70% of the women who appeared in *Playboy* magazine centrefolds between 1978 and 1998 were underweight, i.e. had a BMI less than 18.5 (Katzmarzyk & Davis, 2001). The incidence of eating disorders in the West rose significantly during that period, raising the possibility that cultural pressure to be thin may increase the risk of eating disorders. Others have argued that the spread of Westernisation has led to the spread of eating disorders in primarily urban non-Western cultures such as Egypt (Nasser, 2004).

Becker *et al* (2002) examined the impact of the introduction of television, as a proxy for Westernisation, on the eating habits in a traditional, non-Western community in Fiji. The study prospectively examined the prevalence of eating disorder attitudes and beliefs (measured using the Eating Attitudes Test (EAT–26) self-report questionnaire) before and after the introduction of television to Fiji. This brought with it modern, mainstream US portrayals of women into Fijian homes and was associated with a significantly increased score on the EAT–26 and significantly higher levels of dieting and self-induced vomiting. Seventy-four per cent of the participants reported that they felt too big or fat at least some of the time after the introduction of television. Seventy-seven per cent reported that television had influenced their own body image. Traditional Fijian culture endorsed a fuller body shape and the population was relatively media naive. The authors argue that television's effects may be mediated through the peer environment by influencing community aesthetic ideals and stimulating consumerism. This study suggests that Western media may have a profoundly negative impact on body image and disordered eating attitudes and behaviour, even in traditional societies in which eating disorders have been thought to be rare.

Studies in urban South Asia argue that the influence of Westernisation through globalisation has resulted in the spread of eating disorder to non-Western societies. However, none of these studies formally measured Westernisation. A survey of 369 schoolgirls was conducted in Lahore,

Pakistan, using the EAT–26 and Body Shape Questionnaire (BSQ) in English. Girls who scored highly on either questionnaire were invited for interview. One girl met DSM–III–R criteria for bulimia nervosa and five were diagnosed with a partial syndrome of bulimia nervosa. There were no cases of anorexia nervosa (Mumford *et al*, 2006). In Mumbai, India, a survey of student volunteers found that 13.3% of the 451 volunteers, including men, reported abnormal eating attitudes on EAT–26 (Tendulkar *et al*, 2006). A study examining bulimia nervosa in North India concluded that perhaps the degree of concordance between sociocentric views was important in explaining the low rates of bulimia nervosa in the region. It was thought that expectations of the young females interviewed were linked with those of their families and society in general (Bhugra *et al*, 2000). This looks at the influence of Westernisation (which is closely associated with egocentric societies) from a different perspective. Rather than Westernisation being a risk factor, sociocentric views were proposed to be a protective factor against eating disorders.

In a large UK survey of Bradford schoolgirls, the prevalence of bulimia nervosa was 3.4% among Asian girls, compared with 0.6% in White girls. Among the Asians, high EAT–26 and BSQ scores were associated with a more traditional cultural orientation and not with greater Westernisation (Mumford *et al*, 1991; Furnham & Adam, 2001). The relationship between Westernisation and prevalence of eating disorders is therefore complex. What is common in these contradictory findings is that the individual is exposed to conflicting value systems, be it being Westernised in a largely traditional society or coming from a traditional non-Western background into Western society.

This issue has also been examined from the perspective of acculturation. Acculturation among Asian adolescents in London was associated with higher scores on the Bulimia Investigation Rate, Edinburgh (BITE) questionnaire (Bhugra & Bhui, 2003). However, acculturation levels were not correlated with EAT–26 scores in Korean women in the USA (Jackson *et al*, 2006). More Western-oriented Korean American women scored significantly lower on the EAT–26 than Korean immigrants and native Koreans. Once again, acculturation studies have not yielded consistent results.

It is possible that societal pressure to be thin is not an exclusive Western influence that has spread through globalisation. In analysing symptoms in Japanese adolescent girls with eating disorders, Mukai *et al* (1994) argue that contemporary Japanese society shares many values with Western society, including the thin body standard for attractiveness in women, and this is not necessarily a result of Western influences but is itself a tradition in Japan. This might be true for Eastern European countries as well. For example, one study carried out in Georgia when the country was relatively isolated and shielded from the effects of globalisation found significant levels of anorexia nervosa and bulimia nervosa in women with a fear of fatness (Tchanturia *et al*, 2002).

Family factors

Evidence of occurrence of eating disorders in historical and contemporary cultures in which thinness is not idealised, for example medieval Europe (Vandereycken & van Deth, 1994), Ghana (Bennett *et al*, 2004) and Georgia (Tchanturia *et al*, 2002), suggests that globalisation of the drive for thinness may be neither necessary nor sufficient on its own to explain the presence of eating disorders. Other cultural factors might therefore be equally important.

The family is a structural unit of society and is influenced by traditions and ideals. While for an individual, the family can be a source of support and care, it can also be a continual source of conflict. A study comparing clinical characteristics and phenomenology of anorexia nervosa in Asian and non-Asian adolescents in the USA revealed that Asians were demographically similar to their non-Asian peers but tended to come from higher-income families who were more achievement oriented (Lee & Lock, 2007). In Israel, Israeli-born, secular, Jewish, urban, Ashkenazi (Western-origin) women from families with higher levels of parental education were over-represented among eating disorder clinic attendees (Latzer *et al*, 2008). Higher educational level was significantly associated with risk of an eating disorder among the Malay ethnic group in Singapore (Ho *et al*, 2006). Culturally influenced family factors, such as pressure to achieve, may also therefore increase the risk of developing an eating disorder.

An idiom of distress

Cultural conflict and stress in many forms, be it Westernisation or pressure to succeed, have been associated with risk of disordered eating behaviour. Eating disorders might therefore represent a form of maladaptive coping behaviour, or an idiom through which vulnerable individuals may express their distress. Stress may be related to reduced acceptance of self, disharmony between reality and expectations, or conflicting societal, familial and personal values. Individuals attempting to cope with their cultural identity may use eating disorder as a tool of self-communication (Nasser *et al*, 2001). Cultural factors may influence an individual's choice of idiom of distress. In a US college-based eating disorder screening programme, binge eating was found to be the best predictor of distress in Whites, Hispanics and African–Caribbeans but vomiting was the best predictor of distress in Asians (Franko *et al*, 2007).

Are eating disorders increasing?

A recent article in a UK newspaper was headlined 'Anorexia doubles in a decade' (*Metro*, 2009). However, such claims about anorexia nervosa are not substantiated by thorough epidemiological studies. The article reported that the number of adolescents treated in a specialised unit had doubled in 10 years, but this is clearly not a reliable measure of community prevalence. It is true that an upward trend was observed in the incidence of anorexia nervosa in the UK in the past century until the 1970s. However, between 1988 and 2000 the incidence of anorexia nervosa presenting to primary care was relatively constant, whereas the incidence of bulimia nervosa increased in the early 1990s and then declined somewhat in the late 1990s (Currin et al, 2005). These findings were replicated in a Dutch primary care survey (Hoek et al, 1995; Hoek, 2006). Again, because this was a primary care survey and not a community sample, it is unclear whether the increased incidence of bulimia nervosa reflects a true rise in incidence or a rise in help-seeking behaviour. The timing of the increase coincided with increased media coverage of well-known figures with eating disorders, such as Diana, Princess of Wales, and the authors therefore argue that the increase may at least in part be due to increased help-seeking (the 'Diana Effect'). This view is supported by the fact that a large number of women in their 30s contributed to the peak in incidence, probably representing late presentation of undiagnosed community cases.

Genes

Since the aetiology of the eating disorders is thought to be an interaction between a person's genes and the environment in which they develop (Fairburn et al, 1999), both genetic factors and cultural factors can potentially mediate cultural pathofacilitation. In Curaçao, no cases of anorexia nervosa were identified among the majority Black population, whereas the incidence among the minority mixed and White population was similar to that of the USA (Hoek et al, 2005). This is consistent with absence of anorexia nervosa cases in Black African or Caribbean populations in other US surveys (Striegel-Moore et al, 2003; Taylor et al, 2007). Hispanic Americans have elevated rates of binge eating disorder but low prevalence of anorexia nervosa and bulimia nervosa (Striegel-Moore et al, 2003; Alegria et al, 2007). These differences in prevalence between ethnic groups within the same environment raise the possibility that genetic factors modulate the expression of environmental risk. In Curaçao, the minority mixed-ethnicity and White women who were found to suffer from anorexia nervosa were also caught between the two cultural experiences and were more likely to have studied and travelled abroad (Katzman et al, 2004).

Gender

Studies have consistently shown eating disorders to be far more prevalent in women, but the ratios vary depending on the study. One study reported a relative risk of 40:1 (females:males) for anorexia nervosa and 47:1 for bulimia nervosa (Turnbull et al, 1996). What accounts for this wide variation is poorly understood. Katzman & Lee (1996) hypothesised that women straddling 'two worlds', be they generational, work–family or traditional and modern cultural values, may employ food denial as an instrument for negotiating the transition. It is possible that women who are faced with transgenerational values or are trapped in a state of cultural transition may struggle with their frame of reference. Disordered eating may be an attempt to cope with a sense of disconnection. However, this pathofacilitative explanation may not account for the gender difference in eating disorders on its own. Biological factors such as hormonal exposure and body composition are also likely to play a key role.

It has been questioned whether gender, like culture, can influence the expression of the condition (Regier, 2007). Do women and men express themselves differently? In this context, 'machismo nervosa' has been suggested as a variant of eating disorder in men who engage in body building associated with binge eating, dietary restriction, diuretics, fluid restriction, repeated self-weighing, mirror checking and use of anabolic steroids in an attempt to achieve their ideal shape. They also show high levels of body dissatisfaction, perfectionism, ineffectiveness and reduced self-esteem compared with others, and tend to underestimate their size by 15% (Connan, 1998). Men are more likely to report overeating, whereas women are more likely to report loss of control over eating (Striegel-Moore et al, 2009). Studies of bulimia nervosa found increased prevalence of homosexuality or bisexuality in men with the disorder compared with women. The authors suggested that this higher prevalence is associated with increased emphasis on physical appearance in gay culture (Carlat et al, 1997).

Few studies look into eating disorders in men. It is even less studied across cultures. Studies examining eating disorders in men across different cultures are sparse and there is a lack of well-conducted epidemiological studies. Studies are limited to case series or population surveys in select populations, for example a case series of five men with anorexia nervosa in urban China (Tong et al, 2005). A survey in a selected population in India found a significant proportion of male participants who reported disorder eating (Tendulkar et al, 2006). Overall, there is too little literature on cross-cultural eating disorders in males to conclude anything beyond the fact of their existence.

Service implications

The idea that eating disorders affect only young, White women from affluent backgrounds has long been disproved, but the legacy may live on in the service models we employ. Minority ethnic groups such as South Asians in the UK are at increased risk of bulimia nervosa. However, patients from minority ethnic groups, and males, were under-represented in referrals to specialist eating disorder services in south London (Waller et al, 2009). Similarly, immigrants in the USA and those living a greater percentage of their lifetime in the USA evidenced higher risk for certain eating disorders, whereas rates of treatment utilisation were exceedingly low in this population (Alegria *et al*, 2007). The ethnicity of women described in case vignettes significantly affected the capacity of participants (undergraduate students) to recognise an eating disorder (Gordon *et al*, 2002). This suggests that a lack of cultural sensitivity may be preventing significant numbers of people from accessing effective treatment. Non-fat-phobic anorexia nervosa has been reported to have better prognosis (Lee *et al*, 2003). It would be a missed opportunity for these cases to lie undetected in the community. Greater awareness of the cultural pathoplasticity of eating disorders is essential if we are to achieve equality of access to services.

The other major issue in terms of service organisation is the public health concerns surrounding obesity. Societal pressure to be thin may increase as obesity becomes more prevalent. Indeed, to accommodate ethnic differences in body weight and associated vascular risk, the World Health Organization has adjusted the 'normal range' for BMI from 20–25 to 18.5–25, reducing the window between normalcy and anorexia nervosa (from BMI = 17.5–20 to BMI = 17.5–18.5). It remains to be seen what effect this will have on prevalence of eating disorders. Obesity remains a risk factor for bulimia nervosa and related disorders (Fairburn *et al*, 1997), so an increase in demand for eating disorder services should be anticipated.

Conclusion

Transcultural studies in eating disorders are often faced with methodological problems that make interpretation of results difficult. Primary care surveys are affected by care pathways, help-seeking behaviour and the ability to identify atypical cases. Many of the studies have relied on self-report questionnaires, which are prone to sampling and response bias. The validity of questionnaires such as the EAT-26 in different cultural settings is debatable (King & Bhugra, 1989). Studies looking into risk factors have rarely been of adequate design to establish causality. Studies often screen for 'disordered eating' and do not establish a diagnosis of eating disorder itself. Nonetheless, there is some evidence to support the hypothesis that cultural factors such as Westernisation, acculturation and drive for achievement increase the risk of bulimia nervosa and related disorders. These findings support a pathofacilitative hypothesis for bulimia nervosa. Future studies with more robust design are desirable to overcome these challenges. A focus on the interplay between genes, gender and culture in shaping the expression of eating disorders would be particularly useful.

Few epidemiological studies have examined rates of eating disorder in the general population, with the Curaçao study (Katzman *et al*, 2004; Hoek *et al*, 2005) being a rare exception. However, these studies have demonstrated that eating disorders, particularly anorexia nervosa, occur across diverse cultures and that the notion of eating disorders as a culture-bound syndrome is no longer valid. The evidence of relative stability of the incidence of anorexia nervosa in Europe and the USA supports the pathoplastic model for this disorder. The phenomenology of eating disorders presents a challenge to those preparing DSM–V and has been widely debated (Franko, 2007). Cultural plasticity needs to be considered in understanding and diagnosing eating disorder for DSM–V (Striegel-Moore & Wonderlich, 2007). Weight loss and the impact of this on the human physiology have demonstrable cross-cultural validity, but the BMI threshold for diagnosis and the beliefs associated with the illness are clearly less robust. Diagnostic cross-over between eating disorders over time further adds to the uncertainty about diagnostic classification (Eddy *et al*, 2008). Well-designed, multicentre studies to identify core phenomenology across cultural and ethnic groups around the world are necessary to establish consensus diagnostic criteria.

While we await clarification on diagnosis, greater awareness of atypical forms of eating disorder, together with education to challenge stereotypes in the minds of the public and clinicians, is paramount to reducing barriers to accessing treatment. Awareness of cultural factors and variants within eating disorders is necessary to provide equitable and quality care.

References

Alegria, M., Woo, M., Cao, Z., *et al* (2007) Prevalence and correlates of eating disorders in Latinos in the United States. *International Journal of Eating Disorders*, **40**, S15–S21.

Becker, A. E., Burwell, R. A, Herzog, D. B., *et al* (2002) Eating behaviours and attitudes following prolonged exposure to television among ethnic Fijian adolescent girls. *British Journal of Psychiatry*, **180**, 509–514.

Bennett, D., Sharpe, M., Freeman, C., *et al* (2004) Anorexia nervosa among female secondary school students in Ghana. *British Journal of Psychiatry*, **185**, 312–317.

Berkman, J. M. (1930) Anorexia nervosa, anorexia, inanition and low basal metabolic rate. *American Journal of the Medical Sciences*, **180**, 411.

Bhugra, D. & Bhui, K. (2003) Eating disorders in teenagers in East London: a survey. *European Eating Disorder Review*, **11**, 46–57.

Bhugra, D., Bhui, K. & Gupta, K. R. (2000) Bulimic disorders and sociocentric values in north India. *Social Psychiatry and Psychiatric Epidemiology*, **35**, 86–93.

Caradas, A. A., Lambert, E. V. & Charlton, K. E. (2001) An ethnic comparison of eating attitudes and associated body image concerns in adolescent South African schoolgirls. *Journal of Human Nutrition and Dietetics*, **14**, 111–120.

Carlat, D. J., Camargo, C. A. & Herzog, D. B. (1997) Eating disorder in males: a report on 135 patients. *American Journal of Psychiatry*, **154**, 1127–1132.

Connan, F. (1998) Machismo nervosa: an ominous variant of bulimia nervosa? *European Eating Disorders Review*, **6**, 154–159.

Currin, L., Schmidt, U., Treasure, J., *et al* (2005) Time trends in eating disorder incidence. *British Journal of Psychiatry*, **186**, 132–135.

Eddy, K. T., Dorer, D. J., Franko, D. L., *et al* (2008) Diagnostic crossover in anorexia and bulimia nervosa: issues for DSM–V. *American Journal of Psychiatry*, **16**, 245–250.

Fairburn, C. G. & Bohn, K. (2005) Eating disorder NOS (EDNOS): an example of the troublesome "not otherwise specified" (NOS) category in DSM–IV. *Behaviour and Research Therapy*, **43**, 691–701.

Fairburn, C. G., Welch, S. L., Doll, H. A., *et al* (1997) Risk factors for bulimia nervosa. A community-based case–control study. *Archives of General Psychiatry*, **54**, 509–517.

Fairburn, C. G., Cowen, P. J. & Harrison P. J. (1999) Twin studies and the etiology of eating disorders. *International Journal of Eating Disorders*, **26**, 349–358.

Franko, D. L. (2007) Race, ethnicity, and eating disorders: considerations for DSM–V. *International Journal of Eating Disorders*, **40**, S31–S34.

Franko, D. L., Becker, A. E., Thomas, J. J, *et al* (2007) Cross-ethnic differences in eating disorder symptoms and related distress. *International Journal of Eating Disorders*, **40**, 156–164.

Furnham, A. & Adam, S. S. (2001) Abnormal eating attitudes and behaviours and perceived parental control: a study of white British and British-Asian school girls. *Social Psychiatry and Psychiatric Epidemiology*, **36**, 462–470.

Gordon, K. H., Perez, M. & Joiner, T. E. Jr (2002) The impact of racial stereotypes on eating disorder recognition. *International Journal of Eating Disorders*, **32**, 219–224.

Ho, T. F., Tai, B. C., Lee, E. L., *et al* (2006) Prevalence and profile of females at risk of eating disorders in Singapore. *Singapore Medical Journal*, **47**, 499–503.

Hoek, H. W. (2006) Incidence, prevalence and mortality of anorexia and other eating disorders. *Current Opinion in Psychiatry*, **19**, 389–394.

Hoek, H. W., Bartelds, A. I., Bosveld, J. J., *et al* (1995) Impact of urbanization on detection rates of eating disorders. *American Journal of Psychiatry*, **152**, 1272–1278.

Hoek, H. W., van Hoeken, D. & Katzman, M. A. (2003) Epidemiology and cultural aspects of eating disorders: a review. In *Eating Disorders* (eds M. Maj, K. Halmi, J. J. López-Ibor, *et al*): pp. 75–104. John Wiley & Sons.

Hoek, H. W., van Harten, P. N., Hermans, K. M. E., *et al* (2005) The incidence of anorexia nervosa on Curaçao. *American Journal of Psychiatry*, **162**, 748–752.

Hudson, J., Hiripi, E., Pope, H. Jr, *et al* (2007) The prevalence and correlates of eating disorders in the National Comorbidity Survey Replication. *Biological Psychiatry*, **61**, 348–358.

Jackson, S. C., Keel, P. K. & Lee, Y. H. (2006) Trans-cultural comparison of disordered eating in Korean women. *International Journal of Eating Disorders*, **39**, 498–502.

Katzman, M. A. & Lee, S. (1996) Beyond body image: the integration of feminist and transcultural theories in the understanding of self starvation. *International Journal of Eating Disorders*, **22**, 385–394.

Katzman, M. A, Hermans, K. M. E., Van Hoeken, D., *et al* (2004) Not your "typical island woman": anorexia nervosa is reported only in subcultures in Curaçao. *Culture, Medicine and Psychiatry*, **28**, 463–492.

Katzmarzyk, P. T. & Davis, C. (2001) Thinness and body shape of Playboy centerfolds from 1978 to 1998. *International Journal of Obesity*, **25**, 590–592.

King M. B. & Bhugra, D. (1989) Eating disorders: lessons from a cross-cultural study. *Psychological Medicine*, **19**, 955–958.

Latzer, Y., Vander, S. & Gilat, I. (2008) Socio-demographic characteristics of eating disorder patients in an outpatient clinic: a descriptive epidemiological study. *European Eating Disorders Review*, **16**, 139–146.

Lee, H. & Lock, J. (2007) Anorexia nervosa in Asian-American adolescents: do they differ from their non-Asian peers. *International Journal of Eating Disorders*, **40**, 227–231.

Lee, S. (1993) How abnormal is the desire for slimness? A survey of eating attitudes and behaviours among Chinese undergraduates in Hong Kong. *Psychological Medicine*, **23**, 437–445.

Lee, S., Chan, L. Y. Y. & Hsu, L. K. G. (2003) The intermediate term outcome of Chinese patients with anorexia nervosa in Hong Kong. *American Journal of Psychiatry*, **160**, 967–972.

Metro (2009) Anorexia 'doubles' in a decade. *Metro*, 17 February (http://www.metro.co.uk/news/article.html?Anorexia_%91doubles%92_in_a_decade&in_article_id=541881&in_page_id=34).

Mumford, D. B., Whitehouse, A. M. & Platts, M. (1991) Sociocultural correlates of eating disorders among Asian schoolgirls in Bradford. *British Journal of Psychiatry*, **158**, 222–228.

Mumford, D. B., Whitehouse, A. M. & Choudry, I. Y. (2006) Survey of eating disorders in English-medium schools in Lahore, Pakistan. *International Journal of Eating Disorders*, **11**, 173–184.

Mukai, T., Crago, M. & Shisslak, C. M. (1994) Eating attitudes and weight preoccupation among female high school students in Japan. *Child Psychology and Psychiatry*, **35**, 677–688.

Nasser, M. (2004) Screening for abnormal eating attitudes in a population of Egyptian secondary school girls. *Social Psychiatry and Psychiatric Epidemiology*, **29**, 25–30.

Nasser, M., Katzman, M. A. & Gordon, R. A. (eds) (2001) *Eating Disorders and Cultures in Transition*. Psychology Press.

Prince, R. (1983) Is anorexia nervosa a culture-bound syndrome? *Transcultural Psychiatric Research Review*, **20**, 299–300.

Reiger, D. A. (2007) Diagnosing eating disorder in DSM–V: new nosological perspectives. *International Journal of Eating Disorders*, **40**, S8–S9.

Russell, G. (1979) Bulimia nervosa: an ominous variant of anorexia nervosa. *Psychological Medicine*, **9**, 429–448.

Striegel-Moore, R. H. & Wonderlich, S. (2007) Diagnosis and classification of eating disorders: finding the way forward. *International Journal of Eating Disorders*, **40**, S1.

Striegel-Moore, R. H., Dohm, F. A., Kraemer, H. C., *et al* (2003) Eating disorders in white and black women. *American Journal of Psychiatry*, **160**, 1326–1331.

Striegel-Moore, R. H., Rosselli, F., Perrin, N., *et al* (2009) Gender difference in the prevalence of eating disorder symptoms. *International Journal of Eating Disorders*, **42**, 471–474.

Tareen, A., Hodes, M. & Rangel, L. (2005) Non-fat-phobic anorexia nervosa in British South Asian adolescents. *International Journal of Eating Disorders*, **37**, 161–165.

Taylor, J., Caldwell, C. H., Baser, R. E., *et al* (2007) Prevalance of eating disorder in Blacks in the National Survey of American Life. *International Journal of Eating Disorders*, **40**, S10–S14.

Tchanturia, K., Katzman, M., Troop, N. A., *et al* (2002) An exploration of eating disorders in a Georgian sample. *International Journal of Social Psychiatry*, **48**, 220–230.

Tendulkar, P., Krishnadas, R., Durge, V., *et al* (2006) Study of eating attitudes and behaviours in junior college students in Mumbai, India. *Journal of Child and Adolescent Mental Health*, **18**, 43–48.

Tong, J., Miao, S. J., Wang, J., *et al* (2005) Five cases of male eating disorders in central China. *International Journal of Eating Disorders*, **37**, 72–75.

Tseng, W. S. (2001) *Handbook of Cultural Psychiatry*. Academic Press.

Turnbull, S., Ward, A., Treasure, J., *et al* (1996) The demand for eating disorder care. An epidemiological study using the general practice research database. *British Journal of Psychiatry*, **169**, 705–712.

Vandereycken, W. & van Deth, R. (1994) *From Fasting Saints to Anorexic Girls: The History of Self-starvation*. New York University Press.

Waller, G., Schmidt, U., Treasure, J., *et al* (2009) Ethnic origins of patients attending specialist eating disorders services in a multiethnic urban catchment area in the United Kingdom. *International Journal of Eating Disorders*, **42**, 459–463 .

Part 3

Management issues
in the cultural context

CHAPTER 19

Cross-cultural psychiatric assessment

Dinesh Bhugra and Kamaldeep Bhui

Summary Cultures affect the presentation of psychiatric symptoms, how and where help is sought, and also influence therapeutic engagement. Patients are generally interested in their illness, whereas clinicians are interested in dealing with the disease that patients present with. When assessing patients from other cultures, the clinician must be open-minded and explore symptoms in a culturally sensitive way. This includes a basic awareness of cultural norms and mores, and if the clinician is not aware of these, suitable sources of information must be explored. In this chapter we describe basic principles of assessment and outline good practice points.

Different cultures vary in their perceptions of mental illness (Karno & Edgerton, 1969), which can affect their utilisation of orthodox psychiatric facilities (Padilla *et al*, 1975; Sue, 1977). Mental health services may be seen by people from minority ethnic groups as challenging the value of traditional support systems, reflecting dominant Western cultural values and harbouring implicitly racist psychological formulations. The clinician–patient interaction may become fraught with misunderstandings if the two parties come from different cultural backgrounds and bring distinct cultural expectations to the encounter.

The concept of a core disease process with concentric rings of illness behaviour is a useful one, allowing the clinician to make sense of a diversity of surface phenomena which may all be related to a narrower range of disease categories. Thus, while the patient suffers from an 'illness', the clinician diagnoses and treats a 'disease' (Eisenberg, 1977; Kleinman, 1980). Yet classifications of illness vary across cultures, and individuals often carry such categories with them and use them to make sense of altered functioning. The clinician must identify whether a specific cluster of symptoms, signs and behavioural changes that are demonstrated by the patient are also interpreted consistently by them and their relatives, and how their personalised diagnostic models fit in with the psychiatric models.

Culture and mental illness

Culture can influence mental illness by defining the normal and the abnormal, by implicating domains of aetiological factors, by influencing the clinical presentation and by determining help-seeking behaviour. Cultural mechanisms can provide social support, socially acceptable emotional outlets, cathartic strategies and synchronisation of individual differences, which combine to give a meaningful and consistent world view. Such cultural determinants operate as much within the doctor's field of communication as among patients. The doctor–patient interaction is affected by the training, experience, social class and ethnicity of the doctor and by the experiences, educational and social background and ethnicity of the patient, as well as by shared and non-shared aspects of the economic and political climate. Gender, socioeconomic or educational status, lifestyle, job or professional role may overshadow the ethnic identity of the patient as communication barriers; if cultural variables are overemphasised, the service provider is guilty of stereotyping the patient, whereas if ethnic considerations are underemphasised, the doctor is guilty of insensitivity to influences that may affect the dynamics of the interview (Pedersen & Lefley, 1986).

Cross-cultural competency

Sue (1981) has proposed that minimal cross-cultural competency for counsellors lies in three spheres (which are equally applicable to clinicians). First, the beliefs and attitudinal competency of the doctor, including an awareness of their own cultural heritage, biases and values, feeling comfortable with differences in relationships and acknowledgement of the value of the patient's culturally consistent support structures. Second, knowledge competency: the doctor must understand the social structure of minority groups, possess adequate cultural knowledge about their clients, be competent in generic kills and be aware of institutional barriers that patients encounter. Third, skills competency, including a wide repertoire of verbal and non-verbal responses, and the ability to send and receive verbal and non-verbal messages accurately and appropriately, and exercise institutional intervention skills to change the constellation of existing systems of care if they are inappropriate. Similar skills should be nurtured by those wishing to improve communication with all their patients.

Psychiatric assessment

Assessment interviews should be used as the starting point for understanding a patient's distress and for developing a collaborative therapeutic relationship. However, it is not uncommon that a diagnosis is seen as the final stage in the consultation process. Linguistic difficulties compounded by uncertainty about the idioms of distress, coupled with time restrictions and the quick application of the biomedical models the clinician is used to, may lead to inappropriate conclusions. Some patients (whether for reasons of ethnicity or otherwise) require a longer assessment before a comprehensive management plan can be formulated that represents the optimal intervention for that particular individual.

The principles of quality consultation have been described from a multitude of theoretical frameworks (see Pedersen & Lefley, 1986; Fuller & Toon, 1988). An optimal assessment requires special attention to several contextual factors.

Communication and cultural distance

The principles outlined here are general guidelines for safe and sensitive practice. Before assessing a patient, it is important to find out about their culture, including taboos, rites of passage and religious values. First, the language in which the patient prefers to communicate must be identified. If this is not English, an interpreter must be found who can advise on non-verbal communication as well as identifying idioms of distress and 'emotional' words used by the patient. Gumperz *et al* (1982), for example, have demonstrated clear differences in conversational styles of East Indian English and British English. The former was found to be context-based and the latter more individual. Thus, the fact that there is a common language does not necessarily mean that communication will be adequate. An unstructured 10 minutes of 'emotional orientation', during which idioms of distress and emotional words can be identified, will help to show the direction in which the assessment must proceed (Box 19.1).

Box 19.1   Setting up the assessment

- Scrutinise your limits of competency
- Acknowledge how your skills can be blunted or affected by your culture
- Attend to the patient's limitations
- Know the predominant group in the culture and the patient's attitude to it
- Know the patient's skills and strengths
- Know the family's limits – their language limitations, sense of urgency, realistic capacity to cope and the coping strategies available to them
- Explore the family's skills and strengths – do not denigrate these if they appear idiosyncratic
- Explore the interpreter's role, skills and limitations: meet before the assessment to identify their knowledge of the patient's culture; identify sources of difference (e.g. dialect, tribe, religion, island); agree on the method of joint working (e.g. literal translation or use of interpreter to orient complaints within their cultural context)
- Ask whether the patient and family object to a particular interpreter
- Explain that total confidentiality must and will be observed

---

Essential historical information

Adverse events

Do not assume that life events, adverse or otherwise, have the same significance for patients as they do for you or that they have only the significance described in the literature. Flexible enquiry should elicit the impact of a patient's experiences. Separation from children, for example, may be more traumatic than you might imagine, perhaps with culturally unacceptable implications.

World view

World view is the way in which the clinician and the patient make sense of events, and varies depending on how the two individuals invest their worlds with meaning. As Sue (1981) has cautioned, the clinician or therapist is in danger of imposing or negatively interpreting the patient's world view if they are unaware of the basis for differences.

Other components of world view include group and individual identity and the patient's beliefs, values and cognitive perceptions of their distress and the help being offered. World view and identity can appropriately be ascertained only after several semistructured meetings with patients, family, advocates, and religious and community spokespersons nominated by the patient. For example, the Black American or European world view includes African history and culture and the legacy of slavery and racism. Cheatham (1990) suggests that in Afro-centric culture the individual is emphasised only in terms of others, and this world view is therefore interdependent and holistic, oriented to collective survival. In addition, it emphasises an oral tradition, uses a 'being' time orientation (rather than a 'doing' one), emphasises harmonious blending and cooperation, and stresses respect for certain roles, especially those of elders. A further example is given by Ivey *et al* (1993), who examined North American and Euro-centric views, which divide the world into discrete 'knowable' parts, handle emotions carefully, focus on self-actualisation and independence as goals in life, are oriented towards a linear view of time and stress individuation and difference rather than collaboration. To expect patients from other cultures to fit into these norms is bound to create problems in assessment as well as management.

Acculturation

No culture remains static. Contact with other cultures shapes fresh cultural expectations and behaviour across generations. Acculturation must be seen as a multidimensional phenomenon which reflects the changes individuals go through when they are exposed to a new culture. The emergence of a cultural identity, for example, is a complex process. In one model, individual identity is conceptualised in terms of seven concentric equivalents of psychoanalytic structures, only some of which interact with society and culture (see Hsu, 1985). Jackson (1975) has put forward a five-stage theory to explain the development of 'culture consciousness' in African Americans:

Box 19.2   Assessment of migration

- How long ago migration occurred
- Age of the patient at the time
- Motives for, difficulties in and preparedness for migration
- Reversibility of migration
- Differences between expectation and reality
- Experiences before, during and after arrival
- Migrated alone or in a group
- Attitudes towards new country and culture
- Helpfulness of the new society in adjustment
- Previous similar experiences

---

1   naivety – the individual has no awareness of self, and the colour of their skin (ethnic or cultural identity) plays no role in their life;

2   acceptance – personal identity becomes defined by the 'other'; this process can be passive or active and it often creates inner conflict;

3   resistance and naming – the individual identifies a 'Black' self and its full meaning in a racist society and may feel angry and frustrated;

4   redefinition and reflection – the main developmental task is to establish a firm African American consciousness in its own right;

5   a multiperspective internalisation – the individual is African American and sees this with pride in the self and awareness of the other.

Each of the five stages has an entry, adoption and exit point. An individual's identity is a complexity of interrelated definers of self and group identity and is not readily discernible from the ethnic category applied. Acculturation can be explored by determining features of the migration (Box 19.2) and by focusing on areas such as religious activity, diet and attitudes to traditional patterns of behaviour in the community (Box 19.3). It is important to bear

---

Box 19.3   Assessment of acculturation

- Religion – practice, frequency, who attends and where
- Languages – which are spoken where and with what frequency
- Marriage/family – type, attitudes to marriage, responsibility at home, gender roles, arranged marriages
- Employment – working with others of the same ethnicity, relationship to colleagues, work ethic
- Leisure activities – interests, languages spoken, films, music, preferences
- Food – type, where shopping takes place
- Aspiration and attitudes to self

---

in mind that not all cultures can be pigeonholed into traditional Western European psychoanalytic models of self-identity, and that individual experiences of migration and acculturation may not pass through the same stages or proceed at the same pace.

Psychological/somatic mindedness

Too often, the label of somatisation is applied in a derogatory manner, especially if there is poor communication between patient and clinician.

Although core depressive or psychotic symptoms are often regarded as universal, some see these constructs as disorders consistent merely with the Western world's conceptualisation of distress. Deep psychological reflection common in (parts of) the West appears to be relatively uncommon among the world's cultures and cannot be viewed on an evolutionary basis. India, for example, has a history of inner reflection which predates Western forms by millennia and which exhibits a depth and complexity that makes Western psychology look quite superficial, although it is found in theology and not (necessarily) in medical traditions (Leslie, 1977; Leslie & Young, 1992). In Japan, China and India, internal psychological explanations of suffering are neither sought nor seen as credible (Kleinman, 1980; Reynolds, 1980; Shweder, 1991). Gaines (1995) suggests that somatic experiences and delusions may be more common in societies that do not psychologise distress, which is to say, most cultures of the world.

Previous experiences

Previous experiences with treatments and services give a clue to the future working within the therapeutic relationship. These experiences are as valid for the clinicians as for the patients.

Racism

Patients from ethnic minorities are likely to have experienced discrimination in some fields of daily activity, whether it be open discrimination or suspected prejudicial treatment, on account of skin colour, religion, language, gender, ethnicity or other factors which may well be masked under a broader umbrella. One should not underestimate the impact of such events and invalid assumptions about their personal significance must be avoided. One should ask about such events in a careful, paced, sensitive manner so that the patient may respond accordingly. Even if perceived racist experiences do not directly contribute to the patient's presentation, such reports must be treated with respect; otherwise, the patient may find it difficult to trust the professional with more sensitive information.

Microskills for the clinician

Basic microskills for a clinician include those of attentive listening, influencing, focusing, confrontation and following of non-verbal cues. Patients may interpret the body language of the clinician as an early sign of the therapeutic encounter to be expected. It may be seen as intrusive, threatening or inviting. Eye-contact rituals and the significance attached to patterns of gaze avoidance vary across cultures. The patient may expect evidence of understanding from the clinician and, if this is not clear, may respond in a way that the clinician perceives to be either unduly docile or aggressive (Fuller & Toon, 1988). These form the basis of good clinical practice.

Limitations of standard mental state examinations

If the patient does not share the mental health professional's culture (regardless of skin colour) any symptoms and signs must be appraised critically in a cultural context and the appraisal revised in response to further information. Various cultural, religious and social groups are likely to have different and possibly unique idioms of distress but to list them would suggest that clinicians could and should follow a recipe of cultural assessment based on initial and perhaps erroneous impressions about the impact of cultural, religious and social differences. However, application of diagnostic processes without due attention to sociocultural influences (and cultural context) is likely to meet with numerous pitfalls (Rack, 1982).

Behaviour

Behaviours which to the assessing clinician might appear odd may have a culturally sanctioned role (e.g. speaking in tongues, extreme religiosity, trance and possession). These phenomena can only be evaluated by carefully recording the behaviour, the patient's explanation for it, and the family and the cultural group's response to it. These views, if a sign of illness, may change as the patient recovers and become important signs by which the patients, their carers and others may in future identify a relapse. Unusual behaviour which is not clearly understandable is too readily seen as evidence of psychosis without due attention to the adaptive or coping potential of the behaviour.

Aggression

One of the best documented gender differences is that males (particularly adolescents) are consistently more aggressive than females (Berry et al, 1992), men accounting for a disproportionate number of violent crimes in both industrial and developing nations (Goldstein, 1983). As Berry et al (1992) emphasise, cultural influences affect aggressive behaviour through culturally mediated childhood experiences. Barry et al (1976) reported a gender difference in the deliberate teaching and encouragement of aggression among children from a sample of nearly 150 societies. It has also been suggested that intergender identity developed by younger males because of almost exclusively female child-rearing is corrected either by severe male initiation ceremonies (Whiting et al, 1958) or by males asserting their manliness purely as a 'gender-making' behaviour. Segall et al (1990) propose that hostility, conflict, frustration and anger are all interrelated constructs, but that aggression is behaviour whereas frustration or anger are intent, and the two do not always go together. Aggression is also to be distinguished from assertiveness, the latter being more acceptable in some cultures. The aim here is not to discuss possible aetiological models, but to emphasise that there are important cultural contributions to aggression which need to be taken on board in assessment.

Aggression is too often labelled as a manifestation of psychosis. Potential aggression is difficult to anticipate and the interviewer may err on the side of caution by intervening too early with control and restraint. Early intervention may well jeopardise any future treatment alliance. The only way to assess a potentially aggressive patient is from a position of security regarding one's own safety. Ensure that you are accompanied and encourage a relative or friend of the patient to join you. There may be cultural norms of frustration, conflict resolution and aggression sanctions. Do not be prompted to anticipate an aggressive situation through your own fear of assault and uncertainty about a patient with whom you do not share cultural values, norms and mores.

Hallucinations

Hallucinations are traditionally defined as perceptions that lack sufficient basis in external stimuli even though the patient places their origin in the outside world (Leff, 1988). They are generally considered rare in normal people, but Rees (1971) demonstrated that nearly half of bereaved individuals experience hallucinations of the dead person for years after the loss but that the experience disappears as soon as the individual remembers that the other person is dead. In some cultures, this experience appears to have status value (Cheetham & Cheetham, 1976). In a random sample of the general population in the US state of Florida, young people, Black people and people of lower socioeconomic status were more likely to report hallucinations (Schwab, 1977). There was also a clear link with religious affiliation: among members of the Church of God one-fifth experienced hallucinations, whereas none who belonged to the Jewish faith did.

It is clear that hallucinations and delusions (see below) must be judged in relation to the patient's cultural milieu. The experiences of feeling presence of ancestors and hearing their voices or seeing them after their death are related to cultural norms and expectations. This also relates to concepts of self in which individuals may perceive their existence in relation to other family or extended family members or to the village (Morris, 1994).

Hallucinations were found by Mukherjee et al (1983) to be more frequent among Black people than White. Partly because of this, Black people were more likely to be erroneously diagnosed as having schizophrenia in spite of a preponderance of affective symptoms in their presentations. Ben-Tovim (1987) reported from his own experience in Botswana that, by framing the right questions, it is possible to differentiate between auditory hallucinations (in their psychopathological significance) and culturally normal experiences.

Hallucinations and paranoid thought may be understandable in some communities, where victimisation or persecution in everyday life may be reflected in a cautious approach and suspicious attitude towards strangers (including mental health professionals). The patient may not wish to reveal their true mental state; hence investment of time and repeated contact may be required before trust is established. Stress-induced psychoses may be the underlying cause of the symptoms and must be differentiated from schizophrenia (Rack, 1990). One should confirm exact experiences and consistency, and differentiate hallucinations from illusions and suggestibility states. If the patient uses figures of speech inexactly to articulate their illness experience, the clinician must avoid mistaking this for evidence of hallucination. Mukherjee *et al* (1983) demonstrated that in a sample of Black patients with bipolar affective illness 85% had a previous diagnosis of schizophrenia and a higher than expected proportion had auditory hallucinations. The presence of visual phenomena is especially difficult to place within the standard framework of psychopathology (Al-Issa, 1995).

Delusions

The traditional definition of delusion takes the role of culture and its context into account. As Rack (1990) emphasises, a cardinal rule of psychiatry is that a belief should not be classified as a delusion simply because it is erroneous; it must also be outside the range of normal beliefs for the culture to which the individual belongs. Appreciation of congruence with the patient's own culture is crucial in reaching a diagnosis; it is necessary to understand the culture within which individuals are embedded before deciding whether symptoms or beliefs are pathognomonic of underlying psychiatric disorder. There is some clinical evidence from the Caribbean suggesting that changing religions is often linked with the onset of symptoms – the individual is searching for some level of stability or a haven that may tolerate eccentricities (Bhugra *et al*, 2000).

The form and content of delusions must also be understood. The content is often derived from the patient's cultural milieu and is therefore most liable to be recognised as such by other members of their culture. Ben-Tovim (1987) has presented cases from Botswana in which patients (mostly with schizophrenia) were clearly seen as floridly mentally disturbed by their neighbours and other mental health professionals.

It has been argued that differences in the causes of psychoses, especially schizophrenia, are due to subtypes of the illness. Social and cultural factors strongly influence responses to people who are ill and both directly and indirectly influence the course of illness (Waxler, 1977). Desjarlais *et al* (1995) proposed that where an illness is considered an essential part of the self that cannot be expected to change (e.g. schizophrenia as an illness does not change, although a patient can change as a result of schizophrenia) it is more likely to be chronic. The support of the extended family, linked with their concept of the patient's illness, is likely to affect presentation,

---

Box 19.4 Suggested questions for explanatory models

- What do you call your concern/problem experience? What do others call it?
- What is the cause of your trouble?
- Why do you think it started (now) when it did?
- How do your symptoms affect you and others around you? What problems do they cause?
- How serious is your problem?
- Do you think it will have a long course?
- What do you fear most about your symptoms?
- Do you think treatment is needed for this?
- What treatment do you think might help, and with what results?

(modified from Kleinman, 1980)

---

cooperation and treatment. Thus, an understanding of the concepts of illness held by patients and their families' will be productive (Box 19.4).

Delusions are associated with more than 75 distinct clinical conditions in the USA, including schizophrenia, mania, paranoia, depression (Gaines, 1995). Given the enormous variety and distinctiveness of ideas found in cultures across the world, the criteria by which distinctions are drawn are not easy to grasp (Gaines, 1995). The necessity of knowing the cultural context of the presenting ideation suggests that delusion must be externalised and communicated; it should be unshared and be 'incredible' in a native local context. The determination of delusion requires an internal cultural judgement. As Sims (1995) points out, patients believe their delusions literally and certain delusions may be more common than others, and since the definition is made by an external observer, the evidence needs to be studied carefully.

It is unreasonable to expect the doctor to have an anthropological knowledge of all the belief systems likely to be encountered in a multicultural practice, but the patient's family and advocates, teachers and community leaders, and community or voluntary organisations should provide sufficient sources. It is possible that if the examiner is not clear about related cultural values, a delusional experience may be misattributed. Religious ideas, culturally sanctioned explanations, and spiritual or cosmic explanations must be carefully identified and documented verbatim. Do not just record your impressions. Always consider alternative reasons for a patient's beliefs with their relatives or advocates, and record their responses intact. If a belief is culturally unfamiliar and is coupled with functional impairment or culturally inappropriate behaviour, then it is likely to be a sign of illness.

First-rank symptoms

World Health Organization studies have demonstrated the existence of core symptoms of schizophrenia across cultures, although there is still debate in some anthropological quarters about the validity of such studies. There is considerable concern that first-rank symptoms can occur in other psychiatric states and in the course of culturally sanctioned methods of resolving distress (e.g. passivity, possession, exorcism, delusions of control; Jablensky, 1987). Anecdotal evidence also suggests that some first-rank symptoms are best picked up if a patient's first or preferred language is used for interviewing. Among Asian patients, for example, Schneiderian first-rank symptoms can and do occur in response to stress in people who have no family history of psychosis. As Rack (1990) described, symptom onset is often acute and dramatic, and onset clearly contemporaneous with life events and rapid initial response to treatment should suggest a reactive condition. Desjarlais *et al* (1995) have suggested that outcome of schizophrenia varies across cultures because of a myriad of environmental and psychological factors.

Cognitive assessment

Historical and theoretical aspects of cognition and the role of thought and language are beyond the scope of this chapter (Berry *et al*, 1992). Caroll & Casagrande (1958) have demonstrated that Navajo children, for example, are more likely to use form rather than colour as a basis for the classification of objects. Language is very important in shaping thinking as well as articulating thoughts. Berry *et al* (1992) argue that cognitive processes are likely to be universal but the local cultural meanings of cognitive competence will vary. The underlying theme is that cognitive functioning is related to ecological and cultural contexts – the task is to specify the general life requirements for the group as a whole and then to identify how these are communicated to the developing individual. The eco-cultural approach demands that work of this sort must be accomplished before an individual is assessed. Cultural definitions of 'intelligence' vary and holistic rather than analytic approaches may be valued in some groups (Berry, 1984). The cognitive competence of an individual in a particular culture should thus be conceived of as progress towards culturally valued cognitive norms (Berry *et al*, 1992). The role of literacy, language and education, along with other social and cultural factors, must be remembered before embarking on cognitive assessments. The processes of categorisation, sorting, memory and problem-solving also are affected by culture (Segall *et al*, 1990).

The standard cognitive assessment may yield very little diagnostic psychopathology if used blindly across cultures, especially if the patient's native tongue is different from that of the assessor or the assessment instrument. It is better to get third-party information on memory failure and intellectual decline. If schedules of cognitive assessment are available in the patient's primary language these must be employed bearing in mind the patient's level of education; once again, the help of an advocate or a team member who speaks the patient's first language can be invaluable (Box 19.5).

257

Box 19.5   Good practice points

- Elicit the first language, religion, self-defined ethnicity and identification with cultural groups (for each party concerned)
- Define and redefine terms used by you and the patient to ensure shared understanding
- Identify emotional idioms of distress and develop shared vocabulary with the patient
- Ask for clarification of the unfamiliar
- Assume nothing about the patient
- Do not be judgemental about patterns of communication or domination of the clinical interview by one family member
- Be sensitive to the effects of your actions
- Communicate total confidentiality
- Identify the scenario and setting where the patient may be most comfortable and relaxed (e.g. with family or alone?)
- Be sensitive to religious and social taboos
- Do not ask a child or relative to act as interpreter (unless there is no option)
- Involve patient advocates early, with the patient's consent
- Discuss findings with an independent person familiar with the culture and within the bounds of strict confidentiality

---

Further study

Much has been written on the influence of culture in the assessment of mental health disorders. For further information we recommend any of the texts listed in Box 19.6.

Box 19.6   Sources of further information

Bhugra, D. & Bhui, K. (eds) (2007) *Textbook of Cultural Psychiatry*. Cambridge University Press.

Bhui, K. & Bhugra, D. (eds) (2007) *Culture and Mental Health: A Comprehensive Textbook*. Hodder Arnold.

Cuellar, I. & Paniagua, F. (eds) (2000) *Handbook of Multicultural Mental Health: Assessment and Treatment of Diverse Populations*. Academic Press.

Tseng, W.-S. (2004) *Handbook of Cultural Psychiatry*. Academic Press.

Tseng, W.-S. & Strelzer, J. (eds) (1997) *Culture and Psychopathology: A Guide to Clinical Assessment*. Routledge.

Tseng, W.-S. & Strelzer, J. (2004) *Cultural Competence in Clinical Psychiatry*. American Psychiatric Press.

Conclusion

The patient's model of what a doctor does may be quite different from what you are able to offer. Some ethnic groups have a great respect for health professionals such that they may not confront, question, disagree or point out the problems they are facing. This may manifest later as selective omission of medication, inaccurate reporting of symptoms or consultation with other healers. Sometimes alternative healers are of benefit in treating the illness but some discourage or deter patients from attending standard healthcare services or, more commonly, offer excessive reassurance or promise of miraculous cure, which will encourage patients to disengage from mainstream services.

References

Al-Issa, I. (1995) The illusion of reality or the reality of illusion. Hallucinations and culture. *British Journal of Psychiatry*, **166**, 368–373.

Barry, H., Josephson, L., Lauer, E., *et al* (1976) Agents and techniques for child training: cross-cultural codes 6. *Ethnology*, **16**, 191–230.

Ben-Tovim, D. I. (1987) *Development Psychiatry: Mental Health and Primary Health Care in Botswana*. Tavistock.

Berry, J. W. (1984) Toward a universal psychology of cognitive competence. *International Journal of Psychology*, **19**, 335–361.

Berry, J. W. , Poortinga, Y. H., Segall, M. H., *et al* (1992) *Cross-Cultural Psychology: Research and Applications*. Cambridge University Press.

Bhugra, D., Hilwig, M., Mallett, R., *et al* (2000) Factors in the onset of schizophrenia: a comparison between London and Trinidad samples. *Acta Psychiatrica Scandinavica*, **101**,135–141.

Caroll, J. & Casagrande, J. (1958) The function of language classification in behaviour. In *Readings in Social Psychology* (eds E. Maccoby, T. Newcomb & E. L. Hartley), pp. 18–31. Holt, Rinehart & Winston.

Cheatham, H. (1990) Empowering Black families. In *Black Families* (eds W. H. Cheatham & J. Stewart), pp. 373–393. Transaction Press.

Cheetham, W. S. & Cheetham, R. J. (1976) Concepts of mental illness among the Xhosa people in South Africa. *Australian and New Zealand Journal of Psychiatry*, **10**, 39–45.

Desjarlais, R., Eisenberg, L., Good, B., *et al* (1995) *World Mental Health: Problems and Priorities in Low-Income Countries*. Oxford University Press.

Eisenberg, L. (1977) Disease and illness: distinctions between professional and popular ideas of sickness. *Culture, Medicine and Psychiatry*, **1**, 9–23.

Fuller, J. & Toon, P. (1988) *Medical Practice in a Multicultural Society*. Heinemann.

Gaines, A. D. (1995) Culture-specific delusions: sense and nonsense in cultural context. *Psychiatric Clinics of North America*, **18**, 281–301.

Goldstein, A. (1983) US: Causes, controls and alternatives to aggression. In *Aggression in Global Perspective* (eds. A. Goldstein & M. Segall), pp. 435–474. Pergamon.

Gumperz, J., Aulakh, G. & Kaltman, H. (1982) Thematic structure and progression in discourse. In *Language and Social Identity* (ed. J. Gumperz), pp. 22–56. Cambridge University Press.

Hsu, F. K. (1985) The self in cross-cultural perspective. In *Culture and Self: Asian and Western Perspectives* (eds A. J. Marsella, G. DeVos & F. K. Hsu), pp. 24–55. Tavistock.

Ivey, A. E., Ivey, M. B. & Simek-Morgan, L. (1993) *Counselling and Psychotherapy: A Multicultural Perspective*. Allyn and Bacon.

Jablensky, A. (1987) Multicultural studies and the nature of schizophrenia: a review. *Journal of the Royal Society of Medicine*, **80**, 162–167.

Jackson, B. (1975) Black identity development. *Journal of Educational Diversity and Innovation*, **2**, 19–25.

Karno, M. & Edgerton, R. G. (1969) Perceptions of mental illness in a Mexican–American community. *Archives of General Psychiatry*, **20**, 233–238.

Kleinman, A. (1980) *Patients and Healers in the Context of Culture*. University of California Press.

Kluckhohn, F. & Strodtbeck, F. (1961) *Variations in Value Orientations*. Row Peterson.

Leff, J. (1988) *Psychiatry around the Globe: A Transcultural View*. Gaskell.

Leslie, C. (1977) *Asian Medical Systems*. University of California Press.

Leslie, C. & Young, A. (eds) (1992) *Paths to Asian Medical Knowledge*. University of California Press.

Morris, B. (1994) *Anthropology of the Self: The Individual in Cultural Perspectives*. Pluto Press.

Mukherjee, S., Shukla, S., Woodle, J., *et al* (1983) Misdiagnosis of schizophrenia in bipolar patients: a multi-ethnic comparison. *American Journal of Psychiatry*, **140**, 1571–1574.

Padilla, A. M., Ruiz, R. A. & Alvarez, R. (1975) Community mental health services for the Spanish speaking/surnamed population. *American Psychologist*, **30**, 892–905.

Pedersen, P. B. & Lefley, H. P. (1986) Introduction to cross-cultural training. In *Cross-Cultural Training for Mental Health Professionals* (eds H. P. Lefley & P. B. Pedersen), pp. 5–10. Charles C. Thomas.

Rack, P. (1982) *Culture and Mental Disorder*. Tavistock.

Rack, P. (1990) Psychological/psychiatric disorders. In *Health Care for Asians* (eds B. R. McAvoy & L. J. Donaldson). Oxford University Press.

Rees, W. D. (1971) Hallucinations of widowhood. *BMJ*, **4**, 37–41.

Reynolds, D. (1980) *The Quiet Therapies: Japanese Pathways to Personal Growth*. University Press of Hawaii.

Schwab, M. E. (1977) A study of reported hallucinations in a south eastern country. *Mental Health and Society*, **4**, 344–354.

Segall, M., Dasen, P., Berrey, J., *et al* (1990) *Human Behaviour in Global Perspective*. Pergamon.

Shweder, R. (1991) *Thinking Through Western Cultures*. Harvard University Press.

Sims, A. (1995) *Symptoms of the Mind*. Ballière Tindall.

Sue, D. W. (1981) *Counselling the Culturally Different: Theory and Method*. Wiley.

Sue, S. (1977) Community mental health services to minority groups. *American Psychologist*, **32**, 616–624.

Waxler, N. (1977) Is outcome for schizophrenia better in non-industrial societies? *Journal of Nervous and Mental Diseases*, **167**, 144–158.

Whiting, J. W., Kluckhohn, R. & Anthony, A. (1958) The function of male initiation ceremonies at puberty. In *Readings in Social Psychology* (eds E. Maccoby, T. Newcomb & E. Hartley), pp. 359–370. Rinehart and Winston.

CHAPTER 20

Clinical management of patients across cultures

Dinesh Bhugra and Kamaldeep Bhui

Summary   The primary goals of this chapter are to set down some principles for planning treatment for patients from other cultural backgrounds and to place physical and psychological therapies in a culturally syntonic context. Psychological interventions need to be culturally appropriate in process and content. Ego-centric therapies do not suit all patients. Ethnic matching of the therapist with the patient may not work. Using appropriate language and modified indigenous therapies may improve engagement. Physical interventions will be influenced by cultural expectations of medication. In this chapter we describe the impact of cultural and religious factors on therapeutic adherence and make suggestions for implementing the pharmacotherapy plan. Potential problems are highlighted and suggestions made for managing conflict and confrontation.

Clinical management of patients across cultures challenges the clinician's familiar tried and tested strategies. The relationship between the patient and the psychiatrist is often examined in isolation from a number of premises that both patient and professional bring to the encounter: previous experience of other cultures, contact with less familiar cultures, past experiences and socioeconomic status are some of the determinant influences. There are a number of ways in which the clinician can facilitate therapeutic effectiveness. However, a trusting relationship must first emerge such that the patient has faith in the treatment recommendations. Special difficulties can arise in the context of pharmacological, social, psychotherapeutic and psychological interventions. Community, out-patient, in-patient and emergency settings each require that consideration be given to the context of the assessment and treatment process, as well as the content and immediate outcome. The clinician must plan the assessment and intervention carefully. The rationale and goals of treatment should be discussed and agreed by participants in the therapeutic interaction. Special groups face unique cultural and historical obstacles to receiving healthcare. Basic principles are described in this chapter: psychopharmacology is discussed in greater detail in Chapter 21 and psychotherapy in Chapter 26.

Psychiatry across cultures

Britain is undeniably a multicultural society. The needs of patients from other cultures are becoming paramount in the planning and delivery of psychiatric services. In the preceding chapter we highlighted some of the problems that psychiatrists may come across in the process of assessment; here we will focus on the clinical management of patients from other cultures.

Distress among immigrant communities can be understood in terms of common migration-related themes; yet individual immigrants are heterogeneous in the cause of their problems and in their personalised models of illness, as well as in their appraisal of who in society can act as a help-giver. This diversity is further amplified by the evolving culture of the younger generation. Younger members of Britain's Black communities regard the UK as their home and do not see themselves as immigrants; the use of migration-related models of cross-cultural assessment and management is now less often of help. Psychiatrists generally take account of sociocultural factors in the aetiology and management of psychiatric problems; however, less attention has been directed to those groups who suffer disadvantaged access to healthcare because of societal values and beliefs and the structure of the healthcare system. Despite a general awareness of social and cultural issues, the active engagement of cultural aspects of our patients' presentation is often set aside for pragmatic reasons to do with time and resources.

Principles of management

Clinical management of psychiatric problems is determined by information obtained within the context of health professional–patient interaction. Such a meeting can take place in community, out-patient and in-patient settings. Each of these settings will influence the consultation in terms of degree of crisis, source of referral, immediate resources available to the clinician, the amount of observation data available, and the patient's level of distress or unfamiliarity with the environment. The context of consultations is often not considered but may crucially influence the quality and completeness of the information obtained. Kleinman's (1977, 1988) concepts of category fallacy (making conditions defined by other cultures 'fit' into Western models of diagnosis), idioms of distress (patient expressing subjective concerns with culturally mediated meanings) and explanatory models are worthy of consideration in every therapeutic encounter. Furthermore, the health professional is usually one of many individuals that the patient has 'consulted' in order to return to their previous level of functioning. This is true of members of both majority and minority cultures. The clinician must make every reasonable attempt to understand individual patients' and their families' models of causation of illness and management.

Goals of treatment

Patients are interested in finding out what they should do to alleviate their distress. The purpose of the assessment is to determine not only their explanatory models and idioms of distress, but also to allow shared treatment goals to be identified. Acculturation has been understood largely as a process experienced by the first generation of immigrants, but their children may well also face sociocultural conflict, albeit of a different type. Consequently, treatment options and goals may be differentially received by different generations. In a multicultural society, broad societal pressures, narrower familial expectations, together with different 'help-seeking motivations' and styles of making sense of and dealing with the world all require an integrated individual appraisal. The goals of treatment under such conditions may be broader and may incorporate social interventions to a greater extent than is usual. This is especially the case when there are spiritual or religious objections to medication. Well-intentioned but amateurish, non-indicated or poorly timed interventions may precipitate or even exacerbate psychopathology. For example, if adherence becomes a focus of conflict, it could harm an effective treatment alliance and ultimately result in an exacerbation of symptoms. Any therapeutic efforts need to be sensitive to the unique scenario presented by the patient.

Planning treatment

Basic treatment planning for patients from other cultures is no different from planning for patients who share a greater amount of their cultural attributes with the clinician. However, additional factors to do with language, training, social and cultural rehabilitation and cultural conflicts need to be taken into account. For patients from other cultures, the multidisciplinary team will often require all of its mix of skills; indeed, it may have to evolve new strategies in planning an appropriate treatment package. If language is a problem and bilingual workers are not available, other familiar and trusted (by the patient) community members could be involved. Of course, interpretation, if required, should ideally avoid using a member of the patient's family or social group. Also, the whole process will take longer and become more complex, not least in relation to patient confidentiality.

Treatment planning may be viable only with the active consent and involvement of family members, who could facilitate or impede the clinician's desired pace of progress. The contemporary strength of family ties, expectations and aspirations will all be important. When caught between cultures, the kinship ties of a cultural group may well change according to the local customs and with the passage of time. Clinicians should avoid deploying their own kinship/family systems as normative. Careful scrutiny of local customs and culture is required; such knowledge should be easily accessible from the families themselves as well as from other members of the patient's community. Health professionals ascribed the same ethnicity as a patient may share little with that patient's culture; thus, merely seeking an ethnic match is likely to be inadequate if other aspects of culture are not also considered. Unfortunately, clarification of an individual's cultural expectations is likely to take some time and may not be readily achieved in a convenient single assessment.

Physical treatments

Physical treatment such as drug treatments and electroconvulsive therapy (ECT) carry different symbolic representations depending on past experience and culture. Where the model of illness includes physical causation and physical treatment, problems of adherence may not be as visible an issue but drug dosages and side-effects may well become the factors on which the patient decides to accept or refuse treatment.

Pharmacotherapy

Using pharmacological agents as a first line of management for severe mental illness is a common practice. However, the doses prescribed are often those recommended generally, regardless of ethnic group. Pharmacokinetics vary across ethnicity and culture; a drug may be absorbed, distributed through the body, localised in tissues, metabolised and excreted at different rates by different groups. Age, gender, ethnicity, diet (ingestion of coffee, use of nicotine, etc.) have all been shown to affect levels of drugs in the body. It is known that heavy smokers may need higher doses of antipsychotics and antidepressants, but the role of diet is under-evaluated in clinical therapeutics (see Chapter 21, this volume).

Westermeyer (1989) points out that people from low- and middle-income countries may possess models of drug treatment in accord with their use of aspirin, penicillin or herbal medicine. They might expect a quick response with minimal dosage for a minimal period. Such a conceptualisation of pharmacotherapy will encourage expectations of a rapid response, if not within a few hours then at least a few days, rather than the weeks that antipsychotics or antidepressants may take. If such relief is not forthcoming, patients could discontinue the medication, ask for a different medication or use other medicines in conjunction. A protracted period without relief, the experience of side-effects, dietary restrictions and the way in which psychotropics are prescribed may all lead patients and their families to view psychotropics as problematic unless careful explanation is given and it is clear that this has not been misunderstood (Box 20.1).

Antipsychotics

Studies have shown ethnic differences in the pharmacokinetics of anti-psychotics. When healthy Asian (Japanese, Korean and Chinese Americans) and Caucasian volunteers were given haloperidol, the Asians had significantly higher serum levels and a more pronounced prolactin response compared

---

Box 20.1   Implementing a pharmacotherapy plan

- Clarify the symptoms, diagnosis and indications with the patient and family
- Provide written and oral information on dosage, side-effects and interactions with other substances (especially foods, herbs)
- Start at low dosages and keep a close watch on side-effects
- Involve a family member to act as 'cotherapist'
- Inform the patient of key side-effects and enable them to access the team or their GP in emergencies
- Be aware of cultural patterns which may affect adherence

---

with the Caucasian group. Also, 95% of Asians developed extrapyramidal side-effects within the first 2 weeks, whereas only 60% of Black patients and 67% of Whites did so in the same period. Black in-patients, on the other hand, have shown higher blood levels per milligram dose of chlorpromazine compared with White in-patients (Lin *et al*, 1995).

Antidepressants

Caucasians taking tricyclic antidepressants appear to have lower plasma levels and attain plasma peaks later than Asians (Japanese, Chinese, Korean and those from the Indian subcontinent). These differences are said to be due to a greater incidence of slow hydroxylation among Asians. The evidence of ethnic differences in pharmacokinetics of tricyclics remains inconsistent. Overall, the data suggest that dosages should be carefully individualised over a prolonged period, especially for Asian and African–Caribbean patients.

Lithium

Lithium has been shown to be effective at lower serum levels among Japanese people (Takahashi, 1979; Okuma, 1981). Ethnic differences in red blood cell sodium and lithium levels have been recognised for some time. Taiwanese patients respond well to lithium at serum levels of 0.5–0.79 mmol/1, whereas in patients from Hong Kong these levels are, on average, 0.63 mmol/1. Chinese patients respond to levels around 0.71-0.73 mmol/1, which is lower than the Caucasian sample levels of 0.8-1.2 mmol/1. The precise significance of such pharmacokinetic differences is uncertain.

Culture, diet and pharmacotherapy

Dietary patterns are influenced by the availability of certain kinds of food as well as religious and social taboos. The role of diet has been clearly understood in relation to psychotropic drugs such as monoamine oxidase inhibitors (MAOIs). In cultures in which humoural concepts of 'hot' and 'cold' food are common, patients often see drugs as 'hot' and ask for food prohibitions or additions to contribute to cooling of the excess heat produced by the drugs. It is also likely that some traditional medicines and foods have ingredients that interact with prescribed psychotropic medication. Ethanol metabolism varies tremendously across ethnic groups and the use of alcohol with prescribed medication may produce side-effects that are difficult to understand and manage. Additional factors that in theory could operate on pharmacokinetics include food additives, over-the-counter medication, herbal medication and air pollution (Westermeyer, 1989).

Electroconvulsive therapy

There is some evidence that African–Caribbeans in the UK are given ECT more frequently than the rest of the population, even though they are more likely to be diagnosed with schizophrenia. This discrepancy remains hard to explain: the underlying indications for ECT remain the same whatever the ethnic group. In addition to the fear and the stigma of ECT that might influence any patient, patients from minority ethnic groups who have been victims of discrimination and persecution may see ECT as a further threat. Any approach to patients must be gentle and must include their relatives and families in a full and frank discussion. Reading and audio-visual materials can help patients and families to consider ECT in a more informed way. Meetings with patients who have received ECT in the past (along with the recovered patient's family) can reduce the extreme fear of ECT (Westermeyer, 1989).

Complementary therapies

There are two groups of treatment that the clinicians need to be aware of. First, patients and their families may urge the clinician to offer alternative therapies such as acupuncture, reflexology and aromatherapy. Second, the patient may be taking unprescribed medication – herbs or other substances provided by culturally embedded healing practitioners such as Hakims, Vaids and Unani physicians. Acupuncture may appeal to both patients and service planners as offering relief from mental health problems, although it is unlikely to be a long-term cure for a chronic condition. Temporary systematic relief may not be seen as sufficient reason for delivering such interventions when the financial implications are considered. However, in some individuals this may be the only intervention that affords symptomatic relief and it could form a part of a carefully considered treatment package. Professionals have not established clearly whether acupuncture or any other complementary treatments have a role to play in the relief of depression, anxiety or persistent psychotic symptoms.

Culture, therapy and personality

Murphy (1969, 1972) argued that individual personality traits not only play an important role in treatment response, but also are modified by culture. When culture allows and encourages individuals to be independent, to struggle and take action, there may be a greater readiness to use and hence need medication. On the other hand, where culture encourages individuals to be interdependent and to take healing decisions and actions by group process, less emphasis will be given to medication. Personality traits have been linked with pharmacodynamic as well as pharmacokinetic properties (Westermeyer, 1989). The prognostic value of subjective responses needs to be investigated more thoroughly.

Psychotherapy

Provision of psychological treatments for individuals from other cultures brings with it its own problems. Apart from the language – verbal and conceptual – of psychotherapy, some cultures may find the Western concepts of ego-dependent psychology inappropriate and threatening. In cultures where the individual self remains an integral part of the society and family, individual psychotherapy will not be easily acceptable. Group therapy may also create difficulties, with confidentiality a particular concern.

The quality of the therapy offered, especially if patients do not understand the rationale and have low expectations of it, may play a very important role in its acceptance (Balabil & Dolan, 1992). Service providers have to know the community's attitudes to the processes of healing when planning to provide psychotherapy services (Bhugra, 1993). Potential referrers should be especially curious about an individual's expectations and perceptions of 'talking treatments' and ensure that the faulty appraisal of its potential on the part of the professional is not a barrier to treatment. Ethnic and social oppression will determine the type and intensity of psychopathology, as well as the ability of an individual to share their emotional states with help-providers.

Tyler *et al* (1991) suggest that one of the major problems in psychotherapy is its universalist perspective. This is a congruent process in which the therapist aims to capture the commonality of experience between himself or herself and the patient. Conversely, the particularist view argues that ethnic, racial and cultural variables significantly shape the world view of both the therapist and the patient; hence, any such therapy needs to focus on racial and ethnic issues and especially with ethnic matching of the therapist and the patient (see below). Alternatively, ethnic, racial and cultural values can be transcended in therapy; the focus is then on the skill and experience of the therapist, rather than ethnicity.

Specific models of psychotherapy

Each model brings with it a rationale in which the patient and therapist must believe for the encounter to be effective. From the psychoanalytic body of knowledge the concepts of ego, id and superego have entered common parlance, as have Oedipal complex and 'arrest' at each stage of oral, anal or genital experiences. These concepts are sometimes used without looking

267

at their cultural relevance. The transference–countertransference dyad, which lies at the core of psychoanalytic therapy, produces a unique set of problems when the patient and the therapist have different ethnic and racial identities. Countertransference has to be seen as an experience affected by the individual's cultural knowledge and experiences.

Behavioural therapies can work across cultures, especially because behavioural tasks are observable and measurable. The principles of engagement in a behavioural enterprise may require modification, perhaps with much greater emphasis on explanation. The potential for breaches in the treatment alliance arise from the same sources as in other models of therapy. McCarthy (1988) observes that any attempts to modify behaviour in the direction of the therapist's norms may be deeply offensive and threatening to the patient, and the therapist may risk being offended by culturally determined stereotypes that clash with their beliefs. Attempts to use social skills assessment, assertiveness training, dating behaviour, attitudes to specific problems, and perceived causation of problems are doomed to failure and to increase the discord between the patient and the therapist if they are not handled in an appropriately sensitive manner. Behavioural therapy is focused, needs limited interpreter time, can be used easily to assess improvement, is usually seen as non-threatening and is congenial to various religious philosophies. Cognitive techniques have become a valued part of the armamentarium against depression. However, cognitive models of depression have not been validated across cultures.

Among the social therapies, Westermeyer (1989) includes family therapy, group work, social network reconstruction, acculturation therapy and resocialisation processes. These share the underlying premise that life areas (such as language, occupational skills, family life) are identified and then linked with specific goals and activities depending on individual needs. Mutual support and help groups, art therapies and groups with particular religious leanings can be set up. These may be seen as non-threatening and hence more acceptable. The relationships within such settings allow both the therapist and the patient to progress towards a mutually agreed and acceptable goal at a pace that is 'safe' for both parties. In addition, such approaches work as two-way processes for educating the therapist as well as the patient.

Indigenous therapies

Cuento therapy has been used successfully with Puerto Rican children in New York (Constantino *et al*, 1986). It uses local folk tales to present models of adaptive behaviour, and has been tailored to the bicultural conflict experienced by Puerto Rican children in the USA; results included a clearly marked reduction in anxiety persisting at 1-year follow-up.

The use of models in therapy with patients in India has led to development of theories that put the patient's dilemmas in a socioreligious context, thereby encouraging the individual to seek out appropriate solutions (for review see Lloyd & Bhugra, 1993). Singh & Oberhummer (1980) successfully used a combination of behavioural therapy and karma yoga to treat an Indian women presenting with obsessive ruminations.

For some ethnic groups, the therapist needs to be assertive and directive. In Hindu and Buddhist philosophies, a merging of the self with general fate, mastering of personal ambition and honouring the rights of care and duty to others are essential components of living, and the therapist will need to take all of these into account when planning any psychotherapeutic interventions. The use of vedic rituals for managing addiction and yogic methods for managing anxieties and stress in subgroups of patients now has a universal appeal.

Ethnic matching

Ethnic matching of therapist and patient is not essential. Several studies have indicated that the patient's first experience of the therapist and the therapist's skill and overall experience are more important than relative ethnic identities. As discussed above, rather than focus on the particular school of therapy, the individual therapist needs to transcend the interaction and be able to deal with the patient's problem in a sensitive manner. Ethnic matching is often advocated on the basis that it will allow the patient to be more free in highlighting their problem, but the reality is that the therapist is still often seen as 'one of them' and as being middle-class (Box 20.2).

Management and service development

Thus far we have focused on strategies for treating individual patients. We wish now to draw attention to the larger population perspective of minority ethnic communities. Although individual management is likely to be the most important point of contact between patient and professional, there are inevitable organisational barriers that will make the optimal implementation of strategies difficult and in some instances (because of resource limitations) impossible. This reality highlights the need for

---

Box 20.2 Methods of confrontation without threat

- Be aware of the meaning of conflict in terms of the patient's reference group
- Pose the confrontation as classification
- Diffuse the transference among staff members
- Establish trust and support before confrontation
- Identify the purpose of confrontation and its potential value
- Identify confrontation within the cultural context without challenging religious taboos
- Facilitate confrontation after discussion with family and peers

healthcare providers to build an infrastructure of services, personnel and expertise, which can flexibly respond to changes in a community's demographics. In a rapidly evolving mental health service, a number of reorganisational imperatives are likely to 'trump' the needs of a particular group. Organisations must therefore examine these processes of change and openly state their managerial position on service provision for ethnic minorities. If desirable service structures or staff positions cannot be created for fiscal reasons, for example, this should not deter the overall aim of better service provision for all communities. If budgetary priorities are openly acknowledged, a plan of implementation of immediate, medium-term and long-term service changes can proceed. Training and the generation of expertise about the communities of relevance to each health team should be integral to overall management. Only then will whole communities gain a greater level of trust in the ability of a healthcare system which is at present aversive to many ethnic minorities and used only at times of crisis.

Conclusion

Successful clinical management of patients from other cultural groups relies on the individual therapist's skill, experience and training. Using appropriate models of therapy allows the therapist–patient interaction to work at a level at which both participants feel comfortable. Within such an interaction, physical therapies need to be tailored to culture and ethnicity as well as to clinical needs. Psychoanalytic therapies may well work in some situations, but behavioural and cognitive therapies may be seen as more appropriate and acceptable. In planning any treatment, the involvement of the family and understanding of community norms will allow the therapist to provide culturally sensitive and appropriate therapies whenever and wherever needed. Further reading on this topic is listed in Box 20.3.

Box 20.3 Sources of further information

- Bhugra, D. & Bhui, K. (eds) (2007) *Textbook of Cultural Psychiatry*. Cambridge University Press.
- Bhui, K. & Bhugra, D. (eds) (2007) *Culture and Mental Health: A Comprehensive Textbook*. Hodder Arnold.
- Cuellar, I. & Paniagua, F. (eds) (2000) *Handbook of Multicultural Mental Health: Assessment and Treatment of Diverse Populations*. Academic Press.
- Ng, C. H., Lin, K.-M., Singh, B. S., *et al* (eds) (2008) *Ethno-psychopharmacology: Advances in Current Practice*. Cambridge University Press.
- Tseng, W.-S. & Strelzer, J. (2004) *Cultural Competence in Clinical Psychiatry*. American Psychiatric Press.
- Tseng, W.-S. (2004) *Handbook of Cultural Psychiatry*. Academic Press.
- Tseng, W.-S. (2003) *Clinician's Guide to Cultural Psychiatry*. Academic Press.

References

Balabil, S. & Dolan, B. (1992) A cross-cultural evaluation of expectations about psychological counselling. *British Journal of Medical Psychology*, **65**, 305–330.

Bhugra, D. (1993) Setting up services for ethnic minorities. In *Dimensions of Community Care* (eds M. Weller & M. Muijen), pp. 116–134. Ballière-Tindall.

Constantino, G., Malgady, R. & Regler, R. (1986) Cuento therapy: a culturally sensitive modality for Puerto Rican children. *Journal of Consulting and Clinical Psychology*, **54**, 639–645.

Kleinman, A. (1977) Depression: somatisation and the new crosscultural psychiatry. *Social Science and Medicine*, **11**, 3–10.

Kleinman, A. (1988) *Rethinking Psychiatry: From Cultural Category to Personal Experience*. Free Press.

Lin, K.-M., Poland, R. & Anderson, D. (1995) Psychopharmacology, ethnicity and culture. *Transcultural Psychiatric Research Review*, **32**, 3–40.

Lloyd, K. & Bhugra, D. (1993) Cross-cultural aspects of psychotherapy. *International Review of Psychiatry*, **5**, 291–304.

McCarthy, B. (1988) Working with ethnic minorities. In *New Developments in Clinical Psychology* (ed. F. N. Watts), pp. 122–139. John Wiley & Sons.

Murphy, H. B. M. (1969) Ethnic variations in drug response. *Transcultural Psychiatric Research Review*, **6**, 6–23.

Murphy, H. B. M. (1972) Psychopharmacologie et variations ethno-culturelles. *Confrontation Psychiatrique*, **9**, 163–185.

Okuma, T. (1981) Differential sensitivity to the effects of psychotropic drugs: psychotics vs normals; Asians vs Western populations. *Folia Psychiatrica et Neurologica Japonica*, **35**, 79–81.

Singh, R. & Oberhummer, I. (1980) Behaviour therapy within a setting of karma yoga. *Journal of Behavior Therapy and Experimental Psychiatry*, **11**, 135–141.

Takahashi, R. (1979) Lithium treatment in affective disorders: therapeutic plasma level. *Psychopharmacology Bulletin*, **15**, 32–35.

Tyler, F. B., Broome, D. R. & William, J. E. (1991) *Ethnic Validity, Ecology and Psychotherapy*. Plenum.

Westermeyer, J. (1989) *Psychiatric Care of Migrants: A Clinical Guide*. American Psychological Association.

CHAPTER 21

Ethnic and cultural factors in psychopharmacology

Dinesh Bhugra and Kamaldeep Bhui

Summary In this chapter we highlight some key factors of which clinicians need to be aware in practising psychiatry in ethnically diverse populations. These include pharmacodynamic and pharmacokinetic principles, and their application in pharmacological management of psychiatric conditions. Ethnic differences in pharmacodynamics are most clearly demonstrated in the greater sensitivity to a variety of drugs in Whites than in Asians or in African–Caribbeans.

Barring a few exceptions (such as *rauwolfia serpentina*, a source of reserpine first identified in Asia), most psychiatric medications have been developed in the West, especially the USA, the UK and Europe, and their safety trials have been conducted in these populations. Although these drugs are used all over the world there has been limited research to determine accurate pharmacodynamic and pharmacokinetic profiles across different ethnic groups. Clinicians usually adopt a 'universalist style' (seeing every condition and treatment as similar) of managing psychiatric illnesses, but this appears to neglect the information from the emerging literature that advocates a relativist approach to pharmacotherapy (Lin *et al*, 1995).

A recently recognised key factor in the study of pharmacokinetics is pharmacogenetics: a pharmacogenetic variation according to ethnic group can lead to significant genetically determined modifications of metabolising enzymes (i.e. the pharmacokinetic handling of the drug by the body). This results in differing therapeutic levels and half-lives of drugs and, therefore, variable profiles of their therapeutic and adverse effects. Pharmacogenetic research has uncovered significant differences between ethnic groups related to drug metabolism, clinical effectiveness and side-effect profile (Lee *et al*, 2008).

In addition to ethnobiological determinants of drug response, there are significant cultural factors: the concurrent use of pluralistic health systems, alternative therapies and folk remedies which might support, hinder or complicate pharmacotherapy and treatment adherence.

Ethnicity

General issues

Ethnicity and culture powerfully determine individual pharmacological responses, which are shaped by both environmental and genetic factors (Lin *et al*, 2008). Genetic polymorphism in genes encoding drug metabolising enzymes as well as the putative targets of pharmaceutical agents (e.g. neurotransmitters, receptors and transporters) and environmental factors such as diet and smoking are also likely to be affected by ethnicity and culture.

Definitions of ethnicity and ethnic group classifications provoke considerable discussion and debate. Ethnicity is a social construction and is often invested with greater stability, permanence and biological importance than is justified (Box 21.1). Ethnicity has been defined as colour of skin (e.g. White), nationality (e.g. Indian) and a mixture of the two in the Office of Population Censuses and Surveys (1992) criteria. Definitions of ethnicity can be based at a social level, at an individual identity level or, as is usual in medical practice and research, at a level that recognises a combination of social, cultural and phenotypic similarities rather than genotypic differences. It is the association of phenotypic similarity with pharmacogenetic variations in drug metabolism that render ethnopharmacogenetic variations of clinical importance. The association of phenotypic appearance with culturally distinct health beliefs further emphasises the importance of a biopsychosocial approach. At the identity level, individuals see themselves as belonging to a group with common geographical origins, migratory status, race, language, religion or faith and ties which transcend kinship, neighbourhood and community boundaries. Ethnicity is also linked closely with shared traditions, values, symbols, folk

---

Box 21.1   Definitions of race, ethnicity and culture

Ethnicity – Self or social ascription of belonging to a group with common geographical origins, race, language, religion, etc., which transcends kinship and neighbourhood. Ethnic categories retain a strong racial component. These are ascriptively mobilised by individuals. An ethnic group is a social group characterised by a distinctive tradition and common history maintained within the group across generations.

Race – Largely perceived by appearance and attributed to biological and genetic traits. Racial differences get perpetuated in society because they have cultural significance.

Culture – Shared system of concepts or mental representations established by convention and reproduced by traditional transmission. People live culturally rather than in cultures.

---

music and folk memories. Settlements, food preferences and employment patterns all shape the definition and revision of ethnic identity boundaries. Such a range of features in the definition and understanding of ethnicity reflects a dynamic interaction between biological and sociocultural factors. It is this biopsychosocial interaction that forms the context in which the doctor–patient relationship is located and in which medication is prescribed and taken.

Personality factors

Within any single ethnic group, various social and culturally distinct behaviours, beliefs and social settings are important. Personality is moulded by social and cultural factors. Lin (1996) argues that little is known regarding the potential contribution of cultural and ethnic factors in determining whether particular patients will benefit from a particular treatment.

Culturally determined personality traits such as dependence or independence, orthodoxy or adventurousness, and subjective response all play an important role in pharmacodynamics and pharmacokinetics and need to be studied along with ethnicity (Box 21.2).

The belief of researchers and clinicians alike in the universality of conditions and treatments, and that differences must be due to psychosocial factors only, often leads them to ignore significant and authentic individual variations. Ethnicity and culture might indirectly influence personality traits, which in turn might influence an individual's response to medication. Such a neglect of human biological diversity has been partially responsible for the slow progress of cross-cultural research on biological diversity and factors that affect metabolism of drugs. Such

---

Box 21.2 Pharmacokinetics and pharmacodynamics – definitions

Pharmacokinetics – The study of how a biological organism affects the fate and distribution of a drug. This is determined by four processes – absorption, distribution, metabolism and excretion. The processes of metabolism exhibit substantial cross-ethnic, as well as individual, differences. Height, weight, differences in gastric acidity and percentage body fat are all affected by race and culture and can also affect the pharmacokinetics of drugs.

Pharmacodynamics – The study of the effects of a drug on the person. It refers to the neurotransmitter, neurophysiological, behavioural, psychological and social effects of psychotropic drugs and their mechanisms of action. An interesting and fairly common variation highlighted by Westermeyer (1989) is the flushing response to alcohol which has a variable distribution across races due to differences in enzymes acting on alcohol metabolism. Although the mechanics of alcohol flushing have been well described, the relationships between differences in blood levels, therapeutic responses and dosage are not so well understood, and are a function of more than variable pharmacokinetics.

a 'colour-blind' approach confirms the view that people with divergent
ethnic backgrounds might not differ in their biological responses or
perceptions of drug treatment. This makes patients who complain of
adverse effects and request dosage variations sound as if they are 'non-
compliant' rather than accurately reporting their response to medication.
The use of clinical practice guidelines is escalating, but these originate
from the existing evidence base, most of which has not included patients
from minority ethnic groups. Norms and guidelines based on research on
White populations may have little relevance to the effective treatment of
psychiatric disorders among other ethnic and cultural groups. Individual
personality factors play an important role in help-seeking, in the chosen
models of care and even in treatment adherence.

Environmental factors

Environmental factors (Box 21.3) can affect pharmacogenetics and
associated pharmacokinetics of psychiatric drugs in people from different
ethnic groups. Some of these factors, such as housing and employment,
may even differ across ethnic groups within the same country. Certain
cultural and ethnic groups exposed to specific environmental factors over

---

Box 21.3 Social and environmental factors affecting ethnic differences
in metabolism and efficacy of psychiatric medication

Demographic factors
- Ethnicity
- Age
- Gender

Pharmacogenetic factors
- Enzymic differences

Pharmacokinetic factors
- Enzymic differences
- Dietary habits
- Smoking
- Concurrent drugs

Dietary factors
- Dietary taboos
- Special foods
- Body fat and weight

Environmental factors
- Alternative models
- Alternative drugs
- Healthcare systems
- Prescribing habits

a long period of time can experience adaptations of metabolism, leading to a differential response which could be seen as linked with ethnicity (Smith & Mendoza, 1996).

Westermeyer (1989) has argued that additional factors affecting pharmacokinetics include the use of tobacco, caffeine (in cola, tea and coffee), food additives, over-the-counter medications and herbal remedies, as well as air pollution. Social and family support at a macrolevel and personal factors such as response to stressors can also affect the prognosis and outcome of psychiatric treatment. Lin et al (2008) note that dietary habits affect pharmacokinetics as they change the body's ability to absorb, distribute and metabolise medication and nutrients exert major effects on the expression of many drug-metabolising enzymes. People exposed to stressors while they have low levels of tolerance and social support are more likely to develop mental illness and also to have a poor social and clinical outcome. Alterations in the levels of stress and social support may also change the effective therapeutic dosages of different psychotropic drugs (Lin et al, 1995). For example, high expressed emotion (characterised by frequent criticism, hostility and emotional over-involvement) can affect prognosis and cause relapse even in patients taking antipsychotics. This phenomenon deserves to be studied further.

Various physical diseases can be caused by dietary factors which, in turn, will affect the pharmacodynamics of prescribed drugs. Also, religious rituals and taboos may affect timings of drug-taking and absorption.

Biological factors

Drugs and other foreign substances (xenobiotics) are metabolised by a number of enzymes whose activities, for both genetic and environmental reasons, vary substantially between individuals and across ethnic groups (Lin et al, 1995). Although individual and inter-ethnic differences are substantial, the mechanisms responsible for such variations are not well understood (Lin et al, 1993). There are classic examples of differing drug responses across ethnic groups, and the genetic control of a large number of drug-metabolising enzymes has been established. For example, the cytochrome P-450 (CYP) enzyme system has been linked with the oxidation of several chemotherapeutic agents. More than 20 CYP iso-enzymes exist and each is encoded by a specific gene. Both the phenotypes and genotypes of this enzyme system show clear individual and cross-ethnic variations which have been linked to differential adaptation to divergent environmental exposure, especially diet. Clear diversity is seen for some CYP iso-enzymes, leading to poor or good metabolism. Lin et al (1993) report ethnic variations in these enzymes ranging from 1% in east Asians to 8.1% in Black Americans.

Other enzymes show a similar range of variation. Beta-blockers, for example, are relatively ineffective in treating hypertension in African

Americans but are more effective in Asians, with efficacy in White people falling in between (Dimsdale et al, 1988). Clozapine-induced agranulocytosis has been more commonly observed in Ashkenazi Jews, especially those with a cluster of human leukocyte antigen (HLA) types (Lieberman et al, 1990).

Established ethnic differences in therapeutic effects

Most of the data available on ethnicity and psychopharmacology come from the USA and of all the psychotropic drugs, antipsychotics are most likely to be discussed. Across various ethnic groups additional factors such as smoking, dietary taboos and dietary habits are seen to play a role but are not discussed very often.

Antipsychotics

Cross-racial differences in antipsychotics doses that produce side-effects have been studied extensively in Asian Americans (Japanese, Korean and Chinese Americans). Binder & Levy (1981) reported that 95% of Asian people in their sample had developed extrapyramidal side-effects within 2 weeks of commencing treatment, whereas only 60% of Black patients and 67% of White patients did so. Although the numbers of patients in each group were small, these are significant differences. In a comparison of Chinese and non-Chinese patients taking haloperidol, Jann et al (1989) reported that the Chinese people had higher levels of extrapyramidal side-effects and higher blood plasma levels than the non-Chinese on equivalent dosages. In a similar study, Chang et al (1991) reported reduced haloperidol plasma levels and generally lower steady-state haloperidol ratios in Chinese patients compared with non-Chinese, confirming their earlier findings (Chang et al, 1987) and suggesting that different metabolic factors may be acting.

Asian Americans reportedly have significantly higher serum levels of haloperidol and also a more pronounced prolactin response compared with White patients receiving the same dose. Lower reduced haloperidol:haloperidol ratios in Asian Americans are said to be due to slower rates of reduction and metabolism (Chang et al, 1987; Jann et al, 1989, 1993). It has been hypothesised that the enzyme CYP2D6 plays a crucial role in pathway of such metabolism. Lin et al (1988) demonstrated higher serum haloperidol levels in healthy Americans of Far Eastern ancestry compared with White volunteers, and were able to show in a later study that Asian Americans with schizophrenia responded optimally to significantly lower serum haloperidol concentrations (Lin et al, 1989). Asians have an increased likelihood of carrying genetic polymorphisms that result in significantly lower metabolic clearance rates for drugs that are substrates for CYP enzymes (Lambert & Norman, 2008).This has not been confirmed in other ethnic groups, but if it were the case, then clinicians would need to review their prescribing habits.

Antidepressants

Key differences across different ethnic groups have been indicated for antidepressants as well. A number of studies have reported lower plasma levels of tricyclic antidepressants and later plasma peaks in Whites than in Asians (of Far Eastern ancestry and from the Indian subcontinent) (Allen *et al*, 1977; Lewis *et al*, 1980; Rudorfer *et al*, 1984). These differences have been attributed to a greater incidence of slow hydroxylation among Asians than among White populations (Kilow, 1982). When studying the kinetics of nortriptyline in non-depressed volunteers, Gaviria *et al* (1986) observed that purported hypersensitivity to the drug in their Hispanic volunteers was due to receptor hypersensitivity, as this group responded to lower doses and had more side-effects when taking tricyclic antidepressants. Lin *et al* (1995) confirmed this, although research evidence remains inconsistent. Kishimoto & Hollister (1984) and Rudorfer *et al* (1984) have suggested that Asians metabolise tricyclic antidepressants slowly, but others have not been able to confirm this (Pi *et al*, 1986, 1989; Silver *et al*, 1993).

Two studies from Asia (Yamashita & Asano, 1979; Hu *et al*, 1983) showed that Asian patients with severe depression responded to lower combined concentrations of imipramine and desipramine in comparison with dosages used for White groups. African Americans have been reported to have higher levels of neurological side-effects when taking antidepressants (Escobar & Tuason, 1980), but the mechanisms of such actions are not clear. Lambert & Norman (2008) note that ethnic differences in the pharmacokinetic effects of antidepressants exist and are not dissimilar to the effects of other drugs. Dosages of antidepressants should be carefully individualised over a prolonged period. Intragroup variation in tricyclic pharmacokinetics greatly exceeds intergroup differences, and the slow peak performance in White people may be due to a more rapid hydroxylation in this group.

The data on newer antidepressants (and on atypical antipsychotics) are even scantier regarding dosage measurement and assessment of side-effects across different ethnic groups. It is possible that newer antidepressants such as moclobemide will show greater variation in metabolism compared with other antidepressants because of variations in monoamine oxidase activity across ethnic groups.

Lithium

Ethnic differences in sodium and lithium levels in red blood cells are well recognised (Westermeyer, 1989). Pharmacokinetic differences may exist, but their precise nature and clinical impact have not been identified. Lithium has proved effective at lower blood plasma levels among Japanese patients. Taiwanese patients are maintained at higher plasma levels than Japanese but lower than the Chinese Americans (Chang *et al*, 1991). Taiwanese patients are maintained at lithium levels of 0.5–0.79 mmol/l, whereas Chinese patients had levels of around 0.71–0.73 mmol/l, but in Chinese Americans no pharmacokinetic differences were reported.

Environmental factors such as the weather (hot summers that lead to dehydration) and personal factors such as diet become even more important in the prescription of lithium and the maintenance of individual patients on the drug.

Benzodiazepines

The evidence concerning response to benzodiazepines and their dosages across ethnic groups remains inconclusive. One study found although that Asian Americans cleared diazepam more slowly and had higher serum levels than White Americans, the drug did not demonstrate any significant agonist effects (Ghoneim *et al*, 1981). Other researchers, however, have shown pharmacokinetic differences in two groups, that is, Asian Americans and Caucasians (Kumana *et al*, 1987; Lin *et al*, 1988; Zhang *et al*, 1990). A multi-ethnic study of the effects of adinazolam revealed notably increased clearance, significantly higher concentrations of its metabolites and greater drug effects on psychomotor performance in African Americans as compared with Asian and White volunteers (Ajir *et al*, 1997). The authors attributed this to hepatic oxidation and renal excretion, which may explain the greater drug effect on African Americans despite their higher metabolic capacity for adinazolam.

Other physical treatments

Patients and their carers may use drugs (such as analgesics) and other physical treatments irrespective of indication or need. Often, individuals from minority ethnic groups use pluralistic approaches to help-seeking and it is therefore likely that other drugs, prescribed or non-prescribed, along with other environmental factors, will affect the pharmacokinetics of psychiatric prescriptions. These variations in serum levels of medicines, their metabolism and side-effects may be due to genetic, pharmacokinetic variations, dietary or environmental factors, or variations in the prescribing habits of clinicians (Frackiewicz *et al*, 1997). Dosage studies and the study of adverse effects are only the first steps in understanding the inter-ethnic variations of pharmacological agents.

Non-biological factors

As mentioned earlier, both biological and non-biological factors play a crucial role in responses to medication, but the interaction is less well studied in minority ethnic groups. Cultures differ in the way in which they train their members to be on guard against certain types of mental state and behaviours. Cultural attitudes towards medication are influenced by biology and by psychological and social factors such as stigma (Ng & Klimidis 2008). In collectivist or kinship-based cultures, the role of other members of the family in treatment adherence becomes extremely significant and must be remembered.

Stress

There is no doubt that culture defines sickness, sick role and stress; it also determines protective factors that influence an individual's response to stress. Treatment response is affected by changes in stress levels and in the availability of social support and by conflicts in interpersonal relationships. Continuing stress in refugees and minority ethnic groups may lead individuals to seek relief using complementary medicine (see below), ingesting herbs and even heavy metals that may make drug interactions more likely.

An additional feature related to stress is the gender of the individual, as it affects help-seeking and response to interventions (Dawkins, 1996). Gender roles determine expectations as well as social support. They are affected by culture and ethnicity and may in themselves produce stress, especially if they are in conflict with an individual's culture.

Smoking is a more powerful moderator than any genetic variants in CYPLA2 and is also related to gender (Lambert & Norman, 2008).

Prescription patterns

Prescription patterns (the type of drug prescribed to whom, for what and at what dose) vary widely across cultures. Some variation is due to the availability of certain drugs, and some to local healthcare systems. In addition, beliefs and attitudes on the part of both patient and clinician determine which drugs are prescription only and which can be obtained over the counter. Another key factor is the stereotype of patients that the physician follows. For example, African–Caribbeans given antipsychotics by depot injection might reflect the stereotypical belief that these individuals have problems with treatment adherence.

Treatment adherence

Adherence to medication regimens depends on a number of factors, such as dosage, side-effects, models of illness and beliefs in the healthcare system (Ng & Klimidis, 2008). Many psychiatric patients require long-term treatment with either oral or depot medication. Although treatment packages have been developed for adherence therapy, their success in treating members of minority ethnic groups is not well demonstrated. Divergence in the beliefs of patients and clinicians and communication difficulties have been regarded as the major reasons for ethnic differences in adherence (Lin et al, 1995). It has also been attributed to poor understanding of treatment protocols by some. Educational packages might improve adherence, provided they are culturally appropriate and targeted at appropriate levels.

Complementary medicine

Traditional herbal remedies, whether from medical systems such as the Ayurveda or Unani or simply from herbalists, are used extensively across

---

Box 21.4 Planning pharmacological treatment for patients from minority ethnic groups

Prior to prescribing
- Check diet
- Check religious taboos and rituals
- Check smoking, alcohol and drug use and attitudes to these

While prescribing
- Start at lower dose
- Have low threshold for identifying side-effects/evidence-based
- Adjust dosages regularly if required
- Provide information

After prescribing
- Monitor side-effects
- Check adherence
- Check environmental/dietary factors

---

different ethnic groups. Many of these substances are pharmacologically active and capable of significant interactions with prescribed drugs. Unani medication may also contain large quantities of heavy metals such as gold, silver, tin, copper, barium, lead, mercury, zinc, antimony and iron. In addition to herbal remedies or Unani medications, the Vaid or the Hakim may recommend dietary restrictions that may affect the absorption of food and prescribed medication. Other folklore remedies may be used. Yu (2008) notes that herbal medicines are not without problems: they may cause renal failure, interference with absorption, synergy of therapeutic effects and unwanted effects related to drug metabolism. Several minority ethnic groups also use pluralistic approaches to healthcare and patients or their carers may not volunteer the information to the clinician. Health professionals must ask questions in a sensitive and careful manner (Box 21.4).

Conclusion

Ethnic and cultural considerations are as important for those who conduct drug trials as for those who write out prescriptions. Clinicians must be aware of the differential safety and efficacy of pharmacological agents in people from different ethnic groups. These differences highlight the interaction between biological and cultural factors which may provide a clue to pharmacogenetic effects.

References

Ajir, K., Smith, M., Lin, K.-M., *et al* (1997) The pharmacokinetics and pharmacodynamics of adinazolam: multi-ethnic comparisons. *Psychopharmacology*, 129, 269–270.

Allen, J., Rack, P. & Vaddadi, K. (1977) Differences in the effects of clomipramine on English and Asian volunteers. *Postgraduate Medical Journal*, **53**, 79–86.

Binder, E. & Levy, R. (1981) Extrapyramidal reactions in Asians. *American Journal of Psychiatry*, **138**, 1243–1244.

Chang, S. S., Chen, T.-Y., Lee, C. A., *et al* (1987) Lithium plasma reduced haloperidol/ haloperidol ratios in Chinese patients. *Biological Psychiatry*, **22**, 1406–1408.

Chang, S. S., Jann, M., Hwu, H.-G., *et al* (1991) Ethnic comparison of haloperidol and reduced haloperidol plasma levels: Taiwan Chinese versus American non-Chinese. *Journal of the Formosan Medical Association*, **90**, 572–578.

Dawkins, K. (1996) The interaction of ethnicity, socio-cultural factors and gender in clinical psychopharmacology. *Psychopharmacology Bulletin*, **32**, 283–289.

Dimsdale J., Ziegler M. & Graham R. (1988) The effect of hypertension sodium and race in isopropanol sensitivity. *Clinical and Experimental Hypertension*, **A10**, 747–756.

Escobar, J. & Tuason, V. (1980) Antidepressant agents in a cross cultural study. *Psychopharmacology Bulletin*, **16**, 49–52.

Frackiewicz, E., Stannek, J., Herrara, J., *et al* (1997) Ethnicity and antipsychotic response. *Annals of Pharmacotherapy*, **31**, 1360–1369.

Gaviria, M., Gill, A. & Javaid, J. (1986) Nortriptyline kinetics in Hispanic and Anglo subjects. *Journal of Clinical Psychopharmacology*, **6**, 227–231.

Ghoneim, M., Kortilla, K., Chiang, C.-K., *et al* (1981) Diazepam effects and kinetics in Caucasians and Orientals. *Clinical Pharmacology and Therapeutics*, **29**, 749–756.

Hu, W., Lee, C., Yang, Y., *et al* (1983) Imipramine plasma levels and clinical response. *Bulletin of the Chinese Society of Neurology and Psychiatry*, **9**, 40–49.

Jann, M., Chang, W., Davis, C., *et al* (1989) Haloperidol and reduced haloperidol plasma levels in Chinese vs non Chinese psychiatric patients. *Psychiatry Research*, **30**, 45–52.

Jann, M., Lam, Y. & Chang, W. (1993) Haloperidol and reduced haloperidol plasma concentration in different ethnic populations and inter individual variabilities in haloperidol metabolism. In *Psychopharmacology and Psychobiology of Ethnicity* (eds K.-M. Lin, R. Poland & G. Nakasaki), pp. 133–152. APA Press.

Kilow, W. (1982) Ethnic differences in drug metabolism. *Clinical Pharmacokinetics*, **71**, 373–400.

Kishimoto, A. & Hollister, L. (1984) Nortriptyline kinetics in Japanese and Americans. *Journal of Clinical Psychopharmacology*, **4**, 171–172.

Kumana, C., Lauder, I., Chan, M., *et al* (1987) Differences in diazepam pharmacokinetics in Chinese and white Caucasians. *European Journal of Clinical Pharmacology*, **32**, 211–215.

Lambert, T. & Norman, T. R. (2008) Ethnic differences in psychotropic drug response and pharmacokinetics. In *Ethno-psychopharmacology: Advances in Current Practice* (eds C. H. Ng, K.-M. Lin, B. S. Singh, *et al*), pp. 38–61. Cambridge University Press.

Lee, M.-S., Kang, R.-H. & Hahn, S.-W. (2008) Pharmacogenetics of ethnic populations. In *Ethno-psychopharmacology: Advances in Current Practice* (eds C. H. Ng, K.-M. Lin, B. S. Singh, *et al*), pp. 62–86. Cambridge University Press.

Lewis, P., Rack, P., Vaddadi, K., *et al* (1980) Ethnic differences in drug response. *Postgraduate Medical Journal*, **56**, 46–49.

Lieberman, J., Yunis, J., Egla, E., *et al* (1990) HLA – 1338, DR4, DRW 3 and Clozapine induced agranulocytosis in Jewish patients with schizophrenia. *Archives of General Psychiatry*, **47**, 945–948.

Lin, K.-M. (1996) Psychopharmacology in cross-cultural psychiatry. *Mount Sinai Journal of Medicine*, **63**, 283–284.

Lin, K.-M., Lau, J., Smith, R., *et al* (1988) Comparison of alprazolam plasma levels and behavioural effects in normal Asian and Caucasian male volunteers. *Psychopharmacology*, **96**, 365–369.

Lin, K.-M., Poland, R., Nuccio, I., *et al* (1989) Longitudinal assessment of haloperidol dosage and serum concentrations in Asian and Caucasian schizophrenic patients. *American Journal of Psychiatry*, **146**, 1307–1311.

Lin, K.-M., Poland, R. & Nakasaki, G. (eds) (1993) *Psychopharmacology and Psychobiology of Ethnicity*. APA Press.

Lin, K.-M., Poland, R. & Anderson, D. (1995) Psychopharmacology, ethnicity and culture. *Transcultural Psychiatric Research Review*, **32**, 3–40.

Lin, K.-.M, Chen, C.-H., Yu, S.-H., *et al* (2008) Culture and ethnicity in psychopharmacology. In *Ethno-psychopharmacology: Advances in Current Practice* (eds C. H. Ng, K.-M. Lin, B. S. Singh, *et al*), pp. 27–37. Cambridge University Press.

Ng, C. H. & Klimidis, S. (2008) Cultural factors and the use of psychotropic medications. In *Ethno-psychopharmacology: Advances in Current Practice* (eds C. H. Ng, K.-M. Lin, B. S. Singh, *et al*), pp. 123–134. Cambridge University Press.

Office of Population Censuses and Surveys (1992) *County Monitor*. The Stationery Office (TSO).

Pi, E., Simpson, G. & Cooper, T. (1986) Pharmacokinetics of desipramine in Caucasian and Asian volunteers. *American Journal of Psychiatry*, **143**, 1174–1176.

Pi, E., Tran-Johnson, T., Walker, N., *et al* (1989) Pharmacokinetics of desipramine in Asian and Caucasian volunteers. *Psychopharmacology Bulletin*, **25**, 483–487.

Rudorfer, E., Lam, E., Chang, W., *et al* (1984) Desipramine pharmacokinetics in Chinese and Caucasian volunteers. *British Journal of Clinical Pharmacology*, **17**, 433–440.

Silver, B., Lin, K.-M. & Poland, R. (1993) Ethnicity and pharmacology of tricyclic antidepressants. In *Psychopharmacology and Psychobiology of Ethnicity* (eds K.-M. Lin, R. Poland & G. Nakasaki), pp. 61–89. APA Press.

Smith, M. & Mendoza, R. (1996) Ethnicity and pharmacogenetics. *Mount Sinai Journal of Medicine*, **63**, 285–290.

Westermeyer, J. (1989) *Psychiatric Care of Migrants*. APA Press.

Yamashita, I. & Asano, Y. (1979) Tricyclic antidepressants. *Psychopharmacology Bulletin*, **15**, 40–41.

Yu, X. (2008) Complementary medicine in mental disorders. In *Ethno-psychopharmacology: Advances in Current Practice* (eds C. H. Ng, K.-M. Lin, B. S. Singh, *et al*), pp. 118–122. Cambridge University Press.

Zhang, Y., Reviriego, J., Lou, Y., *et al* (1990) Diazepam metabolism in native Chinese poor and extensive hydroxylators of S-mephenytoin. *Clinical Pharmacology and Therapeutics*, **48**, 496–502.

CHAPTER 22

Communication with patients from other cultures: the place of explanatory models

Kamaldeep Bhui and Dinesh Bhugra

Summary   We discuss the complicated nature of communication between people from different cultural groups, perhaps using a second language. We focus on the fact that mental health practitioners and service users often have in common neither their cultural backgrounds nor their explanatory models of illness. Even in a shared language, communication can be less than optimal as words carry multiple meanings. Consequently, consultations that involve culturally grounded explanatory models of illness challenge the professional. We give examples showing that reconciling different explanatory models during the consultation is a core task for psychiatrists and mental health practitioners working in multicultural settings.

It is nearly two decades since Kleinman (1980) proposed the wider acceptance of the role of explanatory models in the assessment and management of mental disorders. The 'explanatory model' concept was intended to draw on social-anthropological approaches to understanding subjective experiences of distress and to apply them to psychiatric practice (Bhui & Bhugra, 2002). Pleas to recruit 'understanding' and 'empathy' into the clinical method have been with us since Jaspers' early writings on general psychopathology (Broome, 2002). The tension between identifying and understanding abnormalities of mental state persists into current psychiatric practice. Consultations are increasingly regarded, mainly by non-psychiatrists but also by some psychiatrists, as a technological enterprise. Checklists, clinical guidelines, clinical protocols, risk assessment tools, local implementation plans for the National Service Framework, governance requirements, appraisal and CPD portfolios, teaching portfolios and membership of learned institutions all include lists of activities, objectives and achievements. These documents regulate our practice by ensuring that minimum standards are met, and they demonstrate that our work includes more than sound clinical practice. Nonetheless, less attention is now paid to the more human aspects of psychiatry, which rely on sound clinical practice and include 'quality in the clinical method', consultation dynamics, effective history-taking, understanding, empathy and building a therapeutic alliance taking account of transferential and countertransferential issues.

Practising in a multicultural context

Drenan & Swarz (2002) remind us that psychiatric practice in multilingual settings involves various people acting as interpreters, which often leads to different conclusions about the significance of expressions of distress; for example, whether they indicate psychopathology or are culturally grounded and therefore not abnormal. It is often difficult for doctors to realise that family members' own explanation is one of many that patients hold in mind. Furthermore, Williams & Healy (2001) point out that explanatory models are not fixed and stable representations but that they fluctuate and are recruited in a context-dependent manner. This perhaps persuades doctors that explanatory models are not important or influential. Certainly, when actual (observed) behaviour does not map onto reported behaviour (expressed in an explanatory model), this needs to be factored into clinical decision-making. Explanatory models represent the position from which patients may express distress; and they can govern how patients interpret a psychiatric explanation of their problems. Even if patients unconditionally accept the medical perspective, there is still scope for explanatory models to influence adherence to treatment, especially if family, community and some personal explanations are at variance with the medical model.

The process of exploring explanatory models

The concept of explanatory models as it was originally formulated appears to have had little impact on psychiatric practice in general, even though there is now a greater emphasis on user views and satisfaction (chapter 6, this volume). Patients' explanatory models are not fixed and are influenced by the circumstances of their symptoms, but they can influence a physician's assessments (Bhui & Bhugra, 2002; Bhui et al, 2002).

It is the process of exploring with the patient his or her identity and explanatory model that ensures improved understanding and informs the successful negotiation of different world views. This exploration does not require psychiatrists to enter into another culture as a participant observer, a prerequisite for any form of authentic ethnography. Nor does it require them to undergo in-depth psychoanalysis of their own world view. However, they do have to transfer models of mind and functioning from these disciplines into the therapeutic clinical setting. Personal psychotherapy is core to the training of psychiatrists and this may be an appropriate opportunity to begin explorations of cultural differences. It should be remembered, though, that psychotherapeutic theories and practice have their own cultural biases, which are often made manifest in a mismatch at a theoretical, technical or philosophical level (Bhugra & Bhui, 1998, 2002).

> **Box 22.1** The five elements of cultural formulation
>
> - The cultural identity of the individual
> - Cultural explanations of the individual's illness
> - The influence of the patient's psychosocial environment and level of functioning within it
> - Cultural elements in the patient–professional relationship
> - The use of cultural assessment in deciding diagnosis and care
>
> (American Psychiatric Association, 2002)

Cultural formulations

Cultural formulations were introduced into DSM–IV in an attempt to make diagnostic practice more culturally appropriate, relevant and representative. This marked a beginning of the exploration of values in diagnostic criteria, but cannot replace a thorough exploration of the values of patient and professional during the clinical process. The American Psychiatric Association (2002) recommends five elements in the cultural formulation (Box 22.1). The second of these relates to the patient's explanatory model of the illness, and explores cultural factors beyond race and ethnicity. However, in isolation from the other elements, awareness of explanatory models is unlikely to influence the quality of the consultation, the assessment or the management of the patient's distress.

Building on this multilevel approach, a recent review of explanatory models acknowledges the difficulties of striving for a single broadly applicable explanatory law for traditional models in science (Kendler, 2008). Arguing that causal factors have an impact on psychiatric illness at micro- and macrolevels within and outside of the individual and involving processes best understood from biological, psychological and sociocultural perspectives, Kendler advocates a multicausal approach to understanding mechanisms through the concepts of 'decomposition and reassembly'.

Readers might like to explore what further information a cultural formulation might have yielded to influence the management of the young man in the following case history. (For conciseness, the full cultural formulation of Mr B's beliefs is not reproduced here.)

Case history 1

Mr B was an 18-year-old Bangladeshi man under investigation for unexplained physical symptoms by gastroenterological, orthopaedic and general medical services in a teaching hospital. His general practitioner knew that the young man was very distressed and was avoiding school, but could not reassure him. The specialists could find no organic illness. Mr B was seen by two senior psychiatrists (one English and one Indian: no Bangladeshi psychiatrist was then available), and their overall view was that his symptoms were psychosomatic but that his unwillingness to attend psychiatric appointments and failure to communicate with them made it unlikely that he would come to understand why he would not benefit from further physical investigations.

Mr B was eventually seen by another Indian psychiatrist, who found that Mr B spoke English well. Unlike the two previous psychiatrists, the third psychiatrist was able to explore Mr B's problems from the young man's own perspective. During the course of the assessment sessions Mr B revealed that he had first noticed 'stomach noises' in the mosque and had immediately attributed them to an abnormal mass in his stomach – stomach cancer or something equally 'bad'. He became unable to visit the mosque, which distressed both him and his father. Both were concerned that he could not remain active in worship within the local Muslim community, as this would have violated their religious practices. He also admitted that he had palpitations and sweats and became frightened when his stomach made the noises.

The psychiatrist and Mr B acknowledged the latter's belief in this growth in his stomach as both important and disabling, causing much concern to his family. However, the psychiatrist pointed out that there was no evidence of any physical abnormality and recommended an antidepressant, explaining that this fitted into his schema of what was causing Mr B's problems. It was thus explicitly acknowledged that Mr B might have been unfamiliar with this remedy. The young man's belief that there was a mass in his stomach resonated with the phenomenon of *Tharan*, which the psychiatrist had previously encountered among patients of Indian origin. *Tharan* is described as a mass in the stomach, for which the treatment is massage to remove the blockage.

This approach of negotiation without conflict, in which both the psychiatrist and the patient respectfully accepted alternative, perhaps to each unusual, explanatory models led Mr B to accept antidepressant medication, and within 2 weeks he was much less anxious.

The psychiatrist was then able to instigate a series of cognitive–behavioural therapy (CBT) sessions. The CBT was targeted at enabling the young man to return to school and to the mosque, by encouraging response prevention and by cognitively challenging his morbid explanation for the stomach noises (but not challenging his cultural explanation of them). Although Mr B missed 4 of the 16 CBT sessions, he always left a message and followed the behavioural homework tasks. He always came to the clinic with his friends, who waited outside for him. He resumed weekly attendance at the mosque and returned to school, and the stomach noises settled. His explanation of what had led to recovery included regular stomach massage by his father to remove the mass. He thought that the antidepressant medication had helped him, but had no idea whether the CBT had also been useful. Tolerance of his failure to attend all of the CBT sessions, acceptance of his explanations and the psychiatrist's not insisting on taking the credit for recovery enabled Mr B and his father to find a solution that helped relieve their personal, family and social distress.

This case shows how the patient's explanatory models of illness can be creatively used in consultations and need not compete with the psychiatrist's model. One non-confrontational way forward is to work with 'co-constructed illness narratives' (Yeung & Kam, 2008). The psychiatrist does not have to be from the same cultural background to achieve a therapeutic alliance. The case also illustrates that evidence-based interventions can be delivered despite differing explanatory models.

Communication, culture and therapeutic relationships

What is therapeutic in a clinical situation? What makes up a therapeutic relationship? The microskills necessary to maximise the therapeutic alliance and relationship are the cornerstone of sound clinical practice and are exercised during the consultation, when psychiatrist meets patient. Yet less is known about these key aspects of clinical practice than about most pharmacological interventions (McGuire *et al*, 2001). The psychiatrist's primary aim is to gather authentic information, make judgements about psychopathology and then understand how best to make use of this information to achieve the therapeutic goals brought to the consultation by the patients, as well as introduce the psychiatrist's own objectives. This is far from a technical process. So when this complex and value-laden task includes patients from a different cultural background, there is even more potential for miscommunications to enter the discourse.

The problem with words

Acts of speech are often taken for granted as straightforward communications of particular realities. In fact, in a psychiatric setting they are a discourse about individual/private and societal/public issues expressed through languages of distress. The multiple meanings carried by each word, when understood as being reflexively shaped by other words in the same sentence and by the biography of the individual, are also strongly connected with cultural meanings, symbols (social and political), and historical and contemporary narratives. The manifest and latent meanings attached to any word, even in the same language, may differ between patient and clinician. Said, a Christian Palestinian living in exile in New York, writes about communication: 'The language in which we are speaking is his before it is mine. How different are the words home, Christ, ale, master, on his lips and on mine! I cannot speak or write these words without unrest of spirit. His language, so familiar and so foreign, will always before me be an acquired speech' (Said, 1983: p. 48).

A similar position was taken by Lacan (see Nobus, 2000: p. 71). For both the child and the adult, language is most inadequate for the communication of needs, which are more easily expressed symbolically. Even for people who share the same mother tongue, language can lead to miscommunications in symbolic terms. How much more difficult must it be to communicate deep needs in a second language. In a study of Somali refugees, six translators spent at least 40 hours ensuring that the translated instruments used had face and content validity. Clinicians are rarely able to take into account the many factors that influence communication and assessment of emotions across cultures.

Recognising emotions

Despite international research (Shioiri *et al*, 1999) showing that a finite number of emotions are recognised in all societies and cultures (surprise, disgust, fear, anger, contempt, happiness and sadness), the accurate recognition of these emotional states varies with culture and observer (Shioiri *et al*, 1999; Elfenbein & Ambady, 2002, 2003) and becomes more precise the greater the exposure to the culture of the person being assessed. It may be that when psychiatrists assess emotional states across cultures, and even across socioeconomic groups, the emotional content is not fully appreciated. Such fine-grain omissions might account for some of the dissatisfaction felt by patients from minority ethnic groups and perhaps for some of the perceived lower involvement of professionals with such patients. For example, general practitioners in the south London borough of Camberwell reported that they felt less involved in the care of their Black patients, but on examination of the records it was found that they had just as much instrumental involvement with them as they had with their White patients (Bindman *et al*, 1997).

Empathy

Understanding barriers to empathy across cultures sheds light on why psychiatric assessment across cultures is difficult or imprecise. Exploring the explanatory models held by service users may allow a broader exploration of the affects and emotions associated with their own understanding of their problems. Speaking in a second language can have a defensive function (Tesone, 1996); perhaps speaking through some one else's explanatory model serves a similar function, making the other's model seem unreal or unintelligible.

Case history 2

A 24-year-old Bangladeshi man sustained a head injury in a road traffic accident. He presented with impulsiveness and poor judgement; frontal lobe damage was evident on magnetic resonance imaging (MRI). He believed the accident and its consequences to be an act of God. His psychiatrist believed that the young man's behaviour and poor functioning resulted from the head injury. The two could not agree, and the man's family were invited to discuss the reasons for his condition. They also supported the view that God is superordinate and responsible for everything, including the abnormal MRI scan and the young man's symptoms. The mental health team feared that this belief in God would impair the man's ability to adhere to treatment, and were troubled that the family did not accept the medical diagnosis and explanation, which was based on the scan evidence.

This case history illustrates quite distinct but competing explanations for behavioural change. The psychiatrist and mental health team are used to holding a single explanation for events, one that is evidence based and grounded on the scientific foundations of psychiatry. The young man and his family, who have strong religious beliefs, understand the implications of the abnormal scan, but are preoccupied with the broader meaning of the event in terms of the forces they believe to govern the world. Interestingly, they are able to hold competing beliefs without feeling any inner conflict, whereas the mental health team view the family's powerfully held unscientific religious explanations with suspicion.

Differences in religious world view, experiences of health services, expectations of recovery, and lay referral systems in the folk and popular sector may all contribute to the divergence of explanatory models between professionals and patients.

When compromise is difficult

Even if explanatory models differ markedly between professional and patient, it should be possible to reach a compromise quite quickly. By avoiding antagonistic and conflictual styles of consultation and permitting the patient to hold on to their own explanations, the professional should be able to persuade patients that is it OK to 'agree to differ'. This means that members of mental health teams must respect their patients' views just as much as they expect patients to respect theirs.

Sometimes, an impasse is reached where neither side can agree to accept and work with the other's viewpoint. This resembles the quite common situation in which a patient in general medical practice refuses to adopt the sick role. The manner in which this dispute is resolved will be coloured by the values and attitudes of the doctor towards both patients and ill health. Furthermore, differences in education and social class influence ability to negotiate barriers. In cross-cultural consultations it is common for specifically cultural factors also to influence the management of such an impasse (Bhugra & Bhui, 2002). Doctors often feel that the patient's view is exotic, unscientific and, more specifically, embedded in a cultural world view that they do not understand. Such situations often end up as case presentations and spark grand-round debates about how culture influences psychopathology.

Among mental health professionals there is often a fundamental lack of understanding and valuing of foreign or non-psychiatric perspectives. A study in India revealed a wide range of explanatory models for the presence of psychotic symptoms, including, as would be expected, a variety of religious and spiritual beliefs (Saravanan et al, 2007). However, these were noted to be linked with judgements regarding lack of insight, which were not necessarily appropriate: holding a religious or spiritual explanation for psychotic experiences does not automatically mean that insight is lacking. Added to this, the task of reaching consensus with patients is itself loaded with the potential to perpetuate or exacerbate professionals' lack of understanding if mutually agreed rules of discussion and negotiation to build a therapeutic alliance are not prominent. Leff (1988) has described how traditional healers tend to consult in public, with consensus and sanction from the wider community. More specifically, he notes that they skilfully negotiate difference of opinion and attitude using their knowledge of the culture in which they are embedded. Negotiation of differences in world view may be a useful core skill for psychiatrists working in multicultural settings.

Exploring cultural identity with patients allows them to express their culturally determined views, which will have been shaped both by the subculture and the dominant society in which they live. Such an approach is as relevant for White majorities and their subcultural groups as it is for minority ethnic communities, and is therefore of great relevance to services working in increasingly multicultural settings.

References

American Psychiatric Association (2002) *Cultural Assessment in Clinical Psychiatry*. American Psychiatric Publishing.

Bhugra, D. & Bhui, K. (1998) Psychotherapy for ethnic minorities. *British Journal of Psychotherapy*, **14**, 310–326.

Bhugra, D. & Bhui, K. (2002) Is the Oedipal complex universal? Problems for sexual and relationship psychotherapy across cultures. *Sexual and Relationship Therapy*, **17**, 69–86.

Bhui, K. & Bhugra, D. (2002) Explanatory models for mental distress: implications for clinical practice and research. *British Journal of Psychiatry*, **181**, 6–7.

Bhui, K., Bhugra, D. & Goldberg, D. (2002) Causal explanations of distress and general practitioners' assessments of common mental disorder among Punjab and English attendees. *Social Psychiatry and Psychiatric Epidemiology*, **37**, 38–45.

Bindman, J., Johnson, S., Wright, S., *et al* (1997) Integration between primary and secondary services in the care of the severely mentally ill: patients' and general practitioners' views. *British Journal of Psychiatry*, **171**, 169–174.

Broome, M. (2002) Explanatory models in psychiatry. *British Journal of Psychiatry*, **181**, 351–352.

Drenan, G. & Swarz, L. (2002) The paradoxical use of interpreting in psychiatry. *Social Science and Medicine*, **54**, 1853–1866.

Elfenbein, H. A. & Ambady, N. (2002) On the universality and cultural specificity of emotion recognition: a meta-analysis. *Psychological Bulletin*, **128**, 203–235.

Elfenbein, H. A. & Ambady, N. (2003) When familiarity breeds accuracy: cultural exposure and facial emotion recognition. *Journal of Personality and Social Psychology*, **85**, 276–290.

Kendler, K. S. (2008) Explanatory models for psychiatric illness. *American Journal of Psychiatry*, **165**, 695–702.

Kleinman, A. (1980) *Patients and Healers in the Context of Culture*. Thesis. University of California Press.

Leff, J. (1988) *Psychiatry around the Globe: A Transcultural View* (2nd edn). Gaskell.

McGuire, R., McCabe, R. & Priebe, S. (2001) Theoretical frameworks for understanding and investigating the therapeutic relationship in psychiatry. *Social Psychiatry and Psychiatric Epidemiology*, **36**, 557–564.

Nobus, D. (2000) *Jacques Lacan and the Freudian Practice of Psychoanalysis*. Routledge.

Said, E. (1983) *The World, and the Text and the Critic*. Harvard University Press.

Saravanan, B., Jacob, K. S., Johnson, S., *et al* (2007) Belief models in first episode schizophrenia in South India. *Social Psychiatry and Psychiatric Epidemiology*, **42**, 446–451.

Shioiri, T., Someya, T., Helmeste, D., *et al* (1999) Misinterpretation of facial expression: a cross-cultural study. *Psychiatry and Clinical Neuroscience*, **53**, 45–50.

Tesone, J. E. (1996) Multi-lingualism, word-presentations, thing-presentations and psychic reality. *International Journal of Psychoanalysis*, **77**, 871–881.

Williams, B. & Healy, D. (2001) Perceptions of illness causation among new referrals to a community mental health team: explanatory model or exploratory map? *Social Science and Medicine*, **53**, 465–476.

Yeung, A. & Kam, R. (2008) Ethical and cultural considerations in delivering psychiatric diagnosis: reconciling the gap using MDD diagnosis delivery in less-acculturated Chinese patients. *Transcultural Psychiatry*, **45**, 531–552.

CHAPTER 23

Working with patients with religious beliefs

Simon Dein

Summary Mental health professionals in Western societies are generally less religious than their patients and receive little training in religious issues. Using case studies, I discuss issues involved in working with patients who hold religious beliefs: problems of engagement; countertransference; religious and spiritual issues not attributable to mental disorder; problems of differential diagnosis; religious delusions; religion and psychotherapy; psychosexual problems; and religiously oriented treatments. The chapter ends with a discussion of the various ways in which religious themes can be incorporated into mental health work, especially the need to involve religious professionals and develop collaborative patterns of working together.

As part of their everyday clinical practice mental health professionals are likely to encounter patients with religious beliefs or patients who have religious issues. Traditionally, psychiatrists and psychologists have under-emphasised religious issues in their work (Larson, 1986; Lukoff & Turner, 1992; Sims, 1994; Crossley, 1995). Religion is often seen by mental health professionals in Western societies as irrational, outdated and dependency-forming, a view deriving from Freud (1907: p. 25), who saw it as a 'universal obsessional neurosis' (Box 23.1). For similar reasons the topic of religion plays little part in psychiatric training, which may be selected by people of

---

Box 23.1 Antagonism towards religion

Many psychiatrists see religion as:
- primitive
- guilt-inducing
- a form of dependency
- irrational
- having no empirical base

---

a lower level of religiosity than the background population (Shafranske & Malony, 1990; Larson & Larson, 1991; Rubenstein, 1994). It is no wonder that the Danish theologian Hans Kung referred to religion as 'psychiatry's last taboo' (Kung, 1986).

Several studies highlight a 'religiosity gap': psychiatrists are often far less religious than their patients (Kroll & Sheehan, 1981; Neeleman & Lewis, 1994). Both the general public and psychiatric patients report themselves to be more religious and to attend church more regularly than mental health professionals (American Psychiatric Association Task Force, 1975). In fact, a Gallup poll in 1985 indicated that a third of the general population in the USA considered religion to be the most important dimension of their lives, and another third considered it to be very important (Gallup, 1986). Keating & Fretz (1990) report evidence that religious individuals are less satisfied with a non-religious clinician than with a religious one.

There are signs that things may be slowly changing. A number of authors are beginning to stress that mental health professionals should take into account patients' religious and spiritual lives during the psychiatric consultation (Sims, 1994; Crossley, 1995; King & Dein, 1999). Cox (1996: p. 158) argues:

> if mental health services in a multicultural society are to become more responsive to 'user' needs then eliciting this 'religious history' with any linked spiritual meanings should be a routine component of a psychiatric assessment, and of preparing a more culturally sensitive 'care plan'.

Attempts at empirical assessments of the relationships between religion, spirituality and mental health suggest that holding religious beliefs may promote better mental health (Batson & Ventis, 1993; Koenig, 1998; Pargament & Brant, 1998). However, this work is limited to Christianity and Judaism, and there has been little exploration of this topic in other religious groups. Some patients define their problems as spiritual rather than religious; by 'spiritual' they generally mean a transcendent relationship between themselves and a 'higher being' – 'a quality that goes beyond a specific religious affiliation' (Peterson & Nelson, 1987). 'Religion' has been defined as 'adherence to and beliefs and practices of an organised church or religious institution' (Shafranske & Malony, 1990). The distinction between spirituality and religion has been deployed by some contemporary researchers in the field of religion and health (e.g. King et al, 1999).

This chapter is not an overview of the relationship between religion and mental health; rather, it focuses on specific issues involved in working with patients with religious beliefs. In light of my own professional experience, it largely focuses on Judaeo-Christianity, although the same principles apply to working with other religious groups. A major ethical issue when working with patients with religious beliefs is the degree to which psychiatrists should be involved in discussing religious issues. For instance, should a secular psychiatrist become involved in discussing the religious beliefs of a devout Catholic patient, if they impinge on that patient's mental health?

Problems of engagement

A rejecting attitude towards psychiatry is common to many religious groups. There are many reasons for this. First, the stigma of mental illness may affect the marriage prospects of members of religious communities (as in Case study 1 below). Second, in many religious groups, psychiatry and psychology are considered suspect (Greenberg & Witztum, 2001) – both dismiss dogma and God's existence. To turn to a doctor may express a lack of faith in God's ability to help (Peteet, 1981). Third, patients may perceive doctors as at best failing to understand their religious beliefs and at worst ridiculing them; consequently, they may have little faith in medical professionals.

The psychiatrist may overcome this resistance in a number of ways. It may be necessary to use a 'culture broker', someone from the same religious group as the patient who acts as the patient's advocate. Another important technique is to make use of the symbols of the religion that are important to the patient. For instance, some ultra-orthodox Jews (particularly Hasidim, who have little contact with the secular world) may be unaware of current affairs, but can answer questions on familiar topics such as Jewish religious festivals and Bible readings.

Case study 1: The stigma of mental illness

> Sarah, a 50-year-old devout Jew, wrote to her psychiatrist. She had suffered from low mood for some years and had been diagnosed with chronic depression. She took paroxetine regularly but remained anxious much of the time. In her letter, she asked her psychiatrist to provide confirmation that her condition was not hereditary, since she was seeking an arranged marriage for her daughter. She feared that her daughter's marriage prospects would be significantly reduced if anyone knew of her mental illness.

Countertransference problems

Mental health professionals may become angered by patients with religious convictions, arguing that they hold 'primitive' and repressive beliefs that are detrimental to mental health (Case study 2). They may ask themselves how religious patients adhere to their belief systems in the absence of 'empirical' evidence. Greenberg & Witztum (1991) suggest a number of ways in which therapists react to such emotions in themselves:

- with excessive curiosity about the patient, asking many questions about the patient's religious beliefs and practices
- by ignoring cultural influences or tensions and treating the patient as though they belong to the same cultural group as the therapist
- by behaving aggressively towards the patient, becoming angry when the patient refuses to adhere to treatment or accept the therapist's formulation.

Case study 2: Religious convictions and the countertransference

A liaison psychiatrist was asked to see a 60-year-old woman with a fungating breast carcinoma. She was a devout Christian Scientist who had always trusted in God to cure her (Christian Science eschews modern medicine, placing faith in God's ability to heal). Despite 'much persuasion' the woman had refused to accept any surgical intervention. The surgeon who referred her felt that she was 'quite irrational' in stating that God would save her life. He felt angry that she refused what he considered life-saving treatment. The psychiatrist who assessed her felt that she was quite competent to make this decision. There was no evidence that she was depressed or psychotic.

How should religious or spiritual problems be assessed?

How should psychiatrists classify religious or spiritual problems? The new diagnostic category of religious or spiritual problem (V62.89) was included in DSM–IV (American Psychiatric Association, 1994), as part of 'Other conditions that may be a focus of clinical attention', to offset the tendency of mental health professionals to ignore or pathologise such problems. This acknowledgement marks a significant breakthrough (Turner *et al*, 1995).

Common religious problems that may be a focus of clinical attention include questioning and loss of faith, change of religious denomination, conversion to a new religion and intensification of adherence to the beliefs and practices of one's faith. Loss or questioning of faith is a common problem which may be particularly difficult for patients at an early stage of religious development. These problems should be distinguished from functional psychiatric disorders, although they may lead to psychiatric illness. Their resolution generally requires referral to religious professionals.

One particular form of 'religious' conversion is the joining of a new religious movement or cult regarded by the public as oppressive. Although there is little evidence that belonging to such a movement is generally detrimental to mental health (Richardson, 1985; Barker, 1996), it appears that leaving one – often by forcible removal – may result in a number of problems, including agitation, panic attacks, nightmares and repetitive chanting, a phenomenon called 'information disease'. Rarely, religious movements have extremely detrimental effects on their adherents, even to the extent of pushing them to suicide, as did the Branch Davidians in the USA (Dein & Littlewood, 2000). Bogart (1992) reported on psychological problems that may arise when a member of a spiritual group separates from their spiritual teacher; these include agitation, low mood and nightmares.

Although psychiatrists in the UK are rarely asked to see members of new religious movements, they need to be aware of the Information Network Focus on Religious Movements (INFORM), a voluntary organisation that provides information about such movements and that can recommend access to counselling services (www.lse.ac.uk/collections/INFORM; www.inform.ac/infmain.html).

Mystical states

Mystical experiences are common in the UK and the USA, with about a third of people reporting them at some stage of their life (Hay, 1987). These experiences include feelings of unity with the universe and ecstatic states associated with universal love. Although the feelings are transient, they may lead to permanent changes in cognition and lifestyle and may have an emotionally integrative function. It is likely that these states are a normal part of brain function. They may occur spontaneously, be induced by drugs or occur during meditation. Not in themselves symptoms of psychiatric disorder, they can occur in pathological states such as temporal lobe epilepsy and in psychosis, when they are usually associated with an elevation of mood. It is important that psychiatrists respect and differentiate unusual but integrating experiences from those that are distressing or disorganising (Gabbard *et al*, 1982). A negative response to a mystical experience may intensify an individual's sense of isolation and block their efforts to seek assistance in integrating and assimilating the experience. There has been much discussion of the difference between mystical and psychotic states (Clarke, 2001). Generally, there are few problems in differentiating the two phenomena using criteria such as the negative effect on life functioning, loss of volition and loss of insight, which occur in psychosis but not in mystical states (Box 23.2).

Another psychological phenomenon that has been vigorously discussed in the academic literature is the near-death experience – when a person while clinically dead (i.e. without a heartbeat) has the sensation of leaving their body and, characteristically, floating into a tunnel towards a perceived mystical source. It is not attributable to a mental disorder (Basford, 1990; Fenwick & Fenwick, 1995), although anger, depression and isolation may occur following this experience. Generally, however, individuals report beneficial after-effects, including positive attitude and value changes and some personality transformation. However, at times the near-death experience can be associated with negative psychological sequelae.

Box 23.2 Differentiating psychotic states from religious experiences

In psychosis:

- experiences are often very personal
- their details exceed conventional expressions of belief
- in many cases, the only distinguishing feature is the intensity of the belief, with the patient thinking of nothing else
- onset of the beliefs and behaviours marks a change in the patient's life, with a deterioration of social skills and personal hygiene
- episodes often involve special messages from religious figures

---

Case study 3: Near-death experience in delirium

A 50-year-old woman was referred to a psychiatric out-patient clinic following an episode of septicaemia during which she spent 2 weeks in intensive care. Her heart had stopped on two occasions. She described a number of experiences during this time, one of which was a journey to the 'abode of the dead', where she saw corpses lying in coffins who suddenly became animated and spoke to her. At the time she believed herself to be dead. Following recovery, she was preoccupied with these experiences and had difficulty making sense of them; she also developed a morbid fear of death. The psychiatric interview revealed marked anxiety in relation to dying. Diagnostically, it appeared that she had been in a delirious state secondary to hypoxia and septicaemia; this delirium was the likely cause of her near-death experience.

Religious delusions

At times it can be difficult to distinguish religious beliefs from frank delusions. In psychotic disorders there is frequently an overlap between the mental disorder and religious and spiritual problems – especially in manic episodes, which often contain mystical components (Podvoll, 1987). Goodwin & Jamison (1990) have noted the prominence of religious and spiritual concerns in people with bipolar disorder. Religious delusions may be defined as delusions that have a religious content that is not socially acceptable or shared by other religious people. Sims (1992) outlines the criteria for characterising a belief as a religious delusion:

> Both the observed behaviour and the subjective experience conform with psychiatric symptoms. The patient's self description of the experience is recognisable as having the form of a delusion.
> There are other recognisable symptoms of mental illness in other areas of the individual's life, such as delusions, hallucinations, mood or thought disorder.
> The lifestyle, behaviour and direction of the personal goals of the individual after the event or after the religious experience are consistent with the natural history of mental disorder rather than with a personality-enriching experience.

Religious delusions generally are of three types: persecutory (often including the Devil), grandiose (involving messianic beliefs) and belittlement (including beliefs about having committed unforgivable sins). The recorded prevalence of religious delusions varies between studies. In a UK study of people with schizophrenia, Littlewood & Lipsedge (1981) quoted figures of up to 45% in the Black immigrants in their sample, compared with 14% in the White UK-born individuals. Siddle (2000) found a prevalence of 24% in a sample of patients admitted to hospital with a diagnosis of schizophrenia. Religious delusions are found in a number of psychiatric conditions, including depressive and bipolar disorders, schizophrenia and delusional or organic disorders, as Case study 4 demonstrates.

Case study 4: Messianic delusion in organic illness

A 55-year-old African man was admitted to hospital under Section 3 of the Mental Health Act 1983 following severe neglect and odd, disinhibited behaviour. He had previously been given a diagnosis of schizophrenia but had not taken any medication for over 2 years. While on the ward he repeatedly expressed the belief that he was 'God of the universe' and claimed to have supernatural power to heal. He demonstrated no sign of hypomania but a striking degree of apathy and self-neglect. There was no cognitive impairment. Serological tests for syphilis during routine investigation were significantly positive, and a diagnosis of tertiary syphilis was confirmed by lumbar puncture. His delusions responded to a depot medication and intramuscular penicillin. However, his apathy continued to be a problem.

There is some evidence that religious delusions may result in harm to self and others (Field & Waldfogel, 1995): individuals may act on passages from the Bible telling them to pluck out offending eyes or cut off limbs. A study of psychiatric inmates in an American penal institution found that over half of its most dangerous inmates had religious delusions (Scarnati *et al*, 1991).

Case studies 5 and 6 point to the difficulty of differentiating religious beliefs from delusions. The borderline between the two may be unclear, and members of the person's religious community are best able to make the differentiation.

Case study 5: The Devil within?

A 22-year-old woman had become a born again Christian at the age of 15 after attending a service at which a well-known preacher gave a sermon. Although always describing herself as religious, her church attendance fluctuated according to her mood. She suffered from periods of low mood associated with anorexia, and during these episodes she felt hopeless and had marked suicidal ideation. She regularly cut herself as a form of purification. Even when well she expressed the belief that the world is sinful because of the continuing influence of the Devil. Much of her conversation centred on a continuing conflict between the 'powers of good and the powers of evil'. During one episode of severe depression she spoke of the Devil causing her harm and of a constant fight inside her. She took this belief to be literal.

Was this woman's belief in the Devil a normative belief, an overvalued idea or a psychotic delusion?

Case study 6: Mission or psychosis?

A 25-year-old Nigerian woman had arrived in the UK 6 months before her compulsory admission to a psychiatric unit. Following her arrival in Britain she had joined a Pentecostalist church. Over several months her level of religiosity had increased. For 2 weeks prior to admission she had taken to preaching in the street that 'Jesus is our Lord' and 'You will only be saved if you come to Jesus'. For nearly a week she did not sleep and hardly ate. On the day of admission she was involved in a fracas with a passer-by and was taken to hospital under Section 136 of the Mental Health Act.

During her assessment in the accident and emergency department she appeared dishevelled, was overactive, overtalkative and preoccupied with telling the doctor how important it was for him to come to Jesus. When it was possible to interrupt her she admitted to being 'a sister of Christ'. There was no evidence of any other abnormal ideation. She did not believe that she was ill, and held that she was on a mission. She was given 100 mg of chlorpromazine and soon fell asleep.

The following morning she was much calmer and settled. She admitted that her behaviour had been 'over the top', a sentiment shared by members of her church who visited her. By the evening, however, she recommenced talking about 'coming to Christ', upsetting a number of fellow patients. At midnight she went to bed. At 02.00 h the nurse checked on her to find that she had forced open the window in her room on the third floor and jumped to her death. (Adapted from Dein, 2000.)

What was this woman's diagnosis? Was she hypomanic? Manifesting a brief psychosis? Was she in fact psychotic at all?

Spirit possession

There is some – albeit little – recognition of spirit possession in Western society. Bishop Dominic Walker (the co-chair of the Christian Deliverance Study Group) points out that although schizophrenia would seem to be the obvious explanation for people who describe hearing voices or thought insertion, there are cases in which the symptoms disappear 'after the appropriate ministry' (Walker, 1997: p. 3).

Case study 7: Psychosis presenting as possession

A 26-year-old White British man who was not religious was referred to the psychiatric out-patient department with the following history. Two months prior to referral he and a group of friends had been playing with a Ouija board. The following night he started to believe that a spirit had entered him through his rectum and was controlling his behaviour: for instance, the spirit made him move and speak in a certain way.

He sought help from a local church, where he was told this was a psychiatric problem and that he was not really possessed. Although he insisted that he had never believed in spirits in the past, now he was deeply upset by this spirit and just wanted it to go. When interviewed he was visibly distressed but appeared to have no other psychopathological feature. There were no first-rank symptoms. Two exorcisms at a local church by a Church of England minister failed to achieve any improvement. A provisional diagnosis of schizophrenia was made (on account of passivity) and he was prescribed regular antipsychotic medication, which caused stiffness. He failed to return to the out-patient clinic, was not deemed to require detention under the Mental Health Act and was not seen again in the clinic.

It is debatable whether this man did in fact have schizophrenia or whether he was a highly suggestible person, possibly with a dissociative state.

Religious behaviour or obsessional illness?

The relationship between religiosity and obsessional illness has been discussed by a number of authors. A review by Lewis (1998) suggested that religiosity is associated with obsessional traits but not with obsessional neurosis. Similarly, Greenberg & Witztum (2001) pointed out that a review of the prevalence of obsessive–compulsive disorder in people from a variety of cultural backgrounds does not implicate religious background as a causative factor in this disorder. Here the emphasis is on differentiating religious behaviours from obsessional illness, which can be difficult (Box 23.3). Liaison with religious authorities may be necessary in the treatment of religious obsessive–compulsive disorder, since a religious leader may be able to discourage the patient from the performance of religious behaviour.

Case study 8: Excessive religious observance

A 26-year-old man who belonged to a group of ultra-Orthodox Jews presented with a number of problems. Since joining the movement 5 years earlier he had made few friends. Members of the community had remarked that he spent several hours a day in synagogue reciting the daily prayers (far in excess of the time required). During this he would become extremely aroused and at times would shout out the prayers. He prayed at the expense of performing other religious activities such as studying and at the expense of his own personal hygiene. He told other members of the group that it was essential that the prayers were recited perfectly or else they had to be repeated.

I was asked to see him because members of the community felt that he was ill. When I met him he was dishevelled and smelly, with very poor social skills. He was extremely reluctant to talk to me and muttered a few words, one of which sounded like an expletive. I was unable to interview him formally in any depth. Clearly his religious behaviour exceeded what was expected. My impression was that he suffered from a severe obsessional illness. He refused treatment.

Box 23.3 Differences between obsessive–compulsive and religious behaviours

In obsessive–compulsive disorder:

- compulsive behaviours go beyond the 'letter of the law'
- the person is interested only in a specific religious ritual, not in the practice of the religion generally
- the person neglects other aspects of the religion that are not the focus of the obsession
- the ritual typically exemplifies obsessional themes, e.g. cleanliness and checking

(after Greenberg & Witztum, 1991)

Religious ideas in psychotherapy

Patients with religious beliefs may bring up religious ideas and images in therapy. Jungian psychoanalysts emphasise the importance of religion in patients' lives, especially in those over 35 years of age: 'there has not been one whose problem in the last resort was not that of finding a religious outlook on life' (Jung, 1933: p. 229). Freudian and object-relations theories of religion focus on the influence of early relationships on the image of God and the quality of the relationship between the individual and God. For instance, Rizzuto (1992), a psychotherapist in the object-relations tradition, suggests that the image of God is formed from elements originating in early object relations. Spero (1992) demonstrates how religious concepts can change over the course of psychotherapy. Common themes that arise in psychotherapy with patients with religious beliefs concern God being punitive and the perception of having let God down.

Case 9 Psychotherapy and image of God

A 70-year-old man was referred to psychiatric services with a moderate depressive illness associated with marked suicidal ideation. He was being seen as an out-patient and treated with fluoxetine. His history reflected several religious themes. He had been adopted at the age of 3 years; his adoptive mother emotionally and physically abused him, and he was very afraid of her. She punished him almost at whim, and expected his behaviour to be exemplary at all times. At the age of 18 he became a monk, which upset his mother. After spending 5 years in a monastery he decided the life was not for him and married a woman much older than him, who had three children of her own. She died after 12 years of marriage.

Much of his discussion in out-patient therapy centred on how much he had let God down. His image of God was of a 'harsh dictator' who did not tolerate any indiscretion and was keen to punish anyone who failed to keep religious observances to the letter. It soon became obvious that this image of God reflected his relationship with his overpowering and punitive mother. During therapy sessions we looked at his guilt concerning the way he had treated his mother and his extreme anger towards her. Over time his image of God changed to a more benevolent one, as he slowly felt less guilty.

Psychosexual therapies

To date no work has specifically examined the epidemiology of psychosexual problems in specific religious groups. Religious groups may prohibit certain forms of sexual behaviour. For example, masturbation is strongly forbidden by the major world religions. For this reason, patients with religious beliefs may not be able to engage in certain psychosexual therapies such as the Masters & Johnson 'sensate focus' treatment, which deploys masturbation. Psychosexual techniques may have to be modified for these individuals. Owing to gender segregation and the prohibition relating to premarital sexual relations in certain religious communities, some couples may lack knowledge of normal sexual functioning, and an essential part of psychosexual counselling in such cases involves the provision of basic information about this.

Collaboration between psychiatric and religious professionals

At times it may be necessary to enlist the help of a religious professional such as a chaplain or someone influential in a religious organisation. Hospital chaplains in the UK receive some training in mental health through the College of Health Care Chaplains. They may provide help with religious problems such as discussion of the relationship between sin and mental illness, the giving of absolution and prayer. They can give guidelines on the 'normality' of religious beliefs. An issue that is frequently raised is the 'Why me?' question. How can a good God allow a person to suffer? One common answer emphasises that God is with the person in their suffering, consequently engendering hope. Koenig *et al* (2001: p. 450) write:

> Armed with faith, hope, spiritual knowledge, spiritual understanding, spiritual power and perhaps most important, humility, the religious professional is often the most qualified and sometimes the only person who can meet the underlying spiritual and religious needs that give rise to the patient's questions.

Chaplains are increasingly becoming a part of the multidisciplinary team in the UK, a fact justified on the basis that religious and spiritual needs are prevalent among patients with acute and chronic mental illness. They can be involved at all stages of the patient's illness, from diagnosis to discharge planning, and should be available to provide religious or spiritual support or counselling, including helping patients to discover a new spiritual vision for their lives. Religious professionals may be the first 'port of call' for people with mental health problems, and there is a need for collaboration between religious and mental health professionals, especially when dealing with those with serious mental illness. To this extent, religious professionals need to be taught to recognise common psychiatric problems. Likewise, mental health professionals require teaching about problems of a more spiritual nature.

Conclusion

Research is required to examine the prevalence, clinical presentations and relationship to major mental disorders of religious and spiritual problems. Mental health professionals need to be more aware of issues of religion and spirituality in clinical practice, and require education about the major teachings of diverse religious groups (Meyer, 1988). There is a need for more collaboration with religious personnel. Incorporation of religious themes into psychotherapy with religious patients may lead to enhanced efficacy. For example, using religious imagery in cognitive–behavioural therapy with patients with religious beliefs may be more effective than therapy lacking in this imagery (Propst *et al*, 1992). Other therapists have argued for the incorporation of religious values such as confession (Harrison, 1988) and forgiveness (Hope, 1987) into psychotherapy. The value of so doing remains to be demonstrated.

References

American Psychiatric Association (1994) *Diagnostic and Statistical Manual of Mental Disorders (4th edn) (DSM–IV)*. APA.

American Psychiatric Association Task Force (1975) *Psychiatrists' Viewpoints on Religion and Their Services to Religious Institutions and the Ministry*. APA.

Barker, E. (1996) *New Religious Movements: A Practical Introduction*. TSO (The Stationery Office).

Basford, T. K. (1990) *Near Death Experience: An Annotated Bibliography*. Garland.

Batson, C. D. & Ventis, W. L. (1993) *The Religious Experience: A Social, Psychological Perspective*. Oxford University Press.

Bogart, G. (1992) Separation from a spiritual teacher. *Journal of Personal Psychology*, **24**, 1–21.

Clarke, I. (2001) *Psychosis and Spirituality: Exploring the New Frontier*. Whurr.

Cox, J. (1996) Psychiatry and religion: a general psychiatrist's perspective. In *Psychiatry and Religion: Context, Consensus and Controversy* (ed. D. Bhugra). Routledge.

Crossley, D. (1995) Religious experience within mental illness: opening the door on research. *British Journal of Psychiatry*, **166**, 284–286.

Dein, S. (2000) The implications of an anthropology of religion for psychiatric practice. In *Anthropological Approaches to Psychological Medicine: Crossing Bridges* (eds V. Skultans & J. Cox), pp. 172–183. Jessica Kingsley.

Dein, S. & Littlewood, R. (2000) Apocalyptic suicide. *Mental Health, Religion and Culture*, **3**, 109–114.

Fenwick, P. & Fenwick, E. (1995) *The Truth in The Light*. Headline.

Field, H. & Waldfogel, S. (1995) Severe ocular self injury. *General Hospital Psychiatry*, **17**, 224–227.

Freud, S. (1907) Obsessive acts, religious practices. Reprinted (1953–1974) in the *Standard Edition of the Complete Psychological Works of Sigmund Freud* (trans. & ed. J. Strachey), vol. 7. Hogarth Press.

Gabbard, G. O., Twenlow, S. & Jones, P. (1982) Differential diagnosis of altered mind body perceptions. *Psychiatry*, **45**, 361–369.

Gallup, G. (1986) *Gallup Poll: Public Opinion 1985*. Scholarly Resources.

Goodwin, F. & Jamison, K. (1990) *Manic Depressive Illness*. Oxford University Press.

Greenberg, D. & Witztum, E. (1991) Problems in the treatment of religious patients. *American Journal of Psychotherapy*, **45**, 554–565.

Greenberg, D. & Witztum, E. (2001) *Sanity and Sanctity: Mental Health Work Among the Ultra Orthodox in Jerusalem*. Yale University Press.

Harrison, S. M. (1988) Sanctification and therapy: the model of Dante Alighieri. *Journal of Psychology and Theology*, **16**, 313–317.

Hay, D. (1987) *Exploring Inner Space* (2nd edn). Penguin.

Hope, D. (1987) The healing paradox of forgiveness. *Psychotherapy*, **24**, 240–244.

Jung, C. G. (1933) *Modern Man in Search of a Soul*. Harcourt.

Keating, A. M. & Fretz, B. R. (1990) Christians' anticipations about counsellors in response to counsellors' descriptions. *Journal of Counselling Psychology*, **37**, 293–296.

King, M. & Dein, S. (1999) The spiritual variable in psychiatry. *Psychological Medicine*, **28**, 1259–1262.

King, M., Speck, P. & Thomas, A. (1999) The effect of spiritual beliefs on outcome from illness. *Social Science and Medicine*, **48**, 1291–1299.

Koenig, H. G. (1998) Religious beliefs and practices of hospitalised medically ill older adults. *International Journal of Geriatric Psychiatry*, **13**, 213–224.

Koenig, H., McCullough, M. & Larson, D. (2001) *Handbook of Religion and Health*. Oxford University Press.

Kroll, J. & Sheehan, W. (1981) Religious beliefs and practice among 52 psychiatric inpatients in Minnesota. *American Journal of Psychiatry*, **146**, 67–72.

Kung, H. (1986) *Religion: The Last Taboo*. APA Press.

Larson, D. B. (1986) Systematic analysis of research on religious variables in four major psychiatric journals 1978–1982. *American Journal of Psychiatry*, **143**, 329–334.

Larson, D. B. & Larson, S. S. (1991) Religious commitment and health. *Second Opinion*, 27–40.

Lewis, C. A. (1998) 'Cleanliness is next to godliness': religiosity and obsessiveness. *Journal of Religion and Health*, **37**, 49–61.

Littlewood, R. & Lipsedge, R. (1981) Some social and phenomenological characteristics of psychotic immigrants. *Psychological Medicine*, **11**, 289–302.

Lukoff, D. & Turner, R. (1992) To order more culturally sensitive DSN for psycho religious and psycho spiritual problems. *Journal of Nervous and Mental Disease*, **180**, 673–682.

Meyer, M. S. (1988) Ethical principles of psychologists and religious diversity. *Professional Psychology: Research and Practice*, **19**, 486–488.

Neeleman, J. & Lewis, G. (1994) Religious identity and comfort beliefs in three groups of psychiatric patients and a group of medical controls. *International Journal of Social Psychiatry*, **40**, 124–134.

Pargament, K. I. & Brant, C. R. (1998) Religion and coping. In *Handbook of Religion and Mental Health* (ed. H. G. Koenig), pp. 112–128. Academic Press.

Peteet, J. R. (1981) Issues in the treatment of religious patients. *American Journal of Psychotherapy*, **35**, 559–564.

Peterson, E. A. & Nelson, K. (1987) How to meet your clients' spiritual needs. *Journal of Psychosocial Nursing*, **25**, 34–39.

Podvoll, E. (1987) Mania and the risk of power. *Journal of Contemplative Psychotherapy*, **4**, 95–122.

Propst, L., Ostrom, R., Watkins, P., *et al* (1992) Comparative efficacy of religious and non-religious cognitive-behavioural therapy for the treatment of clinical depression in religious individuals. *Journal of Consulting and Clinical Psychology*, **60**, 94–103.

Richardson, J. T. (1985) Psychological and psychiatric studies and new religions. In *Advances in the Psychology of Religion* (ed. L. B. Brown), pp. 209–223. Pergamon.

Rizzuto, A. M. (1992) Afterword. In *Object Relations Theory and Religion: Clinical Applications* (eds M. Finn & J. Gartner), pp. 154–175. Praeger.

Rubenstein, D. (1994) Political attitudes and religiosity levels of Israeli psychotherapy practitioners and students. *American Journal of Psychotherapy*, **48**, 441–454.

Scarnati, R., Madrey, M. & Wise, A. (1991) Religious beliefs and practices among the most dangerous psychiatric inmates. *Forensic Reports*, **4**, 1–16.

Shafranske, E. & Malony, H. M. (1990) Clinical psychologists' religious and spiritual orientations and their practice of psychotherapy. *Psychotherapy*, **27**, 72–78.

Siddle, R. (2000) *Religious Beliefs in Schizophrenia*. PhD thesis. University of Manchester.

Sims, A. C. P. (1992) Symptoms and beliefs. *Journal of the Royal Society of Health*, **112**, 42–46.

Sims, A. (1994) 'Psyche' – spirit as well as mind? *British Journal of Psychiatry*, **165**, 441–446.

Spero, M. H. (1992) *Religious Objects as Psychological Structures: A Critical Integration of Object Relations Theory, Psychotherapy and Judaism*. University of Chicago Press.

Turner, R. P., Lukoff, D., Barnhouse, R. T., *et al* (1995) Religious or spiritual problem: a culturally sensitive diagnostic category in the DSM–IV. *Journal of Nervous and Mental Disease*, **183**, 435–444.

Walker, D. (1997) First aid or last resort. *Chrism: The St Raphael Quarterly*, **34**.

CHAPTER 24

Interpreter-mediated psychiatric interviews

Saeed Farooq and Chris Fear

Summary Language is the essential psychiatric tool for eliciting history and mental state. Both diagnosis and treatment are handicapped if there is no common language between doctor and patient and understanding is facilitated through a third party, who usually has no psychiatric training. Many factors can affect this process, resulting in a convoluted interview and greater potential for misunderstandings and diagnostic errors. Linguistics and the use of interpreters are rarely mentioned in standard psychiatric texts. The different processes of translation and interpretation and their use in psychiatry are explored here. The variety of errors and pitfalls described in the literature are considered. We offer advice on the use of trained and untrained interpreters to minimise errors and make the most of the information available.

> In a language that we know we have substituted for the opacity of sounds the transparency of ideas. But a language that we do not know is a fortress sealed within whose walls the one we love is free to play false, while we, standing outside desperately keyed up in one impotence, can see, can prevent nothing.
>
> Marcel Proust, quoted in Antinucci-Mark (1990)

Language is the principal investigative and therapeutic tool in psychiatry. Interference with communication impairs our ability to assess a patient comprehensively. Nowhere is this more apparent than in the situation where patient and professional are separated by a language barrier, creating a state of dependency on an interpreter, who holds the key to mutual understanding. In today's multiracial society, particularly in larger cities, it is not uncommon to encounter such a situation, where particular skills are required of both interpreter and doctor. Nevertheless, the study of linguistics in relation to psychiatry is rarely mentioned in psychiatric texts, where disorders of communication are often seen as a consequence of disordered attention and the important influences of social cognition and context are ignored (Thomas & Fraser, 1994). A survey of 1000 professionals working in different psychiatric services in Australia found that more than one-third reported having contact, at least on a weekly basis, with patients with whom effective communication was either limited or impossible because of language barriers (Minas *et al*, 1994).

The number of refugees and internally displaced people worldwide is estimated to be 25.1 million, with an unprecedented increase of 2.5 million in 2007 alone (Office of the United Nations High Commissioner for Refugees, 2008). Immigrant populations exhibit a higher incidence of mental illness compared with native populations (Westermeyer, 1989). Moreover, in some countries there are diverse native populations between whom communication is problematic: four entirely different languages are spoken in Pakistan's North-West Province, which has a population of only 10 million or so. Tourists introduce further languages and cultures to the mix. People with different forms of disability may also have specific language difficulties: several different forms of sign language are used around the world by those who have impaired hearing.

A number of studies in English-speaking countries, mostly in medical settings, confirm that patients with limited English experience difficulties in communication and report dissatisfaction with existing interpretation services (Ngo-Metzger *et al*, 2007; Ramirez *et al*, 2008). A systematic review of the evidence has suggested that quality of care is compromised when patients with limited English need, but do not get, interpreters. Even when interpreters are used, errors occur if they are untrained or *ad hoc* (Flores, 2005). Provision of trained professional interpreters and bilingual healthcare providers has been shown to have positive effects on patients' satisfaction, quality of care and outcomes. In a study of 2715 Chinese and Vietnamese patients with limited English proficiency presenting to 11 clinics in the USA, assessments of patients through qualified interpreters gave the same results as assessments by clinicians who spoke their language. However, the patients' rating of overall quality of care was strongly associated with the quality of the interpreter (Green *et al*, 2005).

Eytan *et al* (2002) reported a study that aimed to determine how the use of trained and *ad hoc* interpreters during medical screening interviews affected referral to medical and psychiatric care. The detection of traumatic events and psychological symptoms significantly improved when trained interpreters were used. Adjusted for traumatic events and post-traumatic symptoms, referral to medical care was more frequent when relatives served as *ad hoc* interpreters, whereas interviews conducted through a trained interpreter were not significantly associated with increased referral to medical or psychiatric care. The authors suggested that the verbal communication, dialogue and cultural information provided by trained interpreters increase in importance with the shift from identification of physical symptoms to expression of emotions and psychological suffering, interpreters increasing the sensitivity of detection of psychological distress by acting as 'cultural mediators'. They also proposed that patients were more reluctant to acknowledge psychological suffering in the presence of family members, either to spare them or to avoid stigmatisation. In a study that examined the impact and role of interpreters in videotaped and live diagnostic interviews of psychiatric out-patients, clinicians reported higher confidence in their assessments. They felt that interpreters provided unbiased and accurate information and reported that, without them, patient diagnoses and functioning would have been assessed as less severe (Zayas *et al*, 2007).

Language and symptom recognition

Language has been found to have a significant influence on presenting symptoms. Work with bilingual Spanish patients found more-obvious evidence of psychosis in individuals when they were interviewed in their mother tongue than when they were interviewed in English, their second language (Del Castillo, 1970). In a further study, of bilingual Spanish patients with schizophrenia, interviews that used a single set of questions asked of each patient in both Spanish and English were rated by experienced English- or Spanish-speaking psychiatrists as showing more psychopathology in the part of the interview conducted in Spanish (Marcos *et al*, 1973). A greater frequency of misunderstandings, briefer answers and higher occurrences of speech disturbance were rated in the English section of the interview. From this it has been inferred that bilingual people are more likely to experience psychotic symptoms in their native language, possibly because this allows a freer association of ideas. These studies suggest that, even when the use of the patient's native language is not apparently strictly necessary to ensure understanding, the information gathered from an interview in the native tongue is likely to be more meaningful and to give a clearer representation of the patient's psychopathology.

Interpretation and translation

Many hospitals and local authorities maintain lists of interpreters. Working through an interpreter provides an opportunity for patients to present symptoms in their own language, but it also adds other dimensions to the interview process. It must be remembered that interpretation is a very much more complex process than is word-for-word translation. Rather than the simple substitution of one language for another, it calls for the deciphering of two linguistic codes, each with its own geographical, cultural, historical and linguistic traditions. Furthermore, possible complications introduced by adding two more relationships to the interview (interpreter–patient and interpreter–interviewer) should not be underestimated.

Accuracy of meaning is lost where an unskilled interpreter simply translates. This is well illustrated in the cases of two suicides by Spanish-speaking patients who had been managed by English-speaking psychiatrists working through interpreters. It was concluded that the patients' emotional suffering and despair were underestimated in the interpretation process (Sabin, 1975). The few studies (reviewed below) that have attempted to examine the role of interpreters in psychiatric interviewing have been based largely on analyses of audiotapes of interviews. Although a range of difficulties has been identified, there have been many methodological problems, including a lack of control groups, use of unqualified interpreters and unstructured interviews. Furthermore, the studies failed to relate errors in interpretation to outcome of the interview. These issues were addressed in a study (Farooq et al, 1997) that recognised the following categories of error, specific examples of which appear in Table 24.1.

Omission

In omission, the message is completely or partially deleted by the interpreter. This is more likely to occur in questions about sensitive personal issues such as sex and finances, especially when the interpreter is a family member or has a personal conflict of interest. Even minor omissions may be of considerable importance. In the example in Table 24.1, parts of the message, and the patient's ambivalent response, were not transmitted.

Addition

This is where the interpreter includes in the answer information not expressed by the patient.

Condensation

In condensation, a complicated or lengthy response is simplified and explained, possibly with the use of paraphrase. This is a particular problem when assessing patients whose thoughts are disordered and whose response is incoherent to the interpreter, who is usually a layperson.

Substitution

Substitution refers to the interpreter's replacement of one concept by another. In many such cases, the original question might have been better worded or the interpreter might have sought clarification.

Role exchange

In role exchange, the interpreter takes over the interview, replacing the interviewer's questions with their own.

Closed/open questioning

The way in which the psychiatrist asks the question (making it open or closed) is altered by the interpreter, which may lead to a different answer from the patient. Alternatively, the interpreter may explore the response to the psychiatrist's open question with further closed questions, delivering the results of their own investigation rather than obtaining an accurate response to the original question.

Table 24.1 Examples from the literature of interpreter error

Error category (reference)	Example of error
Omission (Marcos, 1979)	Clinician: 'Do you feel sad or blue; do you feel life is not worth living sometimes?' Interpreter: 'The doctor wants to know if you feel sad or if you like your life.' Patient: 'No. Yes. I know that my children need me. I cannot give up, I prefer not to think about.' Interpreter: 'She says that she loves her children and that her children need her.
Addition (Launer, 1978)	Patient: 'When I go to the toilet, I pass stools with difficulty.' Interpreter: 'He has severe pain when passing stools.'
Condensation (Farooq et al, 1997)	Patient: 'When I was born I have left land, land of India, Handsworth and Bengal. Prime Ministers sign, nations kept fighting, Rajah came to me ...' Interpreter reported this as reflecting grandiose delusions of involvement with the Prime Minister of India to prevent war.
Substitution (Putch, 1985)	In the following example, the interpreter could not translate the word 'allergy' as there is no equivalent in the Navajo language. Physician: 'M., would you ask her if she is allergic to any medication?' Interpreter: 'Does white man's medicine make you vomit?'
Role exchange (Putch, 1985)	In this example, the psychiatrist was preparing to prescribe medication for a Vietnamese patient with a generalised anxiety disorder. Psychiatrist: 'Ask her how long she thinks she will need to take medication.' Interpreter: 'He says you should take this medication for two weeks and then come back and see him.'
Closed/open questioning (Farooq et al, 1997)	Psychiatrist: 'Do you feel happy or sad in your spirits?' Interpreter conveys this accurately. Patient: 'If I am not unhappy or sad ... [pause] ... then I am happy.' Interpreter (without relaying the response): 'Do you feel sad now?' Patient: 'Yes.' Interpreter: 'She is unhappy.'
Normalisation (Marcos, 1979)	Psychiatrist (through interpreter): 'Is there anything that bothers you?' Patient: 'I know, I know that God is with me, I am not afraid, they can't get me ... I am wearing these new pants and I feel protected. I feel good, I don't get headaches any more.' Interpreter: 'He says that he is not afraid, he feels good; he does not have headaches any more.'

Normalisation

This is peculiar to interpreter-mediated psychiatric interviews. The interpreter attempts to make sense of the patient's phenomenology, missing the point of the psychiatric interview.

Problems peculiar to psychiatry

There are more subtle ways in which interpretation may affect the quality of a psychiatric interview. Many questions asked by psychiatrists could be considered to be presumptuous, at best, if presented without the benefit of empathic expression, and this may damage the quality of the rapport or, worse still, provoke a hostile response. In dealing with a lengthy response, background information may be excluded, distorting the context and making the answer appear illogical or tangential, and this can lead the interviewer to consider the possibility that the patient has thought disorder.

Cultural issues are of huge importance in these situations – both those of the patient and of the interpreter. Both Putch (1985) and Westermeyer (1990) give examples of situations in which interpreters actively dissuaded patients from disclosing vital information which was seen as stigmatising their culture or religion. In other situations, patients' views concerning traditional practices and therapy may be withheld in the interests of 'protecting' the patient from medical authorities.

Finally, the indirect nature of an interpreter-mediated interview is an interruption of the process of psychiatric assessment, which combines form and content of speech, facial expressions and bodily movements to reach an impression of mental state. In these circumstances, the process of using an interpreter has been likened to first watching television without sound, then receiving the sound without the pictures, and later trying to combine the two (Kline et al, 1980).

Other sources of error

So far, we have concentrated on sources of error arising from the actions of the interpreter. However, it should be remembered that the clinician's competence and familiarity with the use of interpreters are also extremely important. In the first meeting with a new patient, there is an understandable desire to obtain as much information as possible as quickly as possible to allow an early assessment of mental state. This may lead to the recruitment of the patient's bilingual friends, or even other patients, to help out. It is a widespread misconception that being bilingual automatically qualifies a person to be an interpreter. Apart from confidentiality issues, any deficient linguistic or translating skills of the individual, their lack of understanding of the clinical situation, and of mental health in particular, and their relationship with the patient are likely to magnify any of the errors of interpretation already discussed. Further complications arise from role conflicts (e.g. for a patient's friends or family) or an inadequate understanding of cultural values, as distinct from language.

The process will be further complicated if a clinician speaks quickly, uses long sentences or fails to use layperson's language. Talking to the interpreter about the patient using the third person invites a conversation about them rather than with them, and raises the interpreter from the position of facilitator to participant, distorting the process still further. A clinician conducting an interview involving two or more people with an alien language and culture may feel threatened by the situation and easily become overwhelmed. In such circumstances, the interpreter may lose sight of their role and the situation of 'role exchange' becomes more likely, with the interpreter taking over the interview.

Interviewing through an interpreter is difficult enough in simple history-taking exercises, but the problems experienced in conducting a mental state examination are formidable. Using a methodology which employed both qualitative and quantitative measures, we recorded many errors in translation that muddied the meaning of the verbal responses (Farooq et al, 1997). Interviews were conducted both in English, through an interpreter, and in the patient's own language by a psychiatrist fluent in that language. Errors were also found in the rating of symptoms, which could be minimised by the use of an experienced interpreter.

It has been suggested that unfamiliarity with psychiatric work makes even the most sophisticated medical interpreter an emergency translator (Westermeyer, 1990). In states of anxiety, delusion, depression or thought disorder, patients frequently lose their ability to communicate freely in an acquired language, making an interview with a bilingual patient in their second language unreliable (Marcos et al, 1973). Significant factors affecting this reliability include the age at which the second language was acquired, its day-to-day use at home and work, the patient's attitude to primary and secondary languages and the clinical picture.

Similar considerations should be applied to health professionals who are bilingual, particularly if their second language was acquired in the classroom, as they are likely to use too learned a 'register', the linguistic term defining the social/intellectual level at which a language is pitched. This can result in discomfort, causing a patient to see their own speech as unpolished or rustic and it may interfere with effective communication.

The interpreter in psychiatric practice

For clinician and interpreter to work together effectively, each requires knowledge of the other's style of work and of what can reasonably be expected. This improves with practice, so that the doctor learns to ask translatable questions and the interpreter to render 'nonsensical' responses verbatim. It is important that interviewer and interpreter meet before the interview, to clarify the goals of the psychiatric assessment, the main areas to be assessed and any sensitive issues that are to be explored (e.g. relationships or suicide). It may be necessary to discuss the importance of confidentiality, the need for translation of documents and the problems that can arise if the interpreter tries to 'make sense' of a patient's verbalisations. It should be remembered that an interpreter-mediated interview will take up to twice as long as a standard clinical interview and will require considerable skill and patience from clinician and interpreter alike.

During the interview, addressing the patient directly instead of through the interpreter helps to establish a better rapport and give control of the interview to the clinician. Questions should be planned in advance so as to make the best use of the time available. Long questions, excessive jargon and use of the passive voice will make an interview more difficult. Breaks while the interpreter is speaking to the patient should be used by the clinician to observe the patient's non-verbal behaviour, helping to gain non-verbal clues to the patient's mental state and enabling the next question to be framed more appropriately. Writing notes during these breaks wastes the opportunity to acquire valuable clinical data and should be avoided. A statement that is inconsistent with a patient's non-verbal behaviour should be explored by changing the wording, breaking down the question or asking about a related issue. A post-interview meeting with the interpreter is essential to clarify the interview material and the dynamics of the interaction.

It has been found that these provisions (summarised in Box 24.1), coupled with the use of a qualified and experienced interpreter, minimise the occurrence of qualitative distortions. The process provides a reliable method for making clinical observations and results in a reliable diagnosis (Farooq et al, 1997). However, although this is the standard for which to aim, the reality of clinical practice may require information to be gathered in less than ideal circumstances, greatly magnifying the potential for error.

Box 24.1 Tips for working with an interpreter

- Meet the interpreter before the interview, to explain its purpose and goal
- Speak slowly and clearly
- Use simple, layperson's terms where possible
- Speak to the patient, not the interpreter
- Clarify confusing responses
- Ask for a verbatim translation if the response is still unclear
- Avoid taking notes: concentrate on non-verbal behaviour
- Meet with the interpreter afterwards for feedback
- Ask the interpreter for their impression of the normality of conversation
- Practise

Special considerations

Ad hoc interpreters

Occasionally, a situation is encountered that forces the use of a relative or friend of the patient, or even another patient, as an interpreter. Where possible, these situations should be avoided, given the sensitive and confidential information being captured. Interviews using such interpreters should be confined to essential information and arrangements should be made for a second, more appropriate, interview to be conducted using a qualified interpreter. It must be remembered that the use of such emergency interpreters will greatly increase the number of errors, particularly those involving role conflict and normalisation. Responses such as 'does not know…' or 'talks irrelevantly…' should be explored further to look for errors or psychopathology: in such situations, a verbatim translation should be requested. The interpreter may have their own agenda or insecurities in such settings. During the interview, however, it is important to keep a focus on the patient. Interpreters' questions and insecurities should properly be addressed later.

Where it is not possible to clarify aspects of the patient's mental state, such as where formal thought disorder is suspected and a verbatim trans-lation cannot be given, it is helpful to record the interview on audiotape. This situation may occur however skilled the interpreter is and the recording will allow a more considered view to be taken later, either by the interpreter or by a psychiatrist colleague who is fluent in the language concerned.

Interpreters in psychotherapeutic practice

Psychotherapy relies on language and sociocultural context. Even for bilingual people, psychoanalysis appears to have less benefit in the second language than in the mother tongue (Greenson, 1950), possibly because using the former does not allow access to important areas of the intrapsychic world. Therapists have the difficult task of establishing a trusting therapeutic relationship with the patient in the presence of a 'third party'. Qualitative analysis of interpreter-mediated family therapy sessions in child and adolescent mental health found that important attributes of the process of communication were lost through translation (Raval & Smith, 2003). It was a particular challenge to establish an effective working partnership with the interpreter, which in turn affected the working alliance with the family, and interventions were simplified in consequence. Sadly, the authors missed the point and suggested addressing 'structural inequalities and training issues', without recognising the important dimension of language and cultural misunderstandings. A further study in a similar setting picked up on these issues, advocating the presence of another therapist with a specific interpreting function to improve success (Darling, 2004).

Several studies show the feasibility of conducting psychotherapeutic interventions with the help of interpreters. Interestingly, many studies are with refugees who have been victims of torture, a particularly challenging client group (Abdallah-Steinkopff, 1999; Miller *et al*, 2005). It is possible that cognitive and behavioural techniques, which rely less on empathy and transference, fare better when delivered through interpreters. D'Ardenne *et al* (2007) compared 'routine' clinical outcomes of three groups of people with post-traumatic stress disorder receiving cognitive–behavioural therapy: refugees who required interpreters; refugees who did not require interpreters; and English-speaking non-refugees. All three groups attended a similar number of sessions and showed significant improvements after treatment. Roder *et al* (1997) describe successful use of interpreters in group therapy, a setting that was initially regarded as 'second rate'. Almost all of these studies are based on experience of therapists with limited numbers of patients and lack scientific rigour, in common with literature on working through interpreters in general, but clearly show that the core psychotherapeutic tasks can be performed even in the presence of a language barrier. Tribe (2007) reviews the provision of psychological therapies through interpreters and makes recommendations for therapeutic work with the help of interpreters.

Working with refugees and survivors of torture

Working through interpreters is commonly required with survivors of trauma and torture among refugees in Western countries and among displaced populations. This may pose many challenges. The client may identify the interpreter with perpetrators of the trauma. The experience of torture and trauma can be quite overwhelming and this may trigger responses that are linked with the interpreter's own similar experiences if the interpreter shares the same cultural or ethnic background. Further, it may be a totally new experience for the interpreter to work with victims of trauma and torture. The interpreter may inadvertently alter their interpreting style because they find difficultly in coping with the material. Interpreters may also be influenced by the cultural issues discussed on p. 311, influencing what the patient reveals. Abbasian & Dratcu (2007) have raised the issue of the trust required for a refugee to pass sensitive information through an unknown interpreter. The patient may consider the content of the information compromising or potentially damaging if passed through a third party. In their central London practice these authors encountered the problem of 'interpreters' who appear to have their own political agenda and may breach confidentiality.

In such situations, the importance of pre- and post-interview briefings cannot be overemphasised. The emotionally disturbing nature of the anticipated content of the meeting should be explained. It is important to establish ground rules and manage the expectations of the interpreter.

In smaller communities there is a greater likelihood that the patient will know the interpreter and fear a breach of confidentiality. It is therefore advisable to check that the client is comfortable with the interpreter. The possibility of telephone interpreting should be considered if they are not. Post-interview discussion and debriefing concerning the emotional content of the session may be necessary and the interpreter may require support or counselling.

Conclusion

It has been claimed that transcultural psychiatry is an applied science, converting research-derived concepts into reliable health strategies (Jablensky, 1994). To sustain this position, significant advances are needed in research and in training towards overcoming language barriers in an environment where 80% of psychiatric staff consider that their professional training prepares them 'very little' or 'not at all' for cross-cultural clinical work (Minas *et al*, 1994). Such circumstances demand not only an ability to communicate through an interpreter but also an understanding of an individual's cultural values in a way that has received only limited attention within training programmes for psychiatric staff in multicultural settings (Lefley, 1984). It is essential for psychiatrists to recognise the complexity of the task, particularly the power that interpreters have to control the information being relayed back and forth and thus influence the outcome of the interview (Box 24.2). Interpreters should be selected with care, and supervision by a clinician who is used to working with interpreters is a valuable experience.

Box 24.2   Errors in interpretation

Addition – the interpreter includes information not expressed by the patient

Closed/open questioning – an open question is translated by the interpreter as closed question and vice versa

Condensation – a complicated or lengthy response is shortened, altering its meaning

Normalisation – the interpreter attempts to make sense of and sanitise a bizarre response

Omission – the message is completely or partly deleted by the interpreter

Role exchange – the interpreter takes over the interview, asking his or her own questions

Substitution – one concept is replaced by another

References

Abbasian, C. & Dratcu, L. (2007) Lost in translation. *Psychiatric Bulletin*, **31**, 33.

Abdallah-Steinkopff, B (1999) Psychotherapy of posttraumatic stress disorder in cooperation with interpreters [in German]. *Verhaltenstherapie*, **9**, 211–220.

Antinucci-Mark, G. (1990) Speaking in tongues in the consulting room or the dialect of foreignness. *British Journal of Psychotherapy*, **6**, 375–383.

D'Ardenne, P., Ruaro, L., Cestari, L., *et al* (2007) Does interpreter-mediated CBT with traumatized refugee people work? A comparison of patient outcomes in east London. *Behavioural and Cognitive Psychotherapy*, **35**, 293–301.

Darling, L. (2004) Psychoanalytically-informed work with interpreters. *Psychoanalytic Psychotherapy*, **18**, 255–267.

Del Castillo, J. C. (1970) The influence of language upon symptomatology in foreign born patients. *American Journal of Psychiatry*, **127**, 242–244.

Eytan, A., Bischoff, A., Rrustemi, I., *et al* (2002) Screening of mental disorders in asylum-seekers from Kosovo. *Australian and New Zealand Journal of Psychiatry*, **36**, 499–503.

Farooq, S., Fear, C. F. & Oyebode, F. (1997) An investigation of the adequacy of psychiatric interviews conducted through an interpreter. *Psychiatric Bulletin*, **21**, 209–213.

Flores, G. (2005) The impact of medical interpreter services on the quality of health care: a systematic review. *Medical Care Research and Review*, **62**, 255–299.

Green, A. R., Ngo-Metzger, Q., Legedza, A. T. R., *et al* (2005) Interpreter services, language concordance, and health care quality: experiences of Asian Americans with limited English proficiency. *Journal of General Internal Medicine*, **20**, 1050–1056.

Greenson, R. R. (1950) The mother tongue and the mother. *International Journal of Psychoanalysis*, **31**, 18–23.

Jablensky, A. (1994) Whither transcultural psychiatry? A comment on a project for a national strategy. *Australian Psychiatry*, **2**, 59–61.

Kline, F., Acosta, F. X., Austin, W., *et al* (1980) The misunderstood Spanish-speaking patient. *American Journal of Psychiatry*, **137**, 1530–1533.

Launer, J. (1978) Taking medical histories through interpreters: practice in a Nigerian outpatient department. *BMJ*, **2**, 934–935.

Lefley, H. P. (1984) Cross-cultural training for mental health professionals: effects on the delivery of services. *Hospital and Community Psychiatry*, **35**, 1227–1229.

Marcos, L. R. (1979) Effect of interpreters on the evaluation of psychopathology in non-English-speaking patients. *American Journal of Psychiatry*, **136**, 171–174.

Marcos, L. R., Alpert, M., Urcuyo, L., *et al* (1973) The effect of interview language on the evaluation of psychopathology in Spanish-American schizophrenic patients. *American Journal of Psychiatry*, **130**, 549–555.

Miller K. E., Martell Z. L., Pazdirek L., *et al* (2005) The role of interpreters in psychotherapy with refugees: an exploratory study. *American Journal of Orthopsychiatry*, **75**, 27–39.

Minas, I. H., Stuart, G. W. & Klimidis, S. (1994) Language, culture and psychiatric services: a survey of Victorian clinical staff. *Australian and New Zealand Journal of Psychiatry*, **28**, 250–258.

Ngo-Metzger, Q., Sorkin, D. H., Phillips, R. S., *et al* (2007) Providing high-quality care for limited English proficient patients: the importance of language concordance and interpreter use. *Journal of General Internal Medicine*, **22** (suppl. 2), 324–330.

Office of the United Nations High Commissioner for Refugees (2008) *2007 Global Trends: Refugees, Asylum-seekers, Returnees, Internally Displaced and Stateless Persons*. UNHCR (http://www.unhcr.org/statistics/STATISTICS/4852366f2.pdf).

Putch, R. W. (1985) Cross-cultural communication: the special case of interpreters in health care. *JAMA*, **254**, 3344–3348.

Ramirez, D., Engel, K. G. & Tang, T. S. (2008) Language interpreter utilization in the emergency department setting: a clinical review. *Journal of Health Care for the Poor and Underserved*, **19** (2), 352–362.

Raval, H. & Smith, J. A. (2003) Therapists' experiences of working with language interpreters. *International Journal of Mental Health*, **32** (2), 6–31.

Roder, F., Opalic, P. & Sengun, S. (1997) A psychotherapy group for Turkish patients using an interpreter. *Group Analysis*, **30**, 233–243.

Sabin, J. E. (1975) Translating despair. *American Journal of Psychiatry*, **132**, 197–199.

Thomas, P. & Fraser, W. (1994) Linguistics, human communication and psychiatry. *British Journal of Psychiatry*, **165**, 585–592.

Tribe, R. (2007) Working with interpreters. *The Psychologist*, **20**, 159–161.

Westermeyer, J. (1989) *Psychiatric Care of Immigrants*. American Psychiatric Press.

Westermeyer, J. (1990) Working with an interpreter in psychiatric assessment and treatment. *Journal of Nervous and Mental Disorders*, **178**, 745–749.

Zayas, L. H., Cabassa, L. J., Perez, M. C., *et al* (2007) Using interpreters in diagnostic research and practice: pilot results and recommendations. *Journal of Clinical Psychiatry*, **68**, 6, 924–928.

CHAPTER 25

Treatment of victims of trauma

Gwen Adshead and Scott Ferris

Summary   Not all traumatic events cause post-traumatic stress disorder (PTSD), and people develop PTSD symptoms after events that do not seem to be overwhelmingly traumatic. In order to direct services appropriately, there is a need to distinguish time-limited post-traumatic symptoms and acute stress reactions (which may improve spontaneously without treatment or respond to discrete interventions) from PTSD, with its potentially more chronic pathway and possible long-term effects on the personality. In this chapter, we describe acute and chronic stress disorders and evidence about the most effective treatments.

As the world appears to enter a more uncertain period, attention is being paid to the psychological aftermath of terrorism and natural disasters. However, as the language of PTSD has entered the general lexicon, there is a danger of dilution of the meaning of the term and symptoms. Following the terrorist attack in New York on 11 September 2001, probable PTSD was reported in 7.5% of New Yorkers, many of whom had no direct involvement in the attacks (Galea *et al*, 2003).

Prevalence of PTSD

The prevalence of PTSD within a community will depend to some extent on the prevalence of traumatic events in the life of that community. The National Comorbidity Survey in the USA found the estimated lifetime prevalence of PTSD among adult Americans to be 8%, with women (10%) twice as likely as men (5%) to have PTSD at some point in their lives (Kessler *et al*, 1995). However, this represents only a small portion of those who have experienced traumatic events: 60% of men and 51% of women reported at least one such event. The most frequently reported traumas were witnessing someone being badly injured or killed, being involved in a natural disaster or life-threatening accident, and combat exposure. In this National Comorbidity Survey (which presents the largest data-set and longest follow-up, albeit with retrospective assessments), the rate of PTSD declined at a relatively constant rate over 12 months, with a more gradual decline over 6 years.

Using DSM–IV criteria in a population from Munich, Perkonigg *et al* (2000) found a much lower lifetime incidence of traumatic events: 25% in men and 18% in women. The current rate of PTSD was 1% in males and 2% in females. However, in parts of the world where there have been recent conflicts the rates of PTSD can be as high as 38% (Perilla *et al*, 2002). These data suggest that it is important to consider context when discussing the prevalence of PTSD in the community, since not all 'communities' are the same.

Normal responses to trauma

There is clearly nothing abnormal about feeling bad when bad things happen. It is equally clear that acute psychological stress reactions, however normal, are extremely distressing and uncomfortable. The best analogy is that of the fractured limb: the pain is entirely normal but may be treated nonetheless. In psychiatry, DSM–IV (American Psychiatric Association, 1994) and ICD–10 (World Health Organization, 1992) recognise acute stress reactions as diagnostic entities. The features of normal stress reactions are described in Box 25.1, and DSM–IV criteria for PTSD and acute stress disorder are summarised in Table 25.1. It appears that most people who survive a traumatic event will make a spontaneous, if painful recovery. Only a minority will develop PTSD and related disorders (about 25–40%; Green, 1993). However, the unpleasantness of normal acute

---

Box 25.1   Normal stress reactions after trauma

Short-term effects

- Anticipation phase (often not present): anticipatory anxiety/fear
- Immediate shock, numbness, disbelief
- Acute distress
- Dissociation and denial
- Short-term (1–6 weeks) high levels of arousal
- Intrusive phenomena: thoughts, flashbacks, nightmares
- Poor concentration
- Disturbed sleep, appetite, libido
- Irritability
- Persistent fear and anxiety, especially when reminded of trauma, leading to avoidance behaviour

Long-term effects

- Long-term (6 weeks to 6 months) features described above persist but should decrease in intensity and frequency
- Increased avoidance behaviour
- Irritability is often most persistent
- Substance misuse is common for managing arousal

Table 25.1 Comparison of DSM–IV criteria for PTSD and acute stress disorder

Criterion	PTSD	Acute stress disorder
Stressor criterion	Involves objective and subjective criteria: (a) the person experienced, witnessed or was confronted with threatening, serious events (b) the person's response involved intense fear, helplessness or horror	As for PTSD
Dissociative phenomena	None	At least three of five dissociative symptoms: emotional numbing/detachment, reduced environmental awareness, derealisation, depersonalisation, amnesia
Intrusive phenomena	Persistent re-experiencing in at least one of five ways (e.g. intrusive recollections, dreams, flashbacks, psychological distress)	As for PTSD
Avoidance phenomena	At least three of seven avoidance behaviours (e.g. avoidance of thoughts, feelings or reminders of the trauma, amnesia, decreased interest, feelings of detachment)	As for PTSD
Hyperarousal phenomena	At least two of five possible symptoms: insomnia, irritability, poor concentration, hypervigilance, exaggerated startle response	As for PTSD
Duration	At least 1 month	Lasts from 2 days to 4 weeks
Impairment of social functioning	The symptoms must cause clinically significant distress or social dysfunction	As for PTSD

After American Psychiatric Association (1994).

stress reactions should not be underestimated, and clinicians might need to remind families of this. Recovery is the norm but may be delayed where there is further stress.

Acute stress disorder is a relatively new diagnosis which involves a shorter timescale and the presence of dissociative symptoms (Table 25.1). Studies of survivors of motor vehicle accidents have found rates of acute stress disorder ranging from about 13% (Harvey & Bryant, 1998) to 21% (Holeva *et al*, 2001). Higher rates are found for victims of violence (Classen *et al*, 1998; Elklit, 2002).

Acute stress disorder and PTSD

According to DSM–IV, an individual's diagnosis changes from acute stress disorder to acute PTSD if symptoms persist for more than 1 month. After 3 months of symptoms, the diagnosis changes again to chronic PTSD. There is evidence that a diagnosis of acute stress disorder can identify a significant proportion of people with acute trauma who go on to develop PTSD (around 80%; Harvey & Bryant, 2000). It has been argued that placing greater emphasis on re-experiencing, avoidance and arousal symptoms can further increase the predictive power of these diagnostic criteria. However, there is considerable overlap between acute stress disorder and acute PTSD if the duration criteria are removed, and both are equally predictive of later PTSD, bringing into question the need for a separate diagnosis of acute stress disorder (Brewin *et al*, 2003).

Table 25.1 outlines the DSM–IV criteria for PTSD. The phrase 'outside the range of usual human experience' has now been dropped from the definition. This is in part the result of research which suggests that the perception of fear and threat is crucial in the genesis of PTSD, so that PTSD is possible after events that are common but terrifying (including road traffic accidents and domestic violence).

Risk factors for PTSD

Only a subset of people exposed to trauma develop PTSD, suggesting that certain people are at risk of developing the disorder, whereas others are more resilient. Box 25.2 shows some of the established risk factors for PTSD (McFarlane, 1996). The magnitude and degree of exposure to the stressor influence the risk of developing the disorder. Gender also appears to be significant, with twice the rates of PTSD in women than in men, despite lower reported trauma exposure. Previous personality traits, coping styles and experiences also influence the development of PTSD. Repressive coping style, indicated by low anxiety and high defensiveness, appears to reduce the likelihood of developing PTSD (Ginzburg *et al*, 2002). Other risk factors include previous traumatisation (Smith *et al*, 1990), peri-traumatic dissociative experiences (Birmes *et al*, 2003) and early sensitisation of the hypothalamic–pituitary–adrenal (HPA) axis (Yehuda, 1999, 2002).

In some people PTSD has an unremitting course: more than one-third have a clinical diagnosis of the disorder many years after the onset of their index episode (Kessler *et al*, 1995). The majority of people who do recover from PTSD still report subthreshold symptoms (Ehlers *et al*, 1998). A number of factors have been identified as important in the maintenance of PTSD, including social support and organisational environment. In addition, being divorced and/or widowed, having a lower education and lower income, concurrent family stressors and a low level of psychosocial functioning appear to be important in the maintenance of chronic PTSD (Zlotnick *et al*, 2004).

Box 25.2   Risk factors for PTSD

Aspect of trauma

- Duration and magnitude of exposure to stressor
- Stressors are sudden and/or occur with no warning
- There is multiple loss of life, mutilation or grotesque imagery
- Criminal violence, especially sexual

Experience during trauma

- Perceived own life to be at real risk
- Perceived lack of control of events, intense fear and helplessness
- Perception of grotesque imagery, especially of human remains or children
- Witnessing or carrying out atrocities, e.g. murder, torture
- High levels of dissociative symptoms at the time of the event

Characteristics of the individual

- Previous psychiatric illness or neuroticism
- Previous exposure to trauma, especially childhood trauma
- Previous coping style
- Denial of trauma and/or avoidance
- Female gender
- Previous acute stress reaction

Post-trauma

- Denial of trauma by others or dismissal of experience
- Lack of social support

The development of PTSD is therefore the complex result of the interaction of individual vulnerability and resilience with factors related to the severity of trauma. A fictitious clinical example makes the point. Five men were involved in an aeroplane crash. Superficially, all were exposed to severe life-threatening trauma, involving grotesque imagery (a fellow passenger was decapitated and his mutilated remains spread over the crash site). On the basis of the nature of the trauma alone, one might expect all the survivors to develop PTSD. However, 18 months later, only two of the five had failed to make a reasonable recovery after a normal stress response. Only one man developed PTSD. His subjective experience of the trauma was particularly unpleasant. There was also evidence that his personality put him at risk. The other man who failed to recover did not have PTSD but was chronically anxious in a way that severely affected his work performance. Each man's subjective account of the crash was different, making the point that subjective experience interacts with objective severity to influence the development of psychopathology. It is therefore not possible to state that only extremes of trauma or individual psychological vulnerability lead to the development of PTSD. The relative contributions of past experience and experience of the traumatic event need to be considered during assessment, and have implications for choice of treatment.

Psychopathology and pathophysiology of PTSD

One of the principal debates about PTSD relates to whether it is an anxiety disorder or a mood disorder. Other possible diagnostic categories are dissociative disorders or personality disorders. The rationale for the various positions is detailed in Box 25.3.

Category definition has implications for treatment. Most treatment for PTSD is currently based on symptoms. The pathophysiology of the disorder remains relatively unclear, with research suggesting the involvement of the HPA axis, central monoamine regulation and endogenous opioids. The higher level of cortisol after a trauma might be protective against PTSD, a finding that may shed light on the observed gender disparity (Lamprecht & Sack, 2002). Activation of the HPA axis during acute stress is an adaptive response, but prolonged elevated glucocorticoid concentrations might lead to neuronal degeneration in areas with high densities of corticoid receptors such as the hippocampus. This might be responsible for the

---

Box 25.3   Models of psychopathology in PTSD

Anxiety disorder?

- Fear, anxiety and avoidance behaviour (as with phobias)
- Intrusive phenomena resemble obsessive–compulsive disorder
- Introversion and neuroticism are common personality traits in both PTSD and anxiety
- Some people improve with exposure therapy

Mood disorder?

- Sadness and grief, independent of bereavement
- Comorbidity with depression is very common
- Vegetative symptoms (loss of sleep, appetite, libido) are very similar
- Avoidance, numbing and loss of interest as in mood disorders

Dissociative disorder?

- Flashbacks and amnesia are common

Personality disorder?

- Considerable overlap of symptoms with borderline personality disorder
- Some overlap of symptoms with antisocial personality disorder (antisocial behaviour, irritability)
- Some evidence that trauma can induce personality change

Separate neurophysiological disorder?

- Low monoamine oxidase activity
- Increased excretion of urinary beta-endorphin
- Therapeutic response to serotonergic drugs and drugs that affect the locus ceruleus
- Deregulation of the hypothalamic–pituitary–adrenal axis, resulting in low cortisol levels

reduced hippocampal volume found in people with PTSD (Hull, 2002). The underactivity of the HPA axis which is observed after exposure to chronic stress might increase vulnerability when facing future trauma. In addition to the neurophysiological disturbances exhibited by people with PTSD, there is also evidence of cognitive psychopathology: people with PTSD are more sensitive to percepts indicating threat and respond more vigorously to such cues (Cassiday et al, 1992).

Neuroimaging studies have also contributed to our understanding of the neurobiological changes seen in trauma survivors. In addition to reduced hippocampal volumes, there appears to be hyper-reactivity of the amygdala and reduced activation in the anterior cingulate cortex. These findings might respectively reflect the anxiety symptoms and the reduced extinction of conditioned emotional responses observed in people with PTSD (Damsa et al, 2005).

Post-traumatic stress disorder can present with either predominantly fear-based or shame-based psychological reactions, reflecting conscious and unconscious beliefs and attitudes about the self and the world. It is these schemata that are addressed using psychological therapies, whereas the autonomic effects of anxiety and depression are best addressed with medication.

Other problems post-trauma

It cannot be overemphasised that PTSD is not the only problem that survivors of trauma face. 'Pure' PTSD after trauma is comparatively rare and comorbidity is the norm. Full-blown PTSD is also relatively uncommon and partial PTSD (Stein et al, 1997), in which there are fewer than the required number of DSM–IV avoidance phenomena or hyperarousal phenomena, might be more likely, particularly in a chronic form.

Comorbid Axis I disorders

Depression is the most common co-diagnosis and might be the most common disorder post-trauma. Other psychiatric illnesses post-trauma include anxiety disorders, such as panic disorder or phobic disorders, and substance misuse. These can all lead to more chronic PTSD if not detected and addressed. In particular, the co-occurrence of substance use and anxiety disorders can dramatically reduce the chances of remission (Jacobsen et al, 2001; Zlotnick et al, 2004). Substance misuse might be the primary presenting problem, masking intrusive symptoms of PTSD.

There is now good evidence that PTSD is common in people with severe mental illness such as schizophrenia. Histories of childhood adversity and adult trauma have been commonly reported in people with psychotic disorders (Bebbington et al, 2004). Studies of traumatic experience in community samples have found similar results, which suggests that many people with Axis I disorders might also have either full-blown PTSD or symptoms of PTSD, both of which will amplify other pathology and increase treatment resistance (Mueser *et al*, 1998). These studies suggest that psychiatrists should look for history of trauma and possible post-traumatic pathology in people presenting with severe mental illness or who appear to be making a poor recovery from psychotic episodes.

Comorbid Axis II disorders

Marked changes in personality, in terms of personal interaction with others, might cause more problems than any other disorder post-trauma, especially when they are accompanied by substance misuse or violent behaviour (Southwick & Giller, 1993). The relationship between personality disorder and PTSD is complicated and the diagnosis of complex PTSD can be seen as an attempt to bring together the dichotomy of Axis I (state) and Axis II (trait) symptoms (McLean & Gallop, 2003). A history of childhood trauma is common in adults with personality disorder, particularly borderline or paranoid personality disorder, but is by no means universal.

Childhood abuse appears to be a risk factor for PTSD independently of personality disorder and early trauma (<12 years of age) and it confers an equal risk of depression (Spataro *et al*, 2004). Adults with these personality disorders are more likely to develop PTSD, through a combination of increased exposure to adult trauma (paranoid personality disorder only) and psychological and social vulnerability (Golier *et al*, 2003).

Effects on social systems and support

As in general psychiatric practice, it is important to consider the influence of the disorder on other areas of a person's life, in relation to its effect on the process of recovery and the prognosis. The symptoms of many of the post-traumatic disorders may be troublesome for families and employers, particularly in the first 6–12 months. Families, friends and employers are usually unfamiliar with the timescale of normal recovery, let alone post-traumatic psychiatric illness. Most people do not realise that normal recovery may take 6 months, or longer if there are further stressors, and they might become impatient with survivors, thinking them difficult or weak. Local social support often reduces as press reports of the trauma diminish, and it may seem to healthcare professionals or family members that the trauma happened a long time ago. However, the pathology of PTSD makes the trauma continually real to the survivor (Horowitz, 1973).

The workplace

After experiencing trauma a person may be chronically irritable and withdrawn for weeks, in a way that is alien to them and their families. There is good evidence that marital stress and breakdown increase after traumatic experiences. Work performance may similarly deteriorate because of the person's hypervigilance, accompanying loss of concentration and irritability. However, people often find it impossible to discuss the reasons for this with their employers. Employers may not be sympathetic anyway, especially if the trauma occurred at work (and compensation is being claimed), or where there is a work culture of denial of distress. Examples of this are the emergency or public services, and healthcare professionals. Although the 'macho' culture is changing to some degree, especially in the emergency services, the process is slow, and people may encounter hostility and rejection in their workplace. Contrary to popular assumptions of malingering, compensation claims may not be relevant to the maintenance of PTSD, and their settlement does not appear to influence reported rates of the disorder or return to work following injury (Bryant & Harvey, 2003).

The home

Many major personal disasters are never reported in the press. During peacetime, and between major national disasters, the principal cause of traumatic stress responses is crime, of which the impact on the victim is rarely reported unless it is fatal (Kilpatrick *et al*, 1989). This applies to both men and women. A good example of this is the plight of the families of murder victims. The killer is often a member of the family and relatives must cope with multiple losses. In one case known to us, a woman presented after her husband murdered their daughter to prevent her from telling the mother about his 20-year affair with a family friend. This woman lost not only her daughter and her husband, she also lost her experience of her marriage and the support of a trusted friend. She was also without funds as the husband had been the principal earner and she did not have access to the bank account. The trial did not take place for a year, and the funeral was delayed several times for post-mortem reports for both defence and prosecution.

These social and legal aspects of post-traumatic dysfunction have a profound influence on the management and prognosis of PTSD, and can cause major setbacks in treatment. A man who becomes homeless because of domestic violence related to his post-traumatic irritability may be unable to cooperate with or tolerate a treatment programme. In-patient treatment might be indicated in such instances. People with PTSD as a result of crime have particular problems: not only may they have reminders of the stressor, such as police identification parades or court appearances, they might be at continued risk of further trauma, such as threats from the defendant.

Assessment

Ask the question

It is not always immediately apparent that the presenting complaint is post-traumatic in origin, and it is important to bear the possibility in mind.

Psychiatrists need to be aware that criminal violence is a potent cause of post-traumatic symptoms, and a question about the experience of violent victimisation should now be part of the standard history-taking procedure. This is especially true for people presenting with Axis I disorders, where the experience of victimisation, although not uncommon, might be overlooked (Mueser *et al*, 1998; Bebbington *et al*, 2004). We have found that asking people about their most frightening experience to date is a good way to introduce the subject of experienced trauma. Questions such as 'Have you ever been a victim of crime?' or 'Were you abused as a child?' are less productive because the words 'crime' and 'abuse' mean different things to different people.

There is some evidence that healthcare professionals do not ask enough about trauma, although it seems that patients do not resent this (Friedman *et al*, 1992). People with post-traumatic disorders might find it difficult to describe their experiences and might appreciate a tactful enquiry. In addition, patients may not see their general practitioner (GP) until some time after a traumatic event, so that the importance of an event that might have taken place a year before may be overlooked.

Listen to the answer

Having enquired about trauma, the assessor must be prepared to hear the patient's account. This entails making enough time for the patient to recount it comfortably. If a history of trauma is already known at referral, it may be helpful to suggest to the patient that history-taking takes place in two stages: a general psychiatric history and an account of the trauma and post-traumatic events. This gives the patient some warning and allows them to prepare themselves, reducing anticipatory anxiety. If the trauma is disclosed during the consultation, and the patient wants to give an account of the experience, it is important to allow this to take place. People with post-traumatic disorders are very sensitive to the understandable reluctance of others to hear their story. It might be necessary to let the patient talk for a short time, then negotiate a time for them to return and for the assessment to continue.

It is not advisable to dismiss patients' disclosures of trauma. There is no evidence that patients benefit from being told to 'forget all about it' or 'put it out of your mind'. Intrusive phenomena that cannot be voluntarily excluded are characteristic of PTSD: patients are not actually capable of 'just forgetting'. Dismissal also sends the message that the healthcare professional does not want to hear or does not believe what they are being told. Even when the professional needs to maintain a true scepticism about the patient's account of events (such as in medicolegal work), this does not warrant an unsympathetic manner, which in any case will impede the assessment.

Completing the assessment

Apart from tactfully and sensitively facilitating the patient's disclosure of their experience of the trauma, psychiatric assessment proceeds along usual lines. Interviews with family members might be invaluable for information on the pre-traumatic state of the patient, and might also give an insight into the course of the post-traumatic sequelae. Discussion with the GP and examination of the GP's records may yield more valuable information about the patient's pre-traumatic state, and is essential for medicolegal assessments for PTSD claims.

Key questions in the assessment are outlined in Box 25.4. If the trauma happened only recently (say, in the past 3–6 months) some spontaneous progress may still be made or progress may be augmented with support. Positive signs include the diminishing frequency of nightmares, decreasing use of alcohol and the return of appetite. Spontaneous progress may be retarded by the degree of trauma, simultaneous losses and physical ill health (psychological recovery might not be possible until the physical state of the patient allows it). If they are making progress, then it may be that all they need is pharmacological support for the remaining symptoms, information about the natural course of stress reactions and advice from the GP. The support of community psychiatric nurses may also be useful. Contact details that might be helpful for people with PTSD and their families are given in Box 25.5.

Box 25.4   Key questions in the assessment of post-traumatic disorders

For the clinician

- When did the trauma occur?
- How long has the person had symptoms?
- How have they coped to date?
- What resources do they have to support them?
- Is there a previous history of trauma?
- Is there a history of psychiatric illness pre-trauma?
- Was the trauma risky? (criminal assaults or exposure to grotesque imagery)

For the patient

- What is the most frightening thing that happened to you before this traumatic experience?
- Were you ever frightened of your parents when you were a child?
- Were there any other adults who frightened you when you were a child?
- What was the worst thing about this traumatic experience?
- What is its worst effect on you?

> **Box 25.5**   Contact details for helpful agencies
>
> - National Association of Victim Support Schemes   020 7735 9166
> - Compassionate Friends   0845 123 2304 (help for families after death of a child)
> - Cruse   0844 477 9400 (help for the bereaved)
> - Medical Foundation for the Care of Victims of Torture   020 7697 7777
> - UK Trauma Group   http://www.uktrauma.org.uk (a managed clinical network of UK traumatic stress services)

General practitioners are the obvious professionals to be involved in the management of acute stress reactions. If the patient is referred to psychiatric services while still in the acute phase of response it might be because:

- the GP lacks information about PTSD and needs consultation with the psychiatrist
- the GP/practice counsellor/psychologist has particular concerns because of the nature of the symptoms
- the GP or practice team do not have the time to give support
- the nature of the trauma is particularly serious.

In the early stages, it is useful to consider the risk factors for PTSD and advise both the patient and the GP about them. For example, a man who is the victim of a mugging and who has a history of childhood abuse and previous depression is more at risk of developing PTSD than a man without these risk factors who experiences the same assault. If the trauma is a criminal one, it is important to ascertain the state of any legal proceedings, since this might have an impact on treatment and progress.

People whose traumatic experience took place in the more distant past should be advised that treatment may be less effective. Careful history-taking is necessary to discover why the past trauma seems to be causing distress now, and whether there is a new trauma or a comorbid condition that is relevant. Patients should also be advised that in the early stages treatment can be psychologically painful and distress may be transiently increased as they reduce avoidance and denial.

Treatment of post-traumatic disorders

Once a diagnosis of PTSD has been made, treatment should be vigorous because chronic PTSD is hard to treat. Even if the traumatic events took place some time before (>1 year) it might still be worth trying exposure therapy, if the patient can tolerate it. Antidepressant treatment should also be instituted. However, the prognosis after 1–2 years is not good.

Although the natural history of the disorder is for very gradual improvement over time, the concurrent effects on family and work life continually retard this process. Once chronic PTSD is established, the therapeutic focus may need to be these concurrent problems.

The principal treatment modalities are:

- behavioural and cognitive strategies
- short- and long-term psychological therapies
- medication.

All three may form part of different therapeutic strategies for the same patient over time, depending on the patient's needs. Box 25.6 shows the range of treatments available, the optimal types of therapy for different disorders and their timing. There is no evidence that single one-off debriefing sessions are helpful for treatment or that they reduce the incidence of PTSD after trauma (National Institute for Clinical Excellence, 2005).

Behavioural and cognitive strategies

The rationale for behavioural and cognitive treatments is to break the cycle of intrusion and avoidance described in Horowitz's model of PTSD (Horowitz, 1973). By exposing the patient to their feared memories or their thoughts about the trauma, avoidance is reduced and control over intrusion is introduced. It is likely that exposure to feared memories is an important part of most post-traumatic therapies. Addressing failures in cognitive

---

Box 25.6 Indicated treatments for post-traumatic disorders

Acute stress responses
- Debriefing
- Social supports
- Pharmacological supports, e.g. hypnotics
- Information and advice to families

Acute PTSD
- Exposure therapy may be first-line treatment if intrusive phenomena prominent
- Cognitive therapy
- Brief psychodynamic psychotherapy
- Antidepressants (especially where avoidance prominent)

Chronic PTSD
- Exposure therapy if trauma never discussed
- Cognitive–behavioural approaches may still be effective (group or individual)
- Long-term psychotherapy (group or individual)
- Antidepressants, lithium, carbamazepine

processing of fear responses has also been shown to be effective in PTSD (Resick & Schnike, 1992). Behavioural and cognitive strategies are probably indicated as first-line treatments where there is good psychological health before the traumatic event and when the event itself is discrete.

Psychological therapies

Shame-based PTSD reactions are more common after prolonged childhood trauma, and overlap with the concept of complex PTSD (Herman, 1992) and borderline personality pathology. This type of reaction may be better addressed with shame-based therapies that address the traumatised sense of self through the developing narrative and help restore a sense of meaning (Lindy, 1996). Unlike fear-based therapies, in shame-based therapy the relationship between patient and therapist is likely to be a major part of the therapeutic process. Previous experiences of fear and safety will be relevant to both types of reaction, especially in relation to forming a therapeutic alliance. Therapeutic approaches such as interpersonal and psychodynamic therapy may be helpful. There is little evidence that exposure-based approaches are helpful and they may even exacerbate the problem.

Group psychotherapy may be of particular use when the trauma occurs in a group context, such as occupational settings or public transport. Therapeutic communities have been used principally with combat veterans (Silver, 1986). Brief group work is possible when the group focuses on a particular task, such as in the critical incident stress debriefing model described by Mitchell (1983). Group work may be of particular use after sexual assaults, when shame and guilt may be reduced by making the experience less individual (Roth *et al*, 1988).

Medication

Medication has an important role in the treatment of post-traumatic disorders, both as symptomatic relief and directly addressing pathology. Detailed accounts of the use of various types of medication are given by Davidson (1992) and Stein *et al* (2000). Antidepressants, especially the serotonergic agents, may be helpful, as may tricyclics because of their hypnotic effects. Medication alone is unlikely to be helpful but may be necessary to enable patients to undertake other types of therapy later, and may enhance the efficacy of psychotherapy.

Choosing a treatment

There are particular questions relevant to the selection of treatment.

What is the worst problem at the moment?

Prominent intrusive phenomena suggest exposure therapy as part of a cognitive–behavioural package. If depression and distress are worst, regular supportive therapy sessions plus antidepressants may be most effective.

What supports does this person have?

Many forms of treatment for PTSD are quite stressful. It is therefore important to ensure that the patient will be well supported and that the family are informed about the nature and process of therapy.

What solutions to stress is the patient adopting now?

If a patient is misusing alcohol or drugs as a means of managing their PTSD symptoms this needs to be addressed before any specific PTSD treatment can be implemented. Rarely, patients present with acts of self-harm such as overdose, and these should not be dismissed as 'attention-seeking'.

Efficacy of treatment

A number of studies have addressed the efficacy of treatment for PTSD, although they have tended to focus on psychological treatment. A thorough review by Robertson *et al* (2004) concluded that the evidence is particularly strong for interventions based on cognitive and behavioural therapy, although it is less compelling for other modalities such as acute debriefing interventions. Eye movement desensitisation and reprocessing (EMDR) has always been contentious, in part owing to the seemingly magical nature of the technique – the patient focuses on their traumatic memories while tracking a focal point (often the therapist's finger) in horizontal movements. The evidence base does seem to support its effectiveness, although this is not as strong as for trauma focused CBT (Bisson *et al*, 2007). It remains unclear whether the initiation of saccadic eye movements is an integral therapeutic component of the technique or if it is better conceptualised as an unorthodox form of exposure therapy (Rogers & Silver, 2002).

Psychodynamic psychotherapy and hypnotherapy have intuitive appeal but lack an evidence base, perhaps because of inherent difficulties in standardising such treatments for empirical evaluation. Newer structured psychotherapies such as interpersonal therapy have theoretical promise and await further evaluation. Dialectical behaviour therapy may be useful for complex PTSD when the effects of trauma early in development have led to problems such as dissociation, impulsivity and unstable relationships. However, further clinical trials are needed (Robertson *et al*, 2004).

Two meta-analyses and a systematic review have included studies using 'psychodynamic methods' (Sherman, 1998; Van Etten & Taylor, 1998; Bisson & Andrew, 2005). Psychological therapies appear to be better than psychotropic medication, although both are better than no treatment. Sherman found significant effects for all psychological therapies, particularly behavioural therapy, but no support for one single rationale for therapy. Although there is no clear evidence that any particular class of medication is more effective or better tolerated than any other, the largest trials showing efficacy to date have been with the selective serotonin reuptake inhibitors. There have been negative studies of benzodiazepines, monoamine oxidase inhibitors, antipsychotics, lamotrigine and inositol (Stein *et al*, 2006). There is currently a lack of information about the efficacy of treatment for complex PTSD, which is more common in victims of childhood trauma or chronic interpersonal violence. Given the resemblance of these disorders to borderline personality disorder, there may be some reason for thinking that cognitive approaches to affect and arousal, and therapies that address interpersonal problems, may be most helpful. Interpersonal problems are the most commonly cited reason that patients with complex PTSD seek treatment (Levitt & Cloitre, 2005).

Conclusion

Traumatic events are not uncommon in civilian life. Survivors of traumatic experiences, both large and small scale, are likely to present to general and specialist psychiatric clinics, requiring treatment. Proper diagnosis is essential because treatment for some post-traumatic disorders can be very effective and failure to treat may result in crippling morbidity. There is no evidence to suggest that the majority of people who present with post-traumatic psychopathology are fabricating symptoms for the purposes of compensation. Although this view lingers in the minds of some psychiatrists, 40 years of research suggest that there really are post-traumatic disorders which need and respond to treatment.

References

American Psychiatric Association (1994) *Diagnostic and Statistical Manual of Mental Disorders (4th edn) (DSM–IV)*. APA.

Bebbington, P. E., Bhugra, D., Brugha, T., *et al* (2004) Psychosis, victimisation and childhood disadvantage: evidence from the second British National Survey of Psychiatric Morbidity. *British Journal of Psychiatry*, **185**, 220–226.

Birmes, P., Brunet, A., Carreras, D., *et al* (2003) The predictive power of peritraumatic dissociation and acute stress symptoms for posttraumatic stress symptoms: a three-month prospective study. *American Journal of Psychiatry*, **160**, 1337–1339.

Bisson, J. & Andrew, M. (2005) Psychological treatment of post-traumatic stress disorder (PTSD). *Cochrane Database of Systematic Reviews*, issue 2 (CD003388).

Bisson, J. I., Ehlers, A., Matthews, R., *et al* (2007) Psychological treatments for chronic post-traumatic stress disorder. Systematic review and meta-analysis. *British Journal of Psychiatry*, **190**, 97–104.

Brewin, C. R., Andrews, B. & Rose, S. (2003) Diagnostic overlap between acute stress disorder and PTSD in victims of violent crime. *American Journal of Psychiatry*, **160**, 783–785.

Bryant, R. A. & Harvey, A. G. (2003) The influence of litigation on maintenance of posttraumatic stress disorder. *Journal of Nervous and Mental Disease*, **191**, 191–193.

Cassiday, L., McNally, R. & Zeitlin, S. (1992) Cognitive processing of trauma cues in rape victims. *Cognitive Research and Therapy*, **16**, 283–295.

Classen, C., Koopman, C., Hales, R., *et al* (1998) Acute stress disorder as a predictor of posttraumatic stress symptoms. *American Journal of Psychiatry*, **155**, 620–624.

Damsa, C., Maris, S. & Pull, C. (2005) New fields of research in posttraumatic stress disorder: brain imaging. *Current Opinion in Psychiatry*, **18**, 55–64.

Davidson, J. (1992) Drug therapy of post-traumatic stress disorder. *British Journal of Psychiatry*, **160**, 309–314.

Ehlers, A., Mayou, R. & Bryant, B. (1998) Psychological predictors of chronic post-traumatic stress disorder after motor vehicle accidents. *Journal of Abnormal Psychology*, **107**, 508–519.

Elklit, A. (2002) Acute stress disorder in victims of robbery and victims of assault. *Journal of Interpersonal Violence*, **17**, 872–887.

Friedman, L. S., Samet, J. H., Roberts, M. S., *et al* (1992) Inquiry about victimisation experiences. *Archives of Internal Medicine*, **152**, 1186–1190.

Galea, S., Vlahov, D., Resnick, H., *et al* (2003) Trends of probable post-traumatic stress disorder in New York City after the September 11 terrorist attacks. *American Journal of Epidemiology*, **158**, 514–524.

Ginzburg, K., Solomon, Z. & Bleich, A. (2002) Repressive coping style, acute stress disorder, and posttraumatic stress disorder after myocardial infarction. *Psychosomatic Medicine*, **64**, 748–757.

Golier, J. A., Yehuda, R., Bierer, L. M., *et al* (2003) The relationship of borderline personality disorder to posttraumatic stress disorder and traumatic events. *American Journal of Psychiatry*, **160**, 2018–2024.

Green, B. (1993) Identifying survivors at risk: trauma and stressors across events. In *International Handbook of Traumatic Stress Syndromes* (eds J. Wilson & B. Raphael), pp. 135–144. Plenum.

Harvey, A. G. & Bryant, R. A. (1998) The relationship between acute stress disorder and posttraumatic stress disorder: a prospective evaluation of motor vehicle accident survivors. *Journal of Consulting and Clinical Psychology*, **66**, 507–512.

Harvey, A. G. & Bryant, R. A. (2000) Two-year prospective evaluation of the relationship between acute stress disorder and posttraumatic stress disorder following mild traumatic brain injury. *American Journal of Psychiatry*, **157**, 626–628.

Herman, J. (1992) Complex PTSD: a syndrome in survivors of prolonged and repeated trauma. *Journal of Traumatic Stress*, **5**, 377–391.

Holeva, V., Tarrier, N. & Wells, A. (2001) Prevalence and predictors of acute stress disorder and PTSD following road traffic accidents: thought control strategies and social support. *Behavior Therapy*, **32**, 65–83.

Horowitz, M. (1973) Phase oriented treatment of stress response syndromes. *American Journal of Psychotherapy*, **27**, 506–515.

Hull, A. M. (2002) Neuroimaging findings in post-traumatic stress disorder. Systematic review. *British Journal of Psychiatry*, **181**, 102–110.

Jacobsen, L. K., Southwick, S. M. & Kosten, T. R. (2001) Substance use disorders in patients with posttraumatic stress disorder: a review of the literature. *American Journal of Psychiatry*, **158**, 1184–1190.

Kessler, R. C., Sonnega, A., Bromet, E., *et al* (1995) Posttraumatic stress disorder in the National Comorbidity Survey. *Archives of General Psychiatry*, **52**, 1048–1060.

Kilpatrick, D., Saunders, B. E. & Amick McMullen, A. (1989) Victim and crime factors associated with the development of crime related PTSD. *Behavior Therapy*, **20**, 199–214.

Lamprecht, F. & Sack, M. (2002) Posttraumatic stress disorder revisited. *Psychosomatic Medicine*, **64**, 222–237.

Levitt, J. T. & Cloitre, M. (2005) A clinician's guide to STAIR/MPE. Treatment for PTSD related to childhood abuse. *Cognitive and Behavioral Practice*, **12**, 40–52.

Lindy, J. (1996) Psychoanalytic psychotherapy of post-traumatic stress disorder: the nature of the therapeutic relationship. In *Traumatic Stress: The Effects of Overwhelming Experience on Mind, Body and Society* (eds B. van der Kolk, A. McFarlane & L. Weisaeth), pp. 525–536. Guilford Press.

McFarlane, A. (1996) Resilience, vulnerability and the course of posttraumatic reactions. In *Traumatic Stress: The Effects of Overwhelming Experience on Mind, Body and Society* (eds B. van der Kolk, A. McFarlane & L. Weisaeth), pp. 155–170. Guilford Press

McLean, L. M. & Gallop, R. (2003) Implications of childhood sexual abuse for adult borderline personality disorder and complex posttraumatic stress disorder. *American Journal of Psychiatry*, **160**, 369–371.

Mitchell, J. (1983) When disaster strikes – the critical incident stress debriefing process. *Journal of Emergency Medical Services*, **8**, 36–38.

Mueser, K., Goodman, C. B., Trumbetta, S. L., *et al* (1998) Trauma and PTSD in severe mental illness. *Journal of Consulting and Clinical Psychology*, **66**, 493–499.

National Institute for Clinical Excellence (2005) *The Management of PTSD in Adults and Children in Primary and Secondary Care*. NICE.

Perilla, J. L., Norris, F. H. & Lavizzo, E. A. (2002) Ethnicity, culture, and disaster response: identifying and explaining ethnic differences in PTSD six months after Hurricane Andrew. *Journal of Social and Clinical Psychology*, **21**, 20–45.

Perkonigg, A., Kessler, R. C., Storz, S., *et al* (2000) Traumatic events and post-traumatic stress disorder in the community: prevalence, risk factors and comorbidity. *Acta Psychiatrica Scandinavica*, **101**, 46–59.

Resick, P. & Schnike, M. (1992) Cognitive processing therapy for sexual assault victims. *Journal of Consulting and Clinical Psychology*, **60**, 748–756.

Robertson, M., Humphreys, L. & Ray, R. (2004) Psychological treatments for posttraumatic stress disorder: recommendations for the clinician based on a review of the literature. *Journal of Psychiatric Practice*, **10**, 106–118.

Rogers, S. & Silver, S. M. (2002) Is EMDR an exposure therapy? A review of trauma protocols. *Journal of Clinical Psychology*, **58**, 43–59.

Roth, S., Dye, E. & Liebowitz, V. (1988) Group therapy for sexual assault victims. *Psychotherapy*, **25**, 82–93.

Sherman, J. J. (1998) Effects of psychotherapeutic treatments for PTSD: a meta-analysis of controlled trials. *Journal of Traumatic Stress*, **11**, 413–436.

Silver, S. M. (1986) An inpatient program for PTSD: context as treatment. In *Trauma and its Wake* (vol. 2) (ed. C. Figley), pp. 142–152. Brunner-Mazel.

Smith, E., North, C., McCool, R., *et al* (1990) Acute post-disaster psychiatric disorders: identification of persons at risk. *American Journal of Psychiatry*, **147**, 202–206.

Southwick, S. & Giller, E. (1993) Personality disorders in treatment seeking combat veterans with PTSD. *American Journal of Psychiatry*, **150**, 1020–1023.

Spataro, J., Mullen, P., Burgess, P. M., *et al* (2004) Impact of child sexual abuse on mental health: prospective study in males and females. *British Journal of Psychiatry*, **184**, 416–421.

Stein, D. J., Zungu-Dirwayi, N., van Der Linden, G. J., *et al* (2000) Pharmacotherapy for posttraumatic stress disorder. *Cochrane Database of Systematic Reviews*, issue 4 (CD002795).

Stein, D. J., Ipser, J. C. & Seedat, S. (2006) Pharmacotherapy for post traumatic stress disorder (PTSD). *Cochrane Database of Systematic Reviews*, issue 1 (CD002795).

Stein, M. B., Walker, J. R., Hazen, A. L., *et al* (1997) Full and partial post-traumatic stress disorder: findings from a community survey. *American Journal of Psychiatry*, **154**, 1114–1119.

Van Etten, M. L. & Taylor, S. (1998) Comparative efficacy of treatment for post-traumatic stress disorder: a meta-analysis. *Clinical Psychology in Psychotherapy*, **5**, 126–144.

World Health Organization (1992) *The ICD–10 Classification of Mental and Behavioural Disorders: Clinical Descriptions and Diagnostic Guidelines*. WHO.

Yehuda, R. (1999) Biological factors associated with susceptibility to posttraumatic stress disorder. *Canadian Journal of Psychology*, **44**, 34–39.

Yehuda, R. (2002) Clinical relevance of biological findings in PTSD. *Psychiatric Quarterly*, **73**, 123–133.

Zlotnick, C., Rodriguez, B. F., Weisberg, R. B., *et al* (2004) Chronicity in posttraumatic stress disorder and predictors of the course of posttraumatic stress disorder among primary care patients. *Journal of Nervous and Mental Disease*, **192**, 153–159.

CHAPTER 26

Effective psychotherapy in an ethnically and culturally diverse society

Kamaldeep Bhui and Neil Morgan

Summary   This chapter is aimed at psychotherapists and health practitioners who have not reflected on the role of race, culture and ethnicity in the provision of psychological treatments. We highlight the key issues of importance in engagement, assessment and ongoing therapy, supporting practitioners to reach a stage of pre-competency. Competency will be achieved with additional training, supervision and innovation.

Psychological treatments are an essential part of a comprehensive mental health service, and there have been a number of influential reviews of their effectiveness. Roth & Fonagy (2005), for example, concluded that psychodynamic interventions are helpful for borderline states and that family therapy is useful for eating disorders and in the treatment of children and adolescents. Cognitive–behavioural therapy (CBT) is an effective treatment for anxiety, obsessive–compulsive disorder (OCD) and depression, and in the management of hallucinations and delusions in chronic mental illness (Turkington *et al*, 2006). Expressed emotion work is effective in preventing relapse in schizophrenia (although it is rarely well resourced).

The ability to conduct psychotherapy effectively with racially and ethnically diverse populations is becoming increasingly relevant and is recognised to be important in addressing inequalities, which may also be patterned by differences in age, gender, class and sexual orientation. In this chapter we focus on culture and ethnicity.

Regarding the evidence base, few evaluations of the effectiveness of psychotherapy have included adequate numbers of ethnic groups (Alvidrez *et al*, 1996), and few studies report on adaptations of proven interventions for use by culturally and linguistically unique populations.

In many National Health Service (NHS) psychotherapy departments in the UK large numbers of people are treated, often by a few highly trained senior therapists and by psychiatry, psychology, social work and psychotherapy trainees under supervision. As few training experiences include attention to racial and cultural implications for effective psychotherapy, experienced and trainee therapists alike share the need to develop and adapt their interventions for a society that is increasingly racially and culturally diverse.

Critiques of this subject area tend to emerge from experts in culture, health and illness, and include sociological and anthropological disciplines that use specific methodologies for generation of knowledge. These analyses are often theory rich and not easily accommodated into everyday practice, although they can highlight its limitations. Alternatively, psychotherapists practising in multi-ethnic areas immediately recognise the need for better knowledge and models of work with multi-ethnic populations, but it is difficult to ensure that adaptations of existing psychological interventions are effective. In the absence of both well-established guidelines and an adequate evidence base, we consider here some of the complex issues facing psychotherapists working in multicultural and multiracial populations. The chapter is aimed at practising clinicians rather than researchers in cultural psychiatry or medical anthropology.

Definitions

The language in which cultural, racial and ethnic issues are described is often used imprecisely and this leads to much confusion. In Box 26.1 we offer some working definitions that we have found useful, but acknowledge that these may not capture definitions on which all researchers, social scientists or psychiatrists can agree.

Assessment

In assessing the mental state of patients, clinicians need to take into account cultural variations of psychopathology and they should be aware of the manner in which empathy and communication can be profoundly influenced by racial and ethnic differences between patient and therapist (Elfenbein & Ambady, 2002; Bhui & Bhugra, chapter 22, this volume). Dogra & Karim (chapter 27, this volume) have drawn attention to the possible repercussions of healthcare providers' lack of awareness of cultural differences: lack of knowledge results in inability to recognise the differences; self-protection and denial lead to an attitude in which such differences are seen as insignificant; and universalistic assumptions are reflected in actions (Box 26.1).

In a diverse society, specific religious taboos and cultural values may prevent take-up of psychological treatment, in favour of more understood or culturally congruent approaches. For example, prayer, rituals and the lay referral system may alleviate mental distress without resort to formal systems of healthcare (Kleinman, 1980). In non-Western cultures, there may not be the same emphasis on talk as a form of treatment, or on

Box 26.1 Definitions

Culture Helman (2000) defines culture as a set of guidelines inherited by members of a particular society that tell them how to view the world, how to experience it emotionally and how to behave in relation to other people. Culture is transmitted by symbol, art, ritual and language.

Ethnicity A community whose heritage offers its members important characteristics in common that make it distinct from other communities is said to have a shared ethnicity – ethnicity is a boundary that distinguishes 'us' from 'them'. It includes an appraisal of appearance, subjective identification, cultural and religious affiliation, and social exclusion (Modood *et al*, 1997: p. 13). 'Ethnicity' is now commonly used in place of 'race'.

Race
- Legal usage: in the Race Relations (Amendment) Act 2000 a racial group is a group of people defined by their race, colour, nationality (including citizenship), or ethnic or national origins. Jews, Sikhs, Gypsies and Irish Travellers have been recognised by the courts as racial groups for the purpose of the Act
- Popular usage: in biology, 'race' distinguishes the distinct populations (subspecies) of a species (including the human species). Many regard race as a social construct. Many think it has a genetic basis. The most widely used human racial categories are based on visible traits (especially skin colour, facial features and hair texture), genes and self-identification. Concepts of race, as well as specific racial groupings, vary by culture and over time, and are often controversial, for scientific reasons as well as because of their impact on social identity and 'identity politics'.

Religion Religious and spiritual beliefs and practices are more common in some ethnic groups than in others. Indeed, some faith groups are defined as distinct not along cultural or ethnic lines but because of a reliance on religious and spiritual ways of living.

Identity Identity has cultural, ethnic, religious as well as personal components. Cultural, religious and ethnic identity formation and expression are processes that include conscious and unconscious compromises between aspired, experienced and imposed identities. Such identities are challenged during acculturation.

Acculturation This refers to the gradual physical, biological, cultural and psychological changes that take place in individuals and groups on contact with another cultural group. There is pressure on newcomers to conform to and accommodate the dominant cultural lifestyle. Such pressure is handled differently by different individuals, and 'acculturation stress' can create vulnerability to certain health problems as well as susceptibility to increase in psychological symptoms (Loshak, 2003). Berry (2004) defines four states of acculturation: integration (both the individual's original culture and the dominant culture are valued); separation (the individual's culture is valued and the dominant culture is devalued); assimilation (the dominant culture is valued but the individual's culture is devalued; marginalisation (both the individual's culture and the dominant culture are devalued).

Universalism This is an approach to health and social care that reflects the assumption that, despite specific cultural and historical contexts in which people live, all interventions suit all cultural groups ('one size fits all'). Universalism assumes that assessments, and emergent recommendations and interventions, are universally effective and acceptable.

introspection, exploration or personal disclosure. Recovery may be expected following biomedical forms of treatment such as injection, medication or physical investigations. More directive instructions may be expected, and the absence of a clear duration for treatment and confidence in expected recovery may puzzle those who expect more paternalistic styles of healthcare. Communication between therapist and patient may be affected by previous experiences of help-seeking and carers, by different notions of self–other relations, and by permitted levels of emotional intimacy and disclosure of problems that may not be perceived to be social in origin. Communication may also be influenced by culturally determined expectations of what a therapist, doctor, nurse or social worker is expected to do.

Although these issues are most likely to arise in diverse cultural settings with cultural differences between therapist and patient, they may well also become evident where therapist and patient are from the same ethnic group but belong to different subcultural groups.

If an understanding of each other's expectations is missing, mis-communication can arise and this will affect the patient–therapist relationship. The therapist may not understand why a patient does not adhere to treatment, or perhaps why family decisions and views are as important in healthcare uptake as the decisions of the patient. The patient may end up rejecting the therapist if they feel that the therapist is not able to understand or sustain a thoughtful consideration of the role of culture, race and ethnicity in the recovery process. Akhtar (2006) suggests that the immigrant analyst, and by our inference any therapist, must:

- maintain cultural neutrality toward 'native' patients
- wonder about the patient's motivation for choosing a therapist of different ethnicity
- scan the patient's associations for inter-ethnic clues to deeper transferences
- negotiate the dilemmas posed if analysis is conducted in a language other than one's mother tongue
- avoid shared projections, acculturation gaps and nostalgic collusion.

We propose that these issues are pertinent irrespective of the ethnic match between therapist and patient, or the ethnic origin of the therapist. However, the challenges of creating a therapeutic alliance and empathy across racial and cultural divides may make their practice more difficult.

Cultural perspectives on the meaning of 'therapy'

Mental distress is not always seen as a disease or illness: it might be thought of as an outcome of family or interpersonal dysfunction, or of adverse life events and misfortune, or a consequence of breaches in religious and cultural codes of conduct. In culturally diverse societies, practitioners and services will need to adapt interventions, or deliver them with a discerning and sensitive appreciation of the way a treatment is received.

Tseng (1999) classifies therapies around the world into three types: the culturally embedded (e.g. Zar possession and trance states); those influenced by the culture (e.g. Morita and naikan therapies); and those based on cultural elements found in a mainstream model (e.g. CBT).

Many societies practise indigenous therapies, and immigrants and minority ethnic groups often resort to these more familiar forms of healing. Psychotherapies that are unique to specific societies make use of the cultural fabric of that society, with its associated beliefs and aspirations and ways of seeing the world. Mobilising these cultural beliefs can lead to recovery.

Culturally embedded or influenced therapies of non-Western origin may be of value in Western settings, not only for people from minority ethnic groups but also for individuals from the majority population. First, these therapies may not emphasise a psychological cause or cure, but treatment will include psychological transformation. Second, patients from specific cultures may prefer to use these sorts of therapy, or may be pluralistic in their help-seeking practices and consumption of treatments and cures. Third, patients may wish to pursue a psychotherapeutic solution where they perceive that part of their problem is indeed psychological in nature, and recovery requires that this be specifically treated. Such patients irrespective of their cultural background will need help to use a psychological model of therapy.

In some cases it will be necessary to re-examine the patient's explanatory model of their problems and their previous help-seeking before therapy can begin. The explicit rationale for psychotherapy may need explanation. Compromise and consensus will be required to promote engagement and to nurture a treatment alliance. 'Intercultural therapies' already specifically acknowledge this, and include a process of exploration of different solutions and illness perceptions in a respectful, caring and therapeutic atmosphere. With such an approach, psychotherapeutic models such as CBT, psychodynamic therapy and family therapies have the potential to be used effectively across cultures.

Theoretical, technical and philosophical adaptations

Tseng (2001: pp. 515–595) has outlined the communication issues that must be considered when working across cultures. These include an understanding of the mutual expectations of therapist and patient. Existing interventions may be ineffective not only because of miscommunication and divergent health beliefs, but also because theoretical and technical failures can culminate in non-adherence. For example, attachment theories in the West emphasise the unique relationship first between mother and child, and then father and child, and then between the child and the outside world. In extended family systems in Eastern societies, there may be less immediate reliance on the mother in the postnatal period, with a number of key figures providing care. For the mother this offers practical support, and some physical and emotional relief; for the child it offers multiple attachment figures that are all important for development and are trusted as carers. Of course the level of intimacy may vary: for example, breast-feeding or nappy changing or bathing may be performed by fewer figures. Nonetheless, a theory of attachment that cannot encompass multiple attachments as healthy, as opposed to perceiving these as enmeshed or diffuse or pathological non-attachment to the mother, will need revision. In cross-cultural therapy, theories of psychotherapy will be challenged. If the therapist holds a culturally insensitive theoretical model the patient may fail to engage with or adhere to treatment. Multiple attachments also have implications for development of the self, either as an I-self organised around the individual embodied person or the We-self that reflects a sociocentric self. A sociocentric self is experienced in social groups in which all people are connected, and the self consists of multiple, compatible (and not pathological) selves (or self states). Such theoretical differences will determine how technical aspects of the therapy are managed.

Another example of a potential cross-cultural limitation of Western therapeutic theory is its appropriation of the classical Oedipus myth. This finds expression and use in therapeutic processes but is a culturally influenced theory (Bhugra & Bhui, 2002). The parent–child incest taboo, found in all cultures, institutes the distinction between gender, generations and contact with the external world. In psychoanalytic terms this refers to the triadic Oedipal constellation, but the figures of the triad may vary depending on the culture. For example, in the Indian setting the mother's brother or another 'father' figure may be the rival with whom Oedipal conflicts are resolved; in a matriarchal society this figure may even be female.

Interpreters

The use of interpreters across cultures is described in detail by Farooq & Fear in chapter 24. Here we will consider the impact on emotional communication. Using interpreters is an inevitable necessity if services and interventions are to be offered to linguistic minorities. All information has to be processed through a third person's linguistic-emotional framework before anything is known about the patient. In turn, the patient can learn something of the therapist only through the interpreter. Gestures, smiles and non-verbal behaviour remain important, but steady, slow and carefully taken steps towards mutual understanding are difficult to sustain through an interpreter.

After a lengthier and yet, compared with work with an English speaker, a less revealing process, the therapist may still be faced with theoretical and philosophical uncertainties. Each theoretical concept will need more weighing up and some therapies, for example psychodynamic work, may be impossible, as the necessary level of intimacy may not be easily achieved unless years are dedicated to the task. Even cognitive–behavioural treatments may be undermined if homework and task completion are not understood, or if therapeutic services are seen as part of a medical review process. This is a not uncommon scenario with refugees and asylum seekers, who often find the process of CBT puzzling or anxiety-promoting.

Interpreters may have their own expectations of the situation and understanding of emotional states. They also have different levels of linguistic proficiency. The sensitive timing in the delivery of psychotherapeutic interpretations linking past and present, and patients' disclosure of intimate traumas and precious aspects of self, may all be jeopardised if the interpreter and the therapist are not attuned. Both need to be experienced and perceptive of the quality of their working relationship and their limitations as a professional dyad working with a patient.

Emotional communications across racial and cultural groups are complex and subject to distortion (Bhui & Bhugra, chapter 22, this volume). Involving a third person in this communicative process may further distort knowledge about the other or, given the limited time available for therapy, leave certain possibilities unexplored. One solution is to ensure that bilingual therapists are recruited and trained to meet the needs of the local population, but this does not overcome the failure of theory or skills in negotiating meanings attached to the therapeutic process. These high-level skills cannot be assumed to exist among bilingual people who happen to be therapists, but should be assessed as a competency of therapists needing to work in bilingual settings.

Racial, ethnic or identity matching

There is little empirical evidence that ethnic matching leads to improved outcomes. It may, however, improve engagement and prevent the silent drop out from treatment perceived to be incongruent with the patient's priorities. A Black therapist may have had the same experiences of racism, or social exclusion or migration as a Black patient. This shared experience may be important for some patients to enter a therapy. However, the therapist may differ at other levels, in terms of age, gender, educational level and social class.

Ethnic matching has been proposed as a way of addressing cultural differences, including those of race, language and religion. Just as patients often seek out therapists of the same gender or of a specific age group, they may also seek out therapists they perceive to be more able or confident. These may be from a different ethnic group, but perhaps also from their own ethnic group. Thomas (1992) describes these sentiments as pre-transference phenomena fuelled by fantasy, myth and internal representations of the other, and by popular portrayals of ethnic groups in the social environment. Morgan (1998) described how a Black patient sought out a White therapist and discovered her own internalised racism and denigration of Blackness: she had equated a White therapist with a better therapist.

> **Box 26.2**   Key requirements for inclusive psychotherapy
>
> - The therapist needs to be skilled in exploring racial and cultural identity
> - The therapist must understand that, for some patients, life events with racial elements are part of a social reality that can become an internal representation and emerge in their mental life, fantasy and beliefs
> - The therapist must have the capacity to perceive, apprehend and think through the primitive feelings of aggression, hatred, humiliation and shame that accompany racial encounters, conflicts and enactments
>
> (After Carter, 1995)

Issues of confidentiality can also cause patients to seek therapists who are outside of their cultural group. Yet therapists who do not speak the primary language of the patient may not be able to communicate effectively or conceptualise the patient's distress in words that are meaningful to the patient.

Some patients experience encounters with people from other ethnic groups as traumatic or as experiences that promote anxiety, fear and primitive impulses that together characterise the dynamics of racial thinking.

Some religious minorities feel that therapy with a non-religious therapist or with a therapist from a different religious group would pose insurmountable obstacles (Lowenthal, 1999).

Language apart, it may not be the ethnic or racial group of the therapist that is crucial. Carter (1995) asserts that the identity status of the therapist and the patient, in terms of the extent of exploration of their own cultural identity, determines the basis of a match or mismatch in therapy. He proposes five stages in the development of a mature cultural identity: separated, pre-encounter, encounter, exploration and closure, in which an identity is finally embraced. Within this process a key discovery that a White therapist has to make is that of the role of 'White privilege'. Carter also identified key skills required by therapists practising inclusive therapy, and these are listed in Box 26.2.

Communication and emotion

The role of communication across cultures and the difficulties of knowing the other are discussed by Bhui & Bhugra in chapter 22. The very act of talking about and putting into words deep personal emotional experience formed from the present and the past results in an alienation of the words from the experience (Nobus, 2000). Communication of internal states of mind is difficult even in a shared language. Across languages and cultures, the task must include a slow and paced review of all that is thought to be known and assumed by both the therapist and the patient. Add to this the divergent expectations of what constitutes therapy, especially among recent immigrants, and there is a real potential for a failure of communication. This may undermine any modality of therapy, leading to unexplained drop out of treatment and therefore a lack of effectiveness; what Morgan (1998) has called the 'silence' of race.

In Box 26.3 we make recommendations to support culturally capable practice. These are aimed at developing basic competencies to address some of the very challenging dilemmas that therapists encounter in the consulting room. However, culture and ethnicity may be misunderstood to refer to homogeneous groups. Although these recommendations will help to engage patients, it must be remembered that ethnic and cultural groups can differ in many other ways, influenced by age, gender, class, sexual orientation, preferred language and degree of integration into British society.

The elements of good practice listed in Box 26.3 are often those that are presumed to be helpful; for example, they may be the factors that mediate benefit when ethnic matching is used. An important component of working in multiracial, multi-ethnic and multicultural populations is noticing and managing the 'racial transference'. This may include racial material acting as a vehicle for the expression of transference defence, or drive derivatives or object ties (see Moodley & Palmer, 2006). Race-based transference may

---

Box 26.3 Recommendations for culturally capable practice in psycho-therapy

- Suspend preconceptions about a patient's race, ethnicity and that of their family members
- Recognise that a client may be quite different from other members of their racial ethnic group
- Consider how racial ethnic differences between therapist and client might affect psychotherapy:
  - differences in conceptualisation of mental health and illness
  - differences in conceptualisation of self in relation to family and community
  - differences in communication styles
- Acknowledge that power, privilege and racism might affect interaction with clients.
- When in doubt about the importance of race and ethnicity and treatment err on the side of discussion
- Keep learning about issues of race and ethnicity, and become a mini-ethnographer with patients and the public
- Notice and apprehend the racial transference so that it is of therapeutic value and not simply re-enacted in the consulting room

(adapted from Cardemil & Battle, 2003)

also be an expression of intrapsychic conflict, and involve splitting and projective defences; racial material may reveal a person's own experience of racism, and their racial identity as internalised representations of past and present relationships. Irrespective of modality of therapy, such processes should be identified and managed in the service of recovery. Therapists should be able to work in supervision (individual and group) to engage with and explore primitive emotional reactions to racial material that may lead to enactments by themselves and in their patients.

Conclusion

This chapter has given a brief outline of some key issues facing therapists working in multicultural and multiracial societies (Bhugra & Bhui, 1998). There is a valuable literature on this topic and Box 26.4 lists some further reading. We do not propose major technical adaptations of interventions, but suggest that an essential 'pre-competency' is to notice the expression of culture and race in therapeutic encounters, and to incorporate these expressions within therapeutic processes and thinking, while taking notice of therapeutic structures that may hinder recovery.

Box 26.4 Further reading

Cardemil, E. V. & Battle, C. L. (2003) Guess who's coming to therapy? Getting comfortable with conversations about race and ethnicity in psychotherapy. *Professional Psychology: Research and Practice*, **34**, 278–286.

Darling, L. (2004) Psychoanalytically informed work with interpreters. *Psychoanalytic Psychotherapy*, **18**, 255–267.

Inayat, Q. (2005) Psychotherapy in a multi-ethnic society. *Psychotherapist*, **26**, 7.

Layard, R. (2006) The case for psychological treatment centres. *BMJ*, **332**, 1030–1032. doi:10.1136/bmj.332. 7548.1030.

Neki, J. S. (1975) Guru-chela relationship: the possibility of a therapeutic paradigm. *American Journal of Orthopsychiatry*, **43**, 755–766.

Patel, N., Bennett, E., Dennis, M., *et al* (2000) *Clinical Psychology, Race, and Culture: A Training Manual*. British Psychological Society Books.

Prince, R. (1980) Variations in psychotherapy procedures. In *Handbook of Cross Cultural Psychopathology* (eds T. C. Triandis & J. G. Draguns), vol 6. Allyn & Bacon.

Tesone, J. E. (1996) Multi-lingualism, word-presentations, thing-presentations and psychic reality. *International Journal of Psychoanalysis*, **77**, 871–881.

Wheeler, S. (2006) *Difference and Diversity in Counselling: Contemporary Psychodynamic Perspectives*. Palgrave Macmillan.

References

Akhtar, S. (2006) Technical challenges faced by the immigrant analyst. *Psychoanalytic Quarterly*, **75**, 21–43.

Alvidrez, J., Azocar, F. & Miranda, J. (1996) Demystifying the concept of ethnicity for psychotherapy researchers. *Journal of Consulting and Clinical Psychology*, **64**, 903–908.

Berry, J. W. (2004) Psychology of group relations: cultural and social dimensions. *Aviation, Space, and Environmental Medicine*, **75** (suppl. 1), C52–C57.

Bhugra, D. & Bhui, K. (1998) Psychotherapy for ethnic minorities. *British Journal of Psychotherapy*, **14**, 310–326.

Bhugra, D. & Bhui, K. (2002) Is the Oedipal complex universal? Problems for sexual and relationship psychotherapy across cultures. *Sexual and Relationship Therapy*, **17**, 69–86.

Cardemil, E. V. & Battle, C. L. (2003) Guess who's coming to therapy? Getting comfortable with conversations about race and ethnicity in psychotherapy. *Professional Psychology: Research and Practice*, **34**, 278–286.

Carter, R. (1995) *The Influence of Race and Racial Identity in the Psychotherapy Process: Towards a Racially Inclusive Model*. John Wiley & Sons.

Elfenbein, H. A. & Ambady, N. (2002) On the universality and cultural specificity of emotion recognition: a meta-analysis. *Psychological Bulletin*, **128**, 203–235.

Helman, C. (2000) *Culture, Health and Illness*. Butterworth-Heinemann.

Kleinman, A. (1980) *Patients and Healers in the Context of Culture*. Thesis. University of California Press.

Loshak, R. (2003) Working with Bangladeshi young women. *Psychoanalytic Psychotherapy*, **17**, 52–67.

Lowenthal, K. (1999) Religious issues and their psychological aspects. In *Mental Health Service Provision for a Multicultural Society* (eds K. Bhui & D. Olajide), pp. 54–65. W. B. Saunders.

Modood, T., Berthoud, R., Lakey, J., *et al* (1997) *Ethnic Minorities in Britain*. Policy Studies Institute.

Moodley, R. & Palmer, S. (2006) *Race, Culture and Psychotherapy*. Routledge.

Morgan, H. (1998) Between fear and blindness: the white therapist and the black patient. *Journal of the British Association of Psychotherapists*, **34**, 48–61.

Nobus, D. (2000) *Jacques Lacan and the Freudian Practice of Psychoanalysis*. Routledge.

Roth, A. & Fonagy, P. (2005) *What Works for Whom? A Critical Review of Psychotherapy Research* (2nd edn). Guilford Press.

Thomas, L. (1992) Racism and psychotherapy. Working with racism in the consulting room: an analytical view. In *Intercultural Therapy: Themes, Interpretations and Practice* (eds J. Kareem & R. Littlewood), pp. 146–160. Blackwell Science.

Tseng, W. S. (1999) Culture and psychotherapy: review and practical guidelines. *Transcultural Psychiatry*, **36**, 131–179.

Tseng, W. S. (2001) *Handbook of Cultural Psychiatry*. Academic Press.

Turkington, D., Kingdon, D. & Weiden, P. J. (2006) Cognitive behavior therapy for schizophrenia. *American Journal of Psychiatry*, **163**, 365–373.

CHAPTER 27

Diversity training for psychiatrists

Nisha Dogra and Khalid Karim

Summary Access of clients from minority ethnic groups to appropriate healthcare and the treatment they experience once they gain access are matters of great concern. There have been recent calls for training in cultural diversity to be prioritised for mental healthcare professionals, including psychiatrists. In this chapter we discuss the term 'cultural diversity' and consider its relevance to psychiatrists. We then briefly review some of the training currently available, discussing related issues and problems, including the lack of evaluation. We suggest how psychiatrists may need to change their approach to this subject.

There is considerable concern in countries such as the UK, USA and Canada about the access of people from Black and minority ethnic groups to appropriate healthcare (Dyson & Smaje, 2001). This may reflect real or perceived barriers to services because of disadvantage related to minority status. Several approaches have been proposed to address this problem, one of which has been to increase cultural diversity training for all clinical staff, including psychiatrists. It is the issues surrounding such training that we discuss in this chapter. Since our original article 5 years ago (Dogra & Karim, 2005) the same issues remain pertinent to good clinical practice, and the death of David 'Rocky' Bennett, the subsequent enquiry and the resulting policy remain in the consciousness of the profession. Internationally there have been some attempts to introduce a framework for the training of staff in cultural competence, with most of the literature originating from North America (Fung *et al*, 2008; Lim *et al*, 2008). A simple literature search on cultural competence using Medline reveals number of articles both nationally and internationally from various specialties, but only a few involve mental health. In this update we review some of the literature and present our interpretation of the progress or lack thereof in this area.

Defining concepts

Culture

Culture is not a value-free concept and it is defined in many ways, as are other widely used terms such as ethnicity and race (Bradby, 2003). One cannot dispute that the concept of culture, cultural identity or belonging to a cultural group is a dynamic process involving a degree of active engagement by individuals. It is problematic to assign cultural categories externally and based only on certain characteristics. It must be recognised that individuals make sense of themselves in various ways in relation to the cultural groups with which they themselves identify or are externally identified. Membership of such groups is not always voluntary. How much an individual chooses to identify with a group to which he or she is assigned varies from person to person. Concepts of culture and understanding cultural groups imply understanding of the hierarchies and rules of conduct of those groups.

The concept of identity is closely related to that of culture. Identities can be formed through the cultures and subcultures to which people belong or in which they participate. Frosh (1999: p. 413) described the view that identity draws from culture but is not simply formed by it. Given that the focus of this chapter is cultural diversity in the context of delivering psychiatric services, the definition of culture that we use is consistent with that adopted by the Association of American Medical Colleges. I introduced this definition chapter 16, but repeat it here for readers' convenience:

> Culture is defined by each person in relationship to the group or groups with whom he or she identifies. An individual's cultural identity may be based on heritage as well as individual circumstances and personal choice. Cultural identity may be affected by such factors as race, ethnicity, age, language, country of origin, acculturation, sexual orientation, gender, socioeconomic status, religious/spiritual beliefs, physical abilities, occupation, among others. These factors may impact behaviours such as communication styles, diet preferences, health beliefs, family roles, lifestyle, rituals and decision-making processes. All of these beliefs and practices, in turn can influence how patients and heath care professionals perceive health and illness, and how they interact with one another. (Task Force on Spirituality, Cultural Issues, and End of Life Care, 1999: p. 25.)

This is a patient-centred definition that can be applied to clinical situations. It suggests that individuals draw on a range of resources and, through the interplay of external and internal meanings, construct a sense of identity and unique culture. Patients will themselves define which aspect of their cultural belonging is relevant at any particular time. This may change in different clinical contexts and at different stages of an individual's life, and may also depend on the clinical presentation itself. This is not to underplay the complexity of the term, but to use it in a way that is suitable in the context of healthcare delivery. The academic debate about the meaning of culture is less relevant here than the interplay between culture and identity, which involves the individual's perception. The latter is more relevant in clinical contexts.

Diversity

Although various definitions of culture are offered, less has been written about diversity. One might think that diversity should be a more straightforward term. However, again the word is used imprecisely. In some cases, it means diversity of ethnicity, which is often called 'multiculturalism' (e.g. Culhane-Pera *et al*, 1997; Loudon *et al*, 2001). There is also a perspective that diversity covers the range of groups within society and thus includes groups identified by characteristics other than ethnicity, such as sexual orientation. In other cases, it covers a much broader range of difference, relating to individual characteristics beyond ethnicity.

In this chapter, diversity includes not only race, ethnicity and gender but also ability/disability, education, class and many other differences.

Cultural competence

In the North American medical system, many educational programmes have endeavoured to teach 'cultural competence' as a way of understanding culture. A widely used definition of this (Cross *et al*, 1989: p. 3) states:

> The model called 'cultural competence' ... involves systems, agencies and practitioners with the capacity to respond to the unique needs of populations whose cultures are different than that which might be called 'dominant' or 'mainstream' American. The word culture is used because it implies the integrated pattern of human behaviour that includes communications, actions, customs, beliefs, values and institutions of a racial, ethnic, religious or social group. The word competence is used because it implies having the capacity to function in a particular way: the capacity to function within the context of culturally integrated patterns of human behaviour as defined by the group. While this publication focuses on ethnic minorities of colour, the terminology and thinking behind this model applies to each person – everyone has or is part of a culture.

Although this definition does not emphasise working towards services that are sensitive to an individual patient's needs, it does highlight the needs of groups which may or may not be as homogeneous as is implied.

Cultural competence is a widely used term and it has many other meanings (Henry J. Kaiser Family Foundation, 2003).

Race and ethnicity

There is similar inconsistency in definitions of race and ethnicity (Bradby, 2003). For example, in the USA 'race' is still perceived more as a biological characteristic, whereas in the UK there is greater acceptance that it is a social construct (Dogra & Karnik, 2004). It is also true that the term 'race' is now less accepted in some contexts in the UK, although it is a term that is still widely used, albeit imprecisely and with different meanings.

The problems about even basic terminology remain unresolved. There continues to be confusion about what constitutes cultural competence at an individual level and, more crucially, at an organisational level. Reducing disparities and inequality in the delivery of culturally appropriate services remains a key target for the National Health Service (NHS). Change has at times felt slow, with the Healthcare Commission (now subsumed within the Care Quality Commission) reporting that there had been some progress but that major problems remained (Healthcare Commission, 2007). The monitoring of employment procedures and the publication of 'race equality impact' were key areas for improvement. It is noteworthy that only 9% of NHS trusts had complied with all three publication duties on race equality, whereas there was a much higher compliance on the publication of disability equality schemes.

When it comes to implementation of policy, most of the energy goes into being seen to do the right thing rather than actually doing it. Organisations want to be seen to be complying and the superficial approaches taken by the Healthcare Commission may be compounding rather than helping the problem. A recent publication (Healthcare Commission, 2009) shows that data collection continues to improve (35% of trusts now have data, compared with 9% in 2007) but there is still little on how this affects patient care or patients' experience of and involvement in care. The latter is an issue that the Healthcare Commission highlighted.

How does diversity relate to healthcare delivery?

Although many psychiatrists readily accept that diversity influences use of healthcare services and health outcomes, there is evidence that some regard psychosocial factors as too 'touchy–feely' (Toynbee, 2002). However, there is evidence to suggest that the patients of clinicians who respect different patient perspectives have improved healthcare outcomes, feeling better understood, respected and valued as partners in their own care (Secker & Harding, 2002).

Levinson et al (1997) offered several reasons to justify the teaching of cultural diversity to medical students. They argued that dealing effectively with diversity should improve doctor–patient communication. This can be generalised to postgraduate contexts: if diversity training does make a difference to healthcare outcomes, training should be undertaken throughout a doctor's career. Evidence shows that good communication skills diminish the risk of malpractice: the doctor is better able to identify the patient's problems, which reduces misdiagnoses and misunderstandings. Appreciation of cultural diversity should also increase patients' adherence to treatment regimens and improve outcomes, including patient satisfaction.

DiversityRx is an American clearing house of information on ways to meet the language and cultural needs of minorities, immigrants, refugees and other diverse populations seeking healthcare. In an overview of cultural competence in medical training and practice, they reported that lack of awareness about cultural differences makes it difficult for both providers and patients to achieve the best, most appropriate care. Figure 27.1 shows some of the problems that may arise if clinicians are culturally incompetent or unaware (DiversityRx, 2001a).

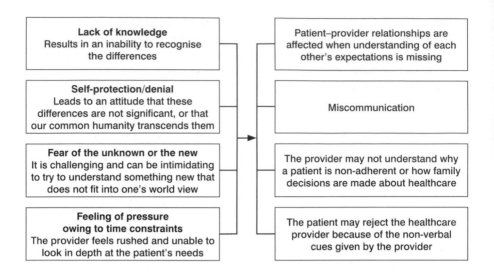

Fig. 27.1 Possible repercussions of healthcare providers' lack of awareness of cultural differences (DiversityRx, 2001*a*).

The National Institute for Mental Health in England (NIMHE) (2003) has highlighted the possibility that people from Black and minority ethnic groups experience inadequate healthcare provision. Williams (1997) argued that when culture is overlooked, incorrect and even harmful decisions may be made. Furthermore, the healthcare provider's ability to engage individuals and families and build on strengths may be limited. DiversityRx (2001*b*) stated that providers may need to ask themselves how they react when confronted with a new situation that does not fit their expectations and whether it provokes feelings of anxiety and discomfort. They also suggested that clinicians consider what is going on within themselves and within their patients. They should ask themselves whether they have useful strategies for clarifying puzzling situations and improving their own and their patients' understanding.

Thom and colleagues found no statistically significant impact of training on physicians' cultural competence, on healthcare processes or outcomes of care (Thom *et al*, 2006). However, they did find that culturally competent physicians had a positive impact on the care of patients with hypertension and/or diabetes.

Diversity training for psychiatrists

Training remains an key factor in addressing the issue of cultural diversity, and the effectiveness of this training is especially important: it must be seen to have an impact on clinical practice. The evidence to date suggests that training has made little difference to patient outcomes or experience.

There is still little evidence that clear frameworks to deliver such training are being utilised. Until recently there has been no framework within which training in diversity has been formally considered for psychiatrists or other healthcare professionals. There has been a tendency to assume that diversity, especially diversity related to ethnicity, inherently leads patients to have different beliefs about mental health and that this should be the focus of exploration (see chapter 22, this volume). Although this may be valuable, it may not reveal the whole picture. Variability within groups is either not recognised or is minimised.

First moves towards a national training programme were published in *Inside Outside* (National Institute for Mental Health in England, 2003: p. 31), which advocated mandatory training in cultural competencies for all professional staff working in mental health. In the same year, an inquiry into the death of a Black man, David 'Rocky' Bennett, in a psychiatric hospital recommended that training the 40 000-strong mental health workforce in cultural competence should become a priority (Department of Health, 2003). In 2004, the NIMHE and the Sainsbury Centre for Mental Health published a document laying down the most important areas in which all staff in mental health services should be trained ('the ten essential shared capabilities'; Hope, 2004). One of these is respecting diversity, which Hope (p. 3) describes as:

> working in partnership with service users, carers, families and colleagues to provide care and interventions that not only make a positive difference but also do so in ways that respect and value diversity including age, race, culture, disability, gender, spirituality and sexuality.

Hope makes specific mention of the discrimination known to exist in many services, pointing out that issues of race and culture require particular attention. Among other things, respect for diversity requires practitioners to understand and acknowledge diversity and to understand the impact of discrimination and prejudice on mental health and mental health services (Hope, 2004: p. 14). Although these are commendable recommendations and evidence-based practice is touched upon, little more is said on the value of such education.

With a clarity often lacking in other documents, the Sainsbury Centre for Mental Health (2002) reviewed the relationship between mental health services and African and Caribbean communities in the UK. In a discussion of the usage of terms and their potential impact on training, the review pointed to the effect of the confusion that exists in healthcare arenas regarding 'cultural diversity', in particular definitions that rely on group-based distinctions. It noted that political rather than educational agendas have often influenced educational programmes. The centrality of issues of 'race' and 'culture' for mental health services should not be underestimated but nor should they be used to reinforce stereotypical views about minority ethnic communities. In some circumstances, the report noted, it is evident that the term 'culture' is used in a similar way to 'race', to denote immutable and fixed physical attributes and/or behaviours. Elsewhere, the term seems to denote a set of shared beliefs or a system of kinship. In the context of mental health this approach is problematic, as an individual's culture needs to be understood for that individual, rather than extrapolated from given generalities. The review felt that this is particularly important, as many 'cultural awareness' courses define or predict the characteristics of certain ethnic groups, along with standard responses by professional workers, by means of overarching generalisations.

Current training and issues raised

When considering the need for an evidence-based approach to medical education, it is clear that evaluation of new programmes needs attention. Many programmes are available, as an internet search will reveal. However, very few claiming to teach cultural diversity have been subject to evaluation beyond subjective student feedback. The exceptions are four studies with undergraduates (Mao et al, 1988; Copeman, 1989; Rubenstein et al, 1992; Dogra, 2001) and two with postgraduates (Culhane-Pera et al, 1997; Majumdar et al, 1999). All used pre- and post-teaching questionnaires and reported some degree of 'positive' change in student perspectives, but there was little follow-up. Only one of these studies was conducted in the UK (Dogra, 2001). This might suggest that, although medical organisations claim to run programmes on cultural diversity, there is little follow-up to ensure that these make any difference. Furthermore, the content of programmes is often variable. Some focus on knowledge acquisition (e.g. Deloney et al, 2000), some on skills (e.g. Majumdar et al, 1999) and some on attitudes (e.g. Sifri et al, 2001). Many attempt to address all three aspects, although their focus varies (e.g. Culhane-Pera et al, 1997; Dogra, 2001). There is evidence that, although many UK medical schools now address this issue at undergraduate level, teaching is fragmented and there is a great deal of uncertainty as to what diversity education actually is (Dogra et al, 2005).

Some study results

Webb & Sergison (2003) reported that child healthcare professionals found race awareness training useful. In a follow-up study, staff commented on how they thought their own behaviour had changed. For example, some used more culturally appropriate pictures in wards and stopped using minors as interpreters. However, there were no objective measures of change.

A systematic review of five interventions to improve cultural competence in healthcare systems that included cultural competence training for healthcare providers was undertaken by Anderson et al (2003). They judged that only one study had a fair quality of execution and therefore concluded that the evidence was insufficient.

The findings of Thom *et al* (2006) suggest that cultural competence is important in healthcare but as yet we have not clarified how physicians can be effectively trained to become culturally competent and how policy relating to this issue can best be framed for medical organisations.

In a survey which included the commissioners of training in NHS mental health trusts, primary care trusts, independent-sector in-patient mental health service providers, a large number of their employees and providers of race equality training, Bennett *et al* (2007) reported significant variation in the training provided. The majority (91%) reported training that was available to employees, and just over two-thirds of staff said that they had attended. In just over half of organisations the training was compulsory. The main reasons for not attending a training programme were that the organisation did not offer one or that the person did not know that training was available. Some discrepancy existed between the percentage of organisations that reported having a formal policy on race equality (96%) and the percentage that the Healthcare Commission (2009) reported (60%). This difference was reflected in the concern that commissioners of training had regarding the commitment that existed in their organisations.

Bennett *et al* comment that although there has been considerable investment in and commitment to race-related training for many years, there is little evidence of any serious attempts to evaluate its effectiveness. The majority of training providers reported that training was evaluated, but mostly they collected only subjective data from participants immediately after sessions, using evaluation forms and questionnaires, verbal feedback and reflection exercises. The authors concluded that evaluation appears to be the area of greatest confusion and least systematic action. It was difficult to evaluate how much the training, as opposed to other measures, led to change, if in fact there was any change at all.

Concerns regarding organisations' attitudes to training in cultural competence have also been reported internationally (Dogra *et al*, 2009). Staff with the lead responsibility for such training in a number of North American healthcare organisations commonly reported a lack of clarity in the implementation of culturally competent care. In addition to the lack of a strategic overview and low priority given to this issue, commonly cited problems included a lack of leadership, difficulties accessing the whole organisation and funding problems.

Significant variations exist in the aims, content, delivery and evaluation of any training provided. In a survey of opinions on cultural diversity training for UK healthcare professionals there was agreement on the main aim – to increase awareness of race and cultural issues – but both employees and training providers were in less agreement on other aims (Bentley *et al*, 2008). The content of training varied widely, apparently influenced by the trainers' perspective or the demands of the commissioning organisation. This may have been compounded by a lack of standards or regulation by a professional body for the trainers. Significantly, the survey demonstrated a wide variation in the teaching of cultural diversity between healthcare professionals and across geographic regions. At present, training programmes are mandatory only for psychiatrists and mental health professionals. Implementation varied significantly in terms of the time devoted to this area, but delivery had some common modalities. These differences emphasise the need for national guidelines on cultural training to the responsible bodies.

There is limited evidence on the effectiveness of cultural competence training and its impact on clinical practice. Bentley *et al* (2008) reported that most employees were positive on many aspects of the training and the majority reported a positive impact on their work. However, less than half felt that the training had a positive impact on service delivery or their organisation. A third of statutory organisations evaluated the training provided, most of them using internal evaluation.

A review of evaluated models of professional education and service delivery found that of 109 potential papers, only nine included an evaluation of a model for improving cultural competence in clinical practice and service delivery (Bhui *et al*, 2007). All the studies were North American and used different methodologies. Not all published their learning and teaching methods, there were differences in definitions and they evaluated different aspects of care and outcomes. More crucially, none of the studies investigated user experiences and outcomes.

A systematic literature review and analysis of interventions designed to improve the cultural competence of healthcare professionals included 34 studies, most of which took place in the USA (Beach *et al*, 2005). There was evidence that cultural competence training improved participants' knowledge, attitudes and skills. There was also some evidence that it affected patient satisfaction, although only three studies investigated this. None of the studies investigated the costs of training. The authors concluded that cultural competence training shows promise in the education of healthcare professionals, but that there is as yet little evidence that it improves patients' adherence to therapy, health outcomes and equity of services across racial and ethnic groups. They suggest that future research should focus on these outcomes and should determine which teaching methods and content are most effective.

Political correctness

In a report mentioned earlier, the Sainsbury Centre for Mental Health (2002) commented on staff concerns that issues of race and culture cannot be freely discussed, implicitly blaming 'political correctness'. The report acknowledges that attempts to address racism and sexism have at times focused on the ridiculous. 'Political correctness' can also be viewed as a tool used by the American political right to discredit the whole process of tackling disparities. Any initiative against racism or sexism is likely to be met with the charge of political correctness by those opposed to change, and it is necessary to achieve a rational balance between outlandish prohibitions on behaviour or language (e.g. black coffee) and reasonable criticism of racism.

The findings of the Sainsbury Centre have been borne out in our own discussions with colleagues about their training experiences. Training is often enforced so that organisations can claim they are complying with legislation, but there is a feeling that there is little commitment to actually changing practice or systems.

Changing how we think

Several issues need consideration if there is a serious intention to review whether or not diversity training influences healthcare outcomes and how psychiatrists can be trained to provide care appropriate to a patient's culture. In the remainder of this section we consider just some of these.

How patients are viewed

First, we need to ask whether information about specific groups is helpful or not. In chapter 1, Kelly highlights studies that have found higher prevalence of particular disorders in particular groups, but there is no evidence to show that having such information influences healthcare outcomes, either for better or worse. Indeed, the information might do more to reinforce stereotypes than to challenge practitioners to question their own biases in decision-making processes. Although public healthcare may be about services to groups of the population, clinical care is about service provision to individuals. We must consider how we tailor public services to individuals' needs. This seems to be a fundamental and yet unresolved issue.

If we consider diversity among patients and use the Association of American Medical College's definition shown near the beginning of this chapter, the focus is on individuals not groups. Ethnicity is only one component of how individuals might choose to define themselves. We need to consider for whose benefit we provide general information about groups with which patients may or may not identify. Individuals should be able to choose how they define themselves, rather than have services define them on the basis of their skin colour or any other characteristic. Publications such as *Addressing Black and Minority Ethnic Health in London* (Department of Health, 1999) imply that the needs of individuals are primarily based on their skin colour. In general, Black people and people from minority ethnic groups are treated as a single homogeneous population. This approach makes assumptions that the experiences of all such individuals are the same and that their skin colour overrides other facets of their individuality. Talking about groups of people reduces patients to lists by which their needs are decided, as opposed to asking them as individuals what their views are. Managing diversity should mean trying to improve access and services for all potential users, not just for those from specific groups. It should also be recognised that equitable care does not mean the same care, as individual needs will be different.

Educational models for teaching cultural diversity

There is criticism that education and training in cultural diversity have largely been driven by government policy and not educational needs or an evidence base (Dogra, 2004b). Nevertheless, the concept of cultural competence discussed earlier has provided an important background to developments in the UK. It might be argued that there are two different models for teaching cultural competence. One is based on a notion of expertise and the other on a notion of sensibility (Dogra, 2004a).

Cultural expertise

An expert may be described as having special skill at a task or knowledge in a subject, so that expertise is the skill or knowledge that the expert possesses (Thompson, 1995). The notion that, through gaining knowledge about 'other' cultures, someone can develop 'cultural expertise' has given rise to educational programmes that try to impart cultural competence, to create 'cultural experts'.

Cultural sensibility

'Cultural sensibility' should not be confused with the more common term 'cultural sensitivity'. In general usage, sensibility (openness to emotional impressions, susceptibility and sensitiveness; Thompson, 1995) relates to a person's moral, emotional or aesthetic ideas or standards. Thus, cultural sensibility is interactional: if one is open to outside experience, one might reflect and change because of that experience. This is not necessarily the case with cultural sensitivity, which is more the quality or degree of being aware of cultural issues and is closer in meaning to cultural expertise. In cultural sensibility, there is no notion of acquiring expertise about others; rather, there is a recognition that we need to be aware of our own perspectives and how they affect our ability to view the perspectives of others with an open mind.

Tables 27.1 and 27.2 show how aspects of culture and diversity training are interpreted from the perspectives of cultural expertise and cultural sensibility (Dogra, 2004a).

Service models

In both teaching and clinical practice too much emphasis on practical matters such as language and use of interpreters may mean that practitioners avoid dealing with difficult personal issues such as questioning their own vulnerabilities, fears, ignorance or prejudices. Very few organisations and individuals set out to plan lower-quality services, but we need to think about why some patients still fail to receive the care they need or value.

Table 27.1 Conceptions of culture from two perspectives

	Cultural expertise	Cultural sensibility
Culture	Culture is an externally recognised characteristic; it is static, unitary and one-dimensional; ethnicity is emphasised	Culture is an internally constructed sense of self; it is dynamic/fluid, multidimensional, diverse/differentiated; ethnicity is one aspect
Difference	Generalises the differences between individuals	Is sensitive to difference
Identity formation	Individuals are shaped by their social world and defined by their culture irrespective of the context	Individuals bring their own meanings and histories to different contexts: meanings may change dependent on the context

After Dogra (2004*a*).

Service models influence the training that is delivered and help to establish who is held responsible for delivering equitable services to all. Some organisations delegate this responsibility to a named individual such as a diversity officer, which appears to absolve everyone else of the need to feel responsible. Legally in the UK it is everyone's responsibility.

In response to a debate about specific services for minority ethnic groups (Bhui & Sashidharan, 2003), Whitley *et al* (2004) raised the issue that the diversity of Canadian society is not captured by the broad ethno-racial categories commonly used in the UK and USA; thus, specialised clinics for each minority group are not feasible in Canada. Provision of ethnicity-specific services in that country is not pursued for practical rather than philosophical reasons.

Robertson *et al* (2000) found that most of the Black services users they interviewed in a UK study did not want an ethnically specific service, but one that all users could access and benefit from. In another UK study, Secker & Harding (2002) reported that service users valued the ability of staff to engage with them and see the world from their perspective and that this was not dependent on ethnic matching.

Bhui (2004) has suggested that the integrationist solution has failed to ensure that generic mental health services are culturally capable or appropriate. However, until there is greater debate about this, training will flounder as there is no consensus on what it is trying to achieve. There is also a danger in assuming that individuals who share the same ethnicity have the same views on issues relating to mental health.

Policies regarding training in cultural diversity

As already mentioned, there is strong evidence that political imperatives rather than educational need or purpose have driven diversity training thus far (Dogra, 2004*b*).

Table 27.2 Two perspectives on conceptions of education in diversity training

	Cultural expertise	Cultural sensibility
Learning process	Acquisition of knowledge	Acquisition of principles (method)
Learning outcomes	Command of body of information and facts	Command of mode of respectful questioning
Expression of learning goals	In terms of skill and competence	In terms of attitudes and self-reflection
Content	Certain Dichotomous Right or wrong	Acknowledges uncertainty Mostly grey areas Not always right or wrong
Cultural focus	Majority view of other cultures is dominant – majority Whites should consider needs of minorities	No focus on particular groups – all individuals should consider needs of others
Role of experts	Some people are experts in understanding cultural perspectives of certain groups and these often become representatives of communities	No one individual has ownership of expertise regarding others with respect to identification of cultural belonging
Organisation of content	To meet demands of local need	To maximise students' learning
Teaching focus	Groups (treats people as groups); is more service-centred	Individuals (views individuals as potentially parts of different groups in different contexts); more patient-centred
Applicability	Learning can only be used for ethnic issues	Learning can apply to any context in which there are differences between the doctor and patient, be related to culture, gender or education
Patient-centredness	Doctor is the expert	Doctor and patient are active partners in care

After Dogra (2004*a*).

It is now essential that policy has an educational priority and that training programmes are developed on a sound evidence base, undergo effective evaluation and have clearly measurable outcomes. (A current educational fashion is 'reflective learning', but there is often little thought given to how this might be measured.) Some of the issues relating to policies regarding diversity training are highlighted in Box 27.1.

Educational bodies may need to take the lead in directing policies in the healthcare sector.

Box 27.1   Policies relating to diversity training

- Training needs to be educationally led and, where possible, evidence based
- The philosophical stance of policies should be transparent and clear
- Diversity has to be an integral part of all aspects of service delivery and diversity training should improve care for all patients
- Policy must be implemented in a meaningful way that improves outcomes
- There is an urgent need to develop measures that can demonstrate that diversity training affects outcomes in mental health

---

In 2001 the Royal College of Psychiatrists held a 2-day workshop to discuss the training required to produce culturally capable psychiatrists. An article arising from this workshop, describing the knowledge skills and attitudes of a well-trained and culturally competent psychiatrist, has been published by Parimala Moodley, then chair of the College's Transcultural Special Interest Group (Moodley, 2002). The core module for basic psychiatric training now includes the competency that trainees be able to perform specialist assessment of patients and document relevant history and examination on culturally diverse patients. There is also a recognition within the document that cultural issues need to be acknowledged and that they may be relevant in many different contexts (Royal College of Psychiatrists, 2009).

The Sainsbury Centre for Mental Health is attempting to establish an evidence base for diversity training, and it is to be hoped that this will inform future policy. There is also a need to direct teaching away from a superficial checklist approach to medical training and to ensure that it delivers health-care professionals who are able to meet the needs of individual patients and their families. Policies might also be more explicit in indicating that the concept of equality applies to everyone and not just to certain minority groups. This does not, of course, minimise the need to address the issue of race equality, which has already been highlighted as a priority.

How can practitioners make a difference?

There is no doubt that organisations need to take responsibility for ensuring they put systems in place that urgently address diversity. However, individual practitioners need to take personal responsibility for their delivery of care. Box 27.2 highlights some questions that practitioners might ask themselves in order to reflect on their practice. We are not suggesting that current practitioners are not thinking about their patients; rather we are reminding everyone that external pressures and our own vulnerabilities affect the care we deliver.

Box 27.2   Reflecting on your practice

- Think about how you view culture and sense of identity given the frameworks presented
- Justify your position in the context of your professional role
- Reflect on your own practice and evaluate how your own views influence the choices you offer your patients
- How often are you genuinely interested in asking individual patients what they might need?
- How often do you assume that the needs of patients are already known on the basis of their diagnosis, ethnicity, gender or any other factor?
- What three things could you do to change your own practice?

Conclusion

There is a need to investigate the steps to be taken to raise the credibility of cultural diversity as a subject within psychiatry and medicine as a whole and to demonstrate the value of diversity training. This is an area in which the links between undergraduate and postgraduate training could be explored to improve the continuity of medical education. Although there appears to be some consistency between educational models, it is not possible to state which model effectively provides the desired outcomes. Implementing and comparing the outcomes of different models of delivering cultural diversity teaching may also help provide the educational clarity that is needed. Different models might meet different learning objectives and it would be helpful for teachers to know this when they are devising educational programmes. Effective instruments for evaluating the outcomes of cultural diversity teaching are urgently needed. It might be possible to derive them from research in other areas, although measuring changes in attitudes and ways of thinking is fraught with difficulties. However, this should not mean that the problem is avoided.

It is now time to implement and evaluate different educational approaches, so that cultural diversity teaching develops rigour and an evidence base. Unless this is done, it will continue to be a path laid with good intentions but one that ultimately fails to educate healthcare providers to meet patients' individual needs irrespective of their background or sense of identity.

We would argue that the lack of effective leadership and any conceptual clarity in this area may be part of the problem. In the UK we are lacking any clear blueprint and many efforts are still undertaken in the absence of clear policy and strategy. This allows complacency and a false belief that we are making progress when in fact little is changing and the significant costs are being minimised. It seems that people are talking the talk but that there is little happening that has been shown to actually improve healthcare. It would be disappointing to find that 5 years from now the situation is still the same.

References

Anderson, L. M., Scrimshaw, S. C., Fullilove, M. T., et al (2003) Culturally competent healthcare systems: a systematic review. American Journal of Preventative Medicine, 24 (3 suppl.), 68–79.

Beach, M. C., Price, E. G., Gary, T. L., et al (2005) Cultural competence: a systematic review of health care provider educational interventions. Medical Care, 43, 356–373.

Bennett, J., Kalathil, J. & Keating, F. (2007) Race Equality Training in Mental Health Services in England: Does One Size Fit All? Sainsbury Centre for Mental Health.

Bentley, P., Jovanovic, A. & Sharma, P. (2008) Cultural diversity training for UK healthcare professionals: a comprehensive nationwide cross-sectional survey. Clinical Medicine, 8, 493–497.

Bhui, K. (2004) Cultural consultation in psychiatric practice: author's reply. British Journal of Psychiatry, 185, 76–77.

Bhui, K. & Sashidharan, S. P. (2003) Should there be separate psychiatric services for ethnic minority groups? British Journal of Psychiatry, 182, 10–12.

Bhui, K., Warfa, N., Edonya, P., et al (2007) Cultural competence in mental health care: a review of model evaluations. BMC Health Services Research, 7, 15.

Bradby, H. (2003) Describing ethnicity in health research. Ethnicity and Health, 8, 5–13.

Copeman, R. C. (1989) Medical students, Aborigines and migrants: evaluation of a teaching programme. Medical Journal of Australia, 150, 84–87.

Cross, T., Bazron, B., Dennis, K. W., et al (1989) Towards a Culturally Competent System of Care. Georgetown University Child Development Center.

Culhane-Pera, K. A., Reif, C., Egli, E., et al (1997) A curriculum for multicultural education in family medicine. Family Medicine, 29, 719–723.

Deloney, L. A., Graham, C. J. & Erwin, D. O. (2000) Presenting cultural diversity and spirituality to first-year medical students. Academic Medicine, 75, 513–514.

Department of Health (1999) Addressing Black and Minority Ethnic Health in London – A Review and Recommendation. Department of Health.

Department of Health (2003) Delivering Race Equality: A Framework for Action. Department of Health.

DiversityRx (2001a) Essentials. DiversityRx (http://www.diversityrx.org/HTML/ESWEL.htm).

DiversityRx (2001b) Why Language and Culture are Important. DiversityRx (http://www.diversityrx.org/HTML/ESLANG.htm).

Dogra, N. (2001) The development and evaluation of a programme to teach cultural diversity to medical undergraduate students. Medical Education, 35, 232–241.

Dogra, N. (2004a) Cultural competence or cultural sensibility? A comparison of two ideal type models to teach cultural diversity to medical students. International Journal of Medicine, 5, 223–231.

Dogra, N. (2004b) The Learning and Teaching of Cultural Diversity in Undergraduate Medical Education in the UK. PhD thesis. University of Leicester.

Dogra, N. & Karim, K. (2005) Training in diversity for psychiatrists. Advances in Psychiatric Treatment, 11, 159–167.

Dogra, N. & Karnik, N. (2004) A comparison between UK and US medical student attitudes towards cultural diversity. Medical Teacher, 26, 703–708.

Dogra, N., Conning, S., Gill, P. S., et al (2005) Teaching of cultural diversity in medical schools in the United Kingdom and Republic of Ireland: cross sectional questionnaire survey. BMJ, 330, 403–404.

Dogra, N., Betancourt, J., Park, E., *et al* (2009) The relationship between drivers and policy in the implementation of cultural competency training in health care. *Journal of the National Medical Association*, **101**, 127–133.

Dyson, S. & Smaje, C. (2001) The health status of minority ethnic groups. In *Ethnicity and Nursing Practice* (eds L. Culley & S. Dyson), pp. 29–66. Palgrave.

Frosh, S. (1999) Identity. In *The New Fontana Dictionary of Modern Thought* (3rd edn) (eds A. Bullock & S. Trombley). HarperCollins.

Fung, K., Andermann, L., Zaretsky, A., *et al* (2008) An integrative approach to cultural competence in the psychiatric curriculum. *Academic Psychiatry*, **32**, 272–282.

Healthcare Commission (2007) *Audit of Equalities Publications 2007*. Healthcare Commission (http://www.cqc.org.uk/publications.cfm?fde_id=110).

Healthcare Commission (2009) *Tackling the Challenge: Promoting Race Equality in the NHS in England*. Healthcare Commission (http://www.cqc.org.uk/publications.cfm?fde_id=11972).

Henry J. Kaiser Family Foundation (2003) *Compendium of Cultural Competence Initiatives in Health Care*. Henry J. Kaiser Family Foundation.

Hope, R. (2004) *The Ten Essential Shared Capabilities: A Framework for the Whole of the Mental Health Workforce*. Department of Health.

Levinson, W., Roter, D. L., Mullooly, J. P., *et al* (1997) Physician–patient communication. The relationship with malpractice claims among primary care physicians and surgeons. *JAMA*, **277**, 553–559.

Lim, R. F., Luo, J. S., Suo, S., *et al* (2008) Diversity initiatives in academic psychiatry: applying cultural competence. *Academic Psychiatry*, **32**, 283–290.

Loudon, R., Ross, N., Gill, P., *et al* (2001) *Making Medical Education Responsive to Community Diversity. Report Prepared by the Department of Primary Care and General Practice and Medical Education Unit*. University of Birmingham.

Majumdar, B., Keystone, J. S. & Cuttress, A. (1999) Cultural sensitivity training among foreign medical graduates. *Medical Education*, **33**, 177–184.

Mao, C., Bullock, C. S., Harway, E. C., *et al* (1988) A workshop on ethnic and cultural awareness for second year medical students. *Academic Medicine*, **63**, 624–628.

Moodley, P. (2002) Building a culturally capable workforce – an educational approach to delivering equitable mental health services. *Psychiatric Bulletin*, **26**, 63–65.

National Institute for Mental Health in England (2003) *Inside Outside: Improving Mental Health Services for Black and Minority Ethnic Groups in England*. Department of Health.

Robertson, D., Sathyamoorthy, G. & Ford, R. (2000) Asking the right questions. *Community Care*, 15 May, 24–25.

Royal College of Psychiatrists (2009) *A Competency Based Curriculum for Specialist Training in Psychiatry: Core Module*. Royal College of Psychiatrists.

Rubenstein, H. L., Bonnie, J. D., O'Connor, B., *et al* (1992) Introducing students to the role of folk and popular health belief systems in patient care. *Academic Medicine*, **67**, 566–568.

Sainsbury Centre for Mental Health (2002) *Breaking the Circles of Fear: A Review of the Relationship between Mental Health Services and African and Caribbean Communities*. Sainsbury Centre for Mental Health.

Secker, J. & Harding, C. (2002) African and African Caribbean users' perceptions of inpatient services. *Journal of Psychiatric and Mental Health Nursing*, **9**, 161–167.

Sifri, R. R., Glaser, K. & Witt, D. K. (2001) Addressing prejudice in medicine during a third-year family medicine clerkship. *Academic Medicine*, **76**, 508.

Task Force on Spirituality, Cultural Issues, and End of Life Care (1999) Task Force report: spirituality, cultural issues and end of life care. In *Report III: Contemporary Issues in Medicine. Communication in Medicine* (eds Association of American Medical Colleges), pp. 26–31. Association of American Medical Colleges.

Thom, D. H., Tiardo, M. D., Woon, L., *et al* (2006) Development and evaluation of a cultural competency training curriculum. *BMC Medical Education*, **6**, 38.

Thompson, D. (ed.) (1995) *The Concise Oxford Dictionary of Current English*. Clarendon Press.

Toynbee, P. (2002) Between aspiration and reality. *BMJ*, **325**, 716.

Webb, E. & Sergison, M. (2003) Evaluation of cultural competence and antiracism training in health services. *Archives of Diseases in Childhood*, **88**, 291–294.

Whitley, R., Kirmayer, L. J. & Jarvis, G. E. (2004) Cultural consultation in psychiatric practice (letter). *British Journal of Psychiatry*, **185**, 76–77.

Williams, C. (1997) Personal reflections on permanency planning and cultural competency. *Journal of Multicultural Social Work*, **5**, 9–18.

CHAPTER 28

Informing progress towards race equality in mental healthcare: is routine data collection adequate?

Peter J. Aspinall

Summary   Collection of ethnicity data in mental health services has long been regarded as unsatisfactory. The Department of Health's 5-year action plan Delivering Race Equality in Mental Health Care seeks to improve this key building block by setting out actions to improve both the quality of information and its analysis and dissemination. However, actions that are tangible and specific are few. The opportunity to improve the quality and coverage of key routine data-sets has not been seized. Moreover, the plan does not mention proposed changes in civil registration (births and deaths) and the coroner service and their potential benefit. This chapter looks at what has been achieved since the 5-year action plan was published and takes stock of progress in this, its fifth and final year. The continuing gaps in the information base justify a stronger emphasis on the processes necessary to bring about change rather than on what ethnic monitoring should provide.

It has long been recognised that the quality, completeness and comprehensiveness of the ethnicity data collected in mental health services are inadequate. This is acknowledged in *Delivering Race Equality in Mental Health Care* (Department of Health, 2005a), which lays out the Department's 5-year action plan for achieving race equality and tackling discrimination in mental health services in England for people in minority ethnic groups. Moreover, this plan for reform – together with the government's formal response to the independent inquiry into the death of David Bennett, which appears in the same document – offers a programme for achieving equality of access, experiences and outcomes for service users from these groups.

A crucial element of this programme and one of its three building blocks is 'better information', including improvements in the monitoring of ethnicity and its analysis and dissemination. The preceding race equality consultation document, dubbed the Framework for Action (Department of Health, 2003a), had invoked practitioners 'to look for outliers' – although not specifying the required tools, such as funnel plots (Spiegelhalter, 2002) and Shewart charts (Mohammed *et al*, 2001), to do so. Among the responses to the 2003 Framework for Action were the criticisms that there were no clear targets, the processes necessary to bring about change were not adequately described, and there was little in the way of direct cross-referencing and building from one policy document to another (Department of Health, 2005a). In this chapter I attempt to assess how successfully the Delivering Race Equality action plan addressed the provision of an information base and analytical resources necessary for the implementation of the programme and evaluate the progress made since its publication.

History of ethnic data collection in the NHS

Over the past two or three decades much of the information collected in the National Health Service (NHS) has not included ethnic group. Where ethnic monitoring has been introduced it has frequently been patchy, resulting in very poor-quality data, including low rates of completeness. On only a few data-sets has a more systematic process of ethnicity data collection been attempted, notably the mandatory recording of ethnic group for hospital in-patients from the mid-1990s and data on the ethnic origin of the NHS non-medical workforce from 1998 and medical workforce from 1991. Nevertheless, until recently, collected information on ethnicity has not commonly been used because of its poor quality.

However, race equality as a matter of governance has gained prominence in the past few years through new legislation requiring public authorities to identify and tackle institutional racism. The Department of Health has adopted mainstreaming as a fundamental principle of its race and equal opportunities work, defining this as a means of automatically considering the race equality dimension of everything that is done. This agenda has resulted in the development of the Race Equality Action Plan for the NHS and an enhanced programme of ethnic-group data collection. The need to monitor the impact of policies and services has also resulted in an improvement in the completeness of existing ethnic-group data collections. In Delivering Race Equality, the Department has indicated that its programme of work will be located within these wider processes of clinical governance, performance management and equal opportunities monitoring.

Statutory/governmental race equality requirements

The main stimulus to instituting and improving ethnic-group data collection, the Race Relations (Amendment) Act 2000, gives public authorities a new statutory duty to promote race equality. This encompasses a general duty to eliminate unlawful racial discrimination and promote equality of opportunity and good race relations. Further, the Act places specific duties on many public (including health) authorities, including the preparation of a race equality scheme and the monitoring of workforce characteristics

Box 28.1   Race equality schemes and ethnicity monitoring

An organisation's race equality scheme should:

- assess whether its functions and policies are relevant to race equality
- monitor its policies to see how they affect race equality
- assess and consult on new policies
- publish the results of these consultations, monitoring and assessments
- ensure that the public has access to the information and services it provides

All public authorities are bound by the duty of employment to monitor by ethnic group their existing staff and job applicants, promotion and training and to publish the results annually.

(Box 28.1). They are therefore required to consider race equality in routine policy-making, service delivery and employment practice and be knowledgeable with respect to how their policies and services affect race equality. Clearly, ethnic monitoring data will be required across all service delivery and other policy areas to demonstrate that the general and specific duties to eliminate unlawful racial discrimination and promote equality of opportunity and good race relations have been met.

The importance of these requirements has been underpinned by the NHS in the Race Equality Action Plan. Its principal aims (listed in Box 28.2) are encompassed in ten specific actions to be delivered that will require monitoring and will be reviewed by an independent expert panel.

Box 28.2   The Race Equality Action Plan

'The NHS and Department of Health must give even greater prominence to race equality as part of our drive to improve health. We must:

- pay greater attention to meeting the service needs of people from ethnic minorities. This will help us to meet the standards both for improved services and health outcomes in the long term and to hit our short term targets
- make race an important dimension of our strategy for the next five years through more focus on helping people with chronic diseases – where morbidity is high amongst people from black and minority ethnic backgrounds – and on health inequalities – where ethnic minority communities are often disadvantaged
- target recruitment and development opportunities at people from different ethnic groups whose skills are often underused. This will assist our drive to recruit more staff, increase our skill base and introduce new working patterns'

(Department of Health, 2004*a*)

Other policy initiatives driving the need for collection of ethnicity data in mental health services include the Department of Health's care standards and planning framework *National Standards, Local Action* (Department of Health, 2004*b*), the National Suicide Prevention Strategy (Department of Health, 2002) and the commitment to equality of access and provision of non-discriminatory services in the National Service Framework for Mental Health and the NHS Plan (Department of Health, 1999*a*, 2000).

Following the publication of guidance on ethnicity data collection (Department of Health, 2007*a*), the main recommendation of the Equalities Review Panel's report of 2007 was that the collection and coordination of equality data be improved. This prompted the Department of Health to establish an Equality Monitoring Group, chaired by the Department's Permanent Secretary. In the same year, the Department of Health (2007*b*: p. 28) could report: 'Patients admitted to hospital are monitored by ethnicity. General practices are required to collect ethnicity data for new patients ... In addition, DH [the Department of Health] is currently looking at how data collection may be improved, for example by ensuring that birth and death registration records ethnicity'.

What has been recommended?

In the years leading up to Delivering Race Equality, improvements in the ethnicity data collected by mental health services – including the Department of Health's Hospital Episode Statistics data-set on hospital in-patients and the data collected by providers of primary care, specialist mental health services and social care – had been recommended by a suite of policy documents (Table 28.1) (Department of Health, 2003*a*, 2005*a*; Patel *et al*, 2003; Sashidharan, 2003). More specifically, mention had been made of: consultation rates; referral rates; hospital admission rates; pathways into care; compulsory admissions, detained patients, Mental Health Act orders, applications to review tribunals, and requests for 'second opinion appointed doctors' (SOADs); diagnosis; treatment regimes, including physical intervention, talking therapies, medication, and use of restraint and seclusion; self-harm and suicide; complaints; violent and racial harassment incidents and deaths of psychiatric in-patients; and workforce monitoring. The range of data to be collected had included information relating to patients (such as ethnic group, spoken language and dialect, and religion) and to where their data are recorded (for example, information systems, patients' record or notes, care plans and assessments).

By any measure this is an ambitious set. In 2006, I assessed how much of this information would be available through current and planned ethnically coded routine data collections (Aspinall, 2006). In the remainder of this chapter, I look at how successfully routine data collections in mental health services have met statutory and governmental race equality requirements as the action plan launched in January 2005 has completed its final year.

Table 28.1 Published recommendations for improving the collection of ethnicity data and related commitments in Delivering Race Equality

Published recommendations	Delivering Race Equality
Ethnic coding on Hospital Episode Statistics (HES) should be improved, using the mental health performance rating indicators, which include an indicator on quality of HES data.[a] Collection of other relevant data – religion, language	No specific information (religion and language included in 2005–2009 Count Me In censuses)
Information about beliefs and practices should be recorded in patient notes[a]	No specific information
To inform planning and commissioning, better-quality ethnic data must be comprehensively collected by providers of primary care, specialist mental health services and social care[a]	No specific information
Black and minority ethnic groups should have greater access to talking therapies (this requires ethnic monitoring to assess outcomes)[a]	No specific information
To inform decisions about appropriate treatment/ services, ethnicity information should be mapped throughout care pathways (primary care, early intervention and assertive outreach teams, crisis services, in-patient care, etc.)[a]	No specific information
The ethnicity, language/dialect and religion of detained patients (hospital in-patients) should be recorded, to inform monitoring of treatment, complaints, use of therapies and activities, violent and racial harassment incidents, self-harm, deaths, use of Mental Health Act, compulsory admissions, seclusion, care and restraint, applications to and outcomes of mental health review tribunals, requests for Mental Health Act Commissioner visits and for second opinion appointed doctors[b]	2005 and subsequent Count Me In censuses include legal status on admission and on the census day, care programme approach level, source of referral, consent status, recorded injury, patient in seclusion, and control and restraint
Services should be staffed by people who represent the community they serve[a] (requiring workforce monitoring)	No information
Every care plan should include details of the patient's ethnic origin and cultural needs[c]	Guidance but not mandatory
The Department of Health should collate and publish annual statistics that include ethnicity on all deaths of psychiatric in-patients[c]	Accepted in principle
Ethnic data on suicide in vulnerable groups are required, to help service planning and delivery: UK death certificates do not currently record ethnicity data and ethnicity is not included in verdicts of coroners' inquests[d,e]	The Department is working towards collecting information on ethnicity by coroners[a]

a. Department of Health (2003a)
b. Patel et al (2003).
c. Norfolk, Suffolk and Cambridgeshire Strategic Health Authority (2003).
d. Sashidharan (2003).
e. Note that the Coroners and Justice Act 2009 did not address the collection of information on ethnicity by coroners.

Equity of access to care

The 2003 Framework for Action accorded particular attention to the provision of equity of access to care and current problems in achieving such access, in response to concerns set out in the preceding consultations. For people from Black and minority ethnic groups these included lower general practitioner (GP) involvement in their care, long delays before they sought a GP's help, higher rates of voluntary admission to hospital, increased risk of compulsory admission, longer stays in hospital and higher readmission rates. The document also noted the urgent need for ethnicity data to be recorded and used to investigate these patterns.

Primary care

The majority of patients with psychiatric disorders – around 90% – are treated in primary care (Goldberg & Huxley, 1992), only a small minority being referred to specialist psychiatric services. Moreover, a significant proportion of routine general practice consultations – estimated at one-quarter (Goldberg & Bridges, 1987) – are for mental health problems. However, there is a dearth of ethnically coded data on patients attending general practices. Ethnic-group data collection is required only for newly registering patients, and the data for existing patients are, in general, sporadic in coverage and of poor quality. Even in London, where targets were set for completeness, recent reviews suggest that primary care trusts are facing considerable challenges in the collection of ethnicity data (North Central London Strategic Health Authority, 2004; Kumarapeli *et al*, 2006). The lack of information on ethnic differences in GP consultation rates for psychiatric disorders is notable. One of the few such studies (Shah *et al*, 2001) used data from the 1991–1992 Fourth National Survey of Morbidity in General Practice. Only 6% of all consultations were for psychiatric disorders, possibly because relatively few inner-city practices participated. The absence of mandatory ethnic data collection for all patients was reflected in primary care databases that derive their data from volunteer practices but is now improving (Box 28.3).

A limited attempt to improve ethnicity recording in general practices has been made under the GP Quality and Outcomes Framework (QOF), in which GPs are rewarded with 1 point if they record the ethnic origin of all new registrants (British Medical Association & NHS Employers, 2006). In England as a whole, 5246 points were achieved for this indicator in 2008–2009, 63.8% of the total points available (as there are 8229 practices). Thus, almost two-thirds of practices achieved 100% ethnic coding for new patient registrations (Health and Social Care Information Centre, 2009). This was substantially the poorest of the 12 QOF 'records' indicators and of all 36 indicators in the 'organisational' domain. Moreover, new registrations may represent only a small proportion of the stock of registered patients at any one time: there is currently no systematic or central reporting of ethnicity recording for all registered patients.

Box 28.3 Primary care databases

The following are the four main UK general practice databases, together covering around 17% of UK general practices:

- The General Practice Research Database (GPRD): ethnically coded (www. gprd.com/home/)
- QRESEARCH: ethnically coded (www.qresearch.org/default.aspx)
- The Health Improvement Network (THIN): not populated with self-ascribed ethnic group (www.thin-uk.com/)
- Doctors Independent Network (DIN): ethnically coded (www.dinweb/about. asp)

See also:

- The Lambeth Datanet Project: ethnically coded (www.raceforhealth.org/ resources/cases_studies/Lambeth/data_collection_to_make_Service- modifications)

Source: Academy of Medical Sciences (2009)

However, a step in this direction has been taken through a new provision for 'directly enhanced services' in England and Scotland. These special services or activities provided by GP practices are negotiated nationally. Practices can choose whether or not to offer such services and they receive payment for any they do provide. Practices are to be rewarded for recording the ethnicity and first language of all patients on their practice list (Scottish Government, 2008; Department of Health, 2009) and not just new registrants. The stated purpose of this recording scheme is to assist contractors, primary care trusts and health boards in assessing the needs of registered patients and in addressing any inequalities in accessing health services and in health outcomes.

The recommendations of a review group convened to investigate why patients from Black and minority ethnic (BME) groups find it more difficult to access GP services than White populations may result in more comprehensive data collection (Lakhani, 2008). They include a recommendation that practices 'collect data as indicated in the national minimum ethnicity dataset' (p. 7) and that the Department of Health 'promote ethnicity data monitoring in primary care and measure progress towards achieving equality' (p. 27). The group argues that: 'The DH should therefore lead development of a minimum national dataset covering ethnicity and first language. The data could be collected locally by primary care trusts and practices who would be able to use it when commissioning services' (p. 27). The Healthcare Commission (now subsumed within the Care Quality Commission) has also recommended that 'collection of ethnicity data about patients should be extended to primary care'

(Healthcare Commission *et al*, 2008: p. 9). Until this happens, the Hospital Episode Statistics data-set could be exploited to monitor GP referrals by ethnic origin (Raleigh, 2008), but there is little current evidence of such use.

Against a suggested standard that variations in primary care consultation rates, referrals to specialist mental health services and use of psychotropic drugs for mental health problems be audited annually by ethnic group (Sashidharan, 2003), Delivering Race Equality recommends only that mental health services should record users' ethnicity, religion and language, offering no specific targets for primary care. This omission is serious, given the primary-care-led nature of the NHS, the commissioning role of primary care trusts and the potential for ethnicity data to link to data on morbidity and prescribing practices. Incentivising the collection of ethnicity data by general practices through the QOF has yielded some results, yet, as mentioned above, less than two-thirds of practices are collecting complete ethnicity information for new registrations (Health and Social Care Information Centre, 2009). Comprehensive recording of ethnicity in primary care awaits further developments, although the new provision under directed enhanced services (Department of Health, 2009) that incentivises practices to record the ethnicity and first language of all their patients may yield results.

Acute in-patient care

Much of the research on ethnic differences in the use of psychiatric services has been carried out in secondary care. Data have been collected on admissions to psychiatric in-patient units since the late 1940s, first as the Mental Health Enquiry, then, following the Korner review in the 1980s, as part of Hospital Episode Statistics (Glover, 2003). The data are available from 1974 to the present day in computerised form, with a break for the years 1987–1990. The advantage of these sources is that coverage is comprehensive, the accumulated number of cases is very large and the data-set has substantial breadth of coverage. However, the availability of ethnically coded data is more limited.

The Mental Health Enquiry data contained information on patients' country of birth (rather than ethnic group) and this was used in a number of studies of patterns of mental illness in immigrants (Cochrane, 1977; Dean *et al*, 1981; Glover, 1987, 1989*a*,*b*; Cochrane & Bal, 1988). Ethnic group was not added to Hospital Episode Statistics until 1 April 1995, such collection now commencing its 16th year. A major drawback from an analytical point of view has been the high proportion of records without a valid ethnic code. In the Hospital Episode Statistics data year 2002–2003, in the 79 primary care and hospital mental health trusts providing in-patient mental healthcare (as defined by the Healthcare Commission), only 61.2% of records (166 822/272 626) had valid ethnic coding, compared with 64.0% (7 609 340/11 877 506) in all the other 324 primary care and hospital NHS trusts (Department of Health, 2005b). However, an analysis by main specialty (learning (intellectual) disability; adult mental illness; child and adolescent psychiatry; forensic psychiatry; psychotherapy; old age psychiatry) shows that, along with nursing, the mental health and illness specialties had the lowest proportion of records with missing ethnic codes (Fitzgerald, 2004).

More recent data show a considerable improvement. Valid coding in the Hospital Episode Statistics had increased from 64% in 2002–2003 to almost 80% in 2004–2005. In 2006–2007, Hospital Episode Statistics admissions specifically for mental health specialties in England numbered 156 999, of which 1.1% (1707) had ethnic group 'not stated' and 4.3% (6674) ethnic group 'invalid' (Healthcare Commission et al, 2008). The Healthcare Commission, and its predecessor the Commission for Health Improvement, has included indicators on ethnicity coding levels in its annual performance assessments of NHS organisations since 2003. This practice is being continued by the Care Quality Commission, the 2008–2009 Annual Health Check including indicators of valid ethnic coding on both Hospital Episode Statistics and the Mental Health Minimum Data Set (MHMDS). It has undoubtedly made a significant contribution to the substantial improvement in coding over recent years.

Some drawbacks remain: notably, the Hospital Episode Statistics do not cover independent-sector providers (and there is no contractual requirement for them to submit these data for their NHS-funded patients). This is important as the proportion of in-patients in independent hospitals has increased steadily during the period 2005–2008, from 10% to 14%. In 2008 it was recommended that submission of Hospital Episode Statistics be made mandatory for all independent providers of in-patient mental health services (Healthcare Commission et al, 2008), a recommendation repeated in the report on the 2009 Count Me In Census.

Relatively little use has been made of ethnically coded Hospital Episode Statistics to investigate hospital in-patient admissions for psychiatric disorders. Bardsley et al (2000) reported proportional admission ratios by ethnic group for the diagnoses of mental/behavioural disorders in Greater London, 1997–1998, showing statistically significant higher ratios for Black Caribbean, Black African and Black Other patients and lower ratios for Indians and Pakistanis. More recent analyses of psychiatric disorders by ethnic group using Hospital Episode Statistics have been prepared by the London Health Observatory (de Ponte & Jacobson, 2007). A very large number of research studies in this setting have generated customised data on the use of mental health services. A strong focus on improving the quality of Hospital Episode Statistics data, through performance indicators in the Care Quality Commission's Annual Health Check, has now produced data that are sufficiently complete to be useful for analytical purposes. The potential utility of the data is substantial and includes the Psychiatric Census, a set of Hospital Episode Statistics records relating to patients who were in hospitals and units for people with a mental illness or learning (intellectual) disability at midnight on the 31 March, which contains additional information useful in analysing the treatment of psychiatric (especially long-term) patients. In addition, the mental category of detained patients is classified using the designations in the Mental Health Act 1983.

Although Hospital Episode Statistics do not provide details of drugs used in hospitals, they are a potential source of data on electroconvulsive therapy (ECT). Unfortunately, there is evidence of substantial under-recording: finished consultant episodes recorded in the Hospital Episode Statistics for 2002 represented only 57% of the Department of Health's survey figure for NHS in-patients treated in that year. Further drawbacks to the utilisation of Hospital Episode Statistics data include the low (but improving) rates of ethnicity coding, the exclusion of the private sector (included in the Department of Health surveys) and the fact that 19% of ECT administrations in the NHS in 2002 were in out-patient settings (Department of Health, 2003b). The ethnic spread of patients receiving ECT in these surveys was broadly similar to the ethnic spread seen in the general population. Clearly, there is substantial scope to improve the quality of the recording of ECT administration in the Hospital Episode Statistics database. The data-set also contains detailed information on diagnosis, admission source, length of hospital stay and discharge destination. Probability algorithms based on critical fields can be used to measure readmission rates. Delivering Race Equality makes no specific recommendations for the Hospital Episode Statistics data-set.

Community services

Specialist community mental health services have expanded following implementation of the National Service Framework for Mental Health but ethnic-group data collection remains poor. A joint review (Commission for Social Care Inspection & Healthcare Commission, 2007) found that 'recording of ethnicity was often lax, and therefore services were not planned'. Although ethnic monitoring of NHS hospital in-patients became mandatory in April 1995, only recently has it been extended to patients in community settings. Collection of ethnic-category information for patients attending accident and emergency and out-patient departments has been mandatory since April 2009 (Information Standards Board for Health and Social Care, 2008). In 2004–2005, only 16.8% of out-patient attendance records had valid and usable ethnicity codes (Dawson, 2006); more recent data are unavailable as provision of ethnic category data is not required for national reporting purposes. The 'standard' contracts for commissioners introduced by the Department of Health include uniform information requirements across both NHS and (NHS-funded) independent healthcare.

The Mental Health Act Commission (2008: p. 138) has stated that it 'will consider ethnic monitoring of all patients subject to formal coercive powers to be an absolute minimum requirement in terms of compliance both with the Race Relations (Amendment) Act 2000 and with general good practice for hospital boards'. It has recommended that ethnic monitoring of patients subject to community treatment orders under the 2007 amendments to the Mental Health Act 1983 should be an explicit mandatory requirement. The Healthcare Commission also recommended that the NHS Information Centre regularly publish data on all supervised community treatment orders under the Mental Health Act in England (both NHS and independent healthcare providers) by the ethnicity of patients (Healthcare Commission *et al*, 2008). However, although the Information Centre has published details of patients subject to supervised community treatment for 1998–99 to 2008–09 through the KP90 aggregate return (Information Centre, 2009), ethnicity is excluded. There are only two sources of published data available on supervised community treatment orders by ethnic group. That published by the Mental Health Act Commission (Mental Health Act Commission, 2009) comprises data from the Count Me In census of patients detained on 31 March 2008 under Section 3 of the Mental health Act (who make up the largest part by far of persons eligible to be placed on supervised community treatment) and requests for second opinion appointed doctor visits to supervised community treatment order patients from the Mental Health Act Commission's own data. The 2009 Mental Health Bulletin also includes for the first time some experimental analysis about supervised community treatment orders by ethnic group from the 2008–2009 MHMDS, although only about half of eligible trusts returned information about supervised community treatment in this first year of the collection (NHS Information Centre, 2009*b*).

Pathways into care

The 2003 Framework for Action looked in detail at this specialist area as one of specific concern for the delivery of race equality. The evidence set out in the consultation document *Inside Outside* (Sashidharan, 2003) and other research showed that people from Black and minority ethnic groups were more likely to experience an aversive pathway into mental health services, with higher rates of compulsory admission to hospital, greater involvement of the legal system and forensic psychiatrists, and higher rates of transfer to medium and high secure facilities. Moreover, such research also indicated lower effectiveness of hospital treatment for these groups, less likelihood that social care and psychological needs would be addressed within care planning and treatment processes, more severe and coercive treatments and lower access to talking treatments. Among the required actions identified by Sashidharan was the mapping of ethnic information throughout care pathways to inform decisions about appropriate treatment and services.

Aversive pathways into specialist mental health services

Only limited ethnicity data are available for monitoring pathways into and out of care. Hospital Episode Statistics provide a potential source on compulsory admissions, although poor ethnic coding limits its usefulness. In addition, data on the ethnicity of detained patients have been monitored in the Mental Health Act offices since 1 April 2002. By the end of 2003 the Mental Health Act Commission had concluded that mental healthcare commissioners must pay more attention to collecting ethnicity data on care pathways, with checks run by chairpersons of commissioner visiting teams and team managers and guidance given to commissioners when completing the form (Mental Health Act Commission, 2003). One difficulty has been the high percentage of 'ethnicity not known' cases: 6.7% (2102/31528) in 1996–1997, 4.3% (1505/35057) in 1997–1998, 3.3% (1204/36301) in 1998–1999 and 11.2% (5029/45053) in 1999–2000 (Mental Health Act Commission, 2001).

More recent returns from Mental Health Act Commission questionnaires continue to show incomplete responses but indicate some improvement over the past few years, with ethnicity 'not stated' for 6.7% of admissions under the Mental Health Act in 2003–2004, 7.3% in 2004–2005, 5.9% in 2005–2006 and 3.2% in 2006–2007 (Mental Health Act Commission, 2008). The quality of ethnicity data for restricted patients may improve under an initiative of the Ministry of Justice's Mental Health Unit, although a written request to hospitals had yielded data on only three-quarters of this patient population by 2007 (Ministry of Justice, 2007). The Ministry of Justice plans to publish these and more recent data in the future. Better quality data are available from the Count Me In censuses (discussed on pp. 388–389), but they provide only a snapshot of services on the census day. In their latest report (Mental Health Act Commission, 2009), the Commission cites ethnicity data for patients detained in hospital at 31 March 2008 from this source: only 1.1% of 16152 patients having ethnicity not stated/recorded. As for supervised community treatment orders, the Healthcare Commission recommended that the NHS Information Centre regularly publishes data on all detentions under the Mental Health Act in England (both NHS and independent healthcare providers) by the ethnicity of patients (Healthcare Commission et al, 2008): as noted, the Information Centre's published data in the KP90 annual returns excludes ethnicity.

The Mental Health Act Commission (2001) also highlighted the high proportion of Black and minority ethnic patients seeing a second opinion appointed doctor (28.3%) and requesting commissioner support (31.0%). Middleton (2002) analysed the sociodemographic characteristics of some 20000 detained patients who received second opinion visits administered by the Mental Health Act Commission between July 1995 and February 1997 and reported that individuals from minority ethnic groups were over-represented among younger patients compared with population-based statistics. The National Institute for Mental Health in England, the Care

Services Improvement Partnership and the Mental Health Act Commission have all recommended ethnic monitoring of mental health review tribunal appeals and their outcomes. The Mental Health Act Commission (2008) recently added that this should include all applications (including those that are withdrawn or where the patient is discharged before the hearing) and should identify the Mental Health Act section under which patients are detained. The Mental Health Act Commission has again recommended the publication of this data in its 13th biennial report for 2007–09.

Treatments

The ways in which aversive care pathways influence the nature of treatment and its outcome highlighted in the 2003 Framework for Action are poorly documented. However, other sources suggest, for example, that Black and minority ethnic groups are over-represented in the receipt of ECT (Alexander, 1999) and are more likely to be given 'physical' treatments (drugs and ECT) than their White counterparts (Mind, 2002). How ethnic monitoring can be applied to the use of such treatments is unclear.

Medication

There are no routinely collected ethnically coded data on prescribing that enable the quality of in-patient prescribing for psychiatric patients to be monitored (Paton & Lelliott, 2004). National Health Service prescription charts are not standardised, each NHS trust using its own individual prescribing system (Barber et al, 2003), and ethnicity tends to be recorded in medical case notes rather than on these charts. The need for this information has been raised by concerns over inappropriate and excessive administration of medication to individuals detained under the Mental Health Act (African and African–Caribbean patients are at increased risk), sometimes without adequate medical authorisation and contrary to guidelines in the British National Formulary (BNF). Mind's written evidence to the Joint Committee on Human Rights expresses particular concern about the simultaneous prescription of several different drugs (polypharmacy) at high doses and the higher doses of medication administered to African–Caribbean men, describing 'a clear pattern of African Caribbean male patients in secure psychiatric settings who have died having been given emergency sedative medication which exceeded BNF levels or due to polypharmacy' (House of Lords & House of Commons, 2004: para. 187).

Expert evidence to the inquiry into the death of David Bennett raised similar concerns about the over-medication of Black patients (Norfolk, Suffolk & Cambridgeshire Strategic Health Authority, 2003). The Joint Committee on Human Rights argued that such administration to patients from some minority ethnic groups 'remains statistically unproven', but if established, would be discriminatory and in breach of the European Convention on Human Rights unless the difference is objectively justified in regard to the needs of the patient. It recommended that health authorities monitor prescription of medication to detained patients 'having regard to ethnicity' and take steps to address any discrepancies found.

The evidence base on this matter is limited, much of it being based on US studies. The Royal College of Psychiatrists' consensus statement on high-dose antipsychotic medication reported that there is evidence that African and African–Caribbean patients 'may be prescribed higher doses of antipsychotics and more often receive depot preparations and conventional antipsychotics than second-generation antipsychotics' (Royal College of Psychiatrists, 2006: p. 18). A 1-day census involving 3576 psychiatric in-patients prescribed antipsychotic medication (nearly half of whom were detained under the Mental Health Act) revealed that the effect of ethnicity was not significant for polypharmacy or the prescription of high-dose (exceeding BNF limits) medication (Lelliott et al, 2002). In an investigation of the prescribing of two widely used atypical antipsychotics, clozapine and olanzapine, Taylor (2004) found that for clozapine the dosage and extent of antipsychotic co-prescription did not differ significantly between ethnic groups; for olanzapine, however, co-prescription was significantly more common in Black (33%) than in White in-patients (20%; $P = 0.023$). In these studies, ethnicity was not recorded on about 10% of the prescription charts. A more recent study involving 153 patients – 60% of whom were detained – at the Maudsley, Bethlem and Lambeth hospitals in London found no statistical differences in the dose, type or number of antipsychotics prescribed for Black and for White patients (Connolly et al, 2007).

In its review of NHS acute in-patient mental health services, the Healthcare Commission (2008) found no significant differences between White British patients and patients from Black and minority ethnic groups in relation to medication prescribed above BNF limits during their first week in hospital. The Mental Health Act Commission similarly found little evidence of disproportionate use of medication at supra-BNF levels within the Black detained population compared with the detained population as a whole (Mental Health Act Commission, 2008). Black patients for whom second opinion appointed doctors had been requested were not statistically more likely to be prescribed supra-BNF levels of medication than patients in the White British group, although Black patients account for a relatively high proportion of requests for second opinion authorisation for medication to be given without the patient's consent.

Psychological therapies

It is often claimed that people from Black and minority ethnic communities are much less likely to be referred for psychological therapies, although there are few published studies and the quality of evidence is not high (McKenzie et al, 1995; Bhugra & Bahl, 1999). In an inner-London study, Lawson & Guite (2005) reported that only 15% of the clients of the primary care counselling service were from Black and minority ethnic groups, compared with 23% of the population, although 47% of clients of private sector and 40% of clients of voluntary sector providers of psychological therapies were from such groups. There is a lack of data on such therapies in key routine data-sets such as the Hospital Episode Statistics and the Count Me In censuses, and most of our knowledge is based on research samples. The Healthcare Commission's NHS patient surveys of community mental health services, which are being continued by the Care Quality Commission, ask about medication and talking therapies in the previous year (and whether the respondent wanted a talking therapy), but the low response rate for minority ethnic groups (Raleigh et al, 2007) and the consequent small number of responses for some of these groups is a limitation. A community mental health survey for 2006–2007 found service users in the White Other and Black/Black British groups were less likely than those in the White British group to say that they received talking therapies if they wanted them (Department of Health & Healthcare Commission, 2008).

This continues to be an information gap. For example, the Care Services Improvement Partnership (CSIP) stated in the consultation for the NHS Information Centre's Mental Health Information Review that 'data relating to psychological therapies should be broken down according to ethnic origin and level of therapy' and that 'inclusion of prescription information would also provide a better picture of treatment provided' (NHS Information Centre, 2008a: p. 12). However, it is being addressed by a new data-set: the Improving Access to Psychological Therapies (IAPT) Data Set. Currently being developed for implementation in 2011, ethnicity will be mandatory for the IAPT Minimum Data Set and optional for the Full Data Set (but recommended as good practice) (Improving Access to Psychological Therapies Team, 2008).

Delivering Race Equality does not robustly endorse ethnic monitoring with respect to these treatment modalities, indicating only that 'commissioners and service providers should consider whether it would help local service development to monitor ethnicity in relation to specific aspects of service treatment and care, for example: use of different categories of medication – novel antipsychotics, high dose prescribing, etc.; ... take-up of psychological therapies' (Department of Health, 2005a: p. 66). No guidance is offered on mechanisms for ethnic monitoring or the appropriate point(s) in the care pathway at which it should be carried out. Such advice does not accord with the earlier recommendation that: 'organisations should have information capable of being analysed by ethnicity on ... the use of seclusion, physical interventions and medication' (p. 45).

The patient's experience

Delivering Race Equality's 5-year action plan identifies increased satisfaction with services as one criterion for assessing success by 2010. This would be measured in terms of reduced fear of mental healthcare and services among people from Black and minority ethnic communities and a service deemed by them to be more responsive to their values. The main source of information on patient experience is the Healthcare Commission's annual national NHS patient surveys on users of mental health services in the community (services that provide care to people in psychiatric outpatient clinics or through a local community mental health team). This programme was started in 2004 by the Healthcare Commission and has run for 5 consecutive years (2004–2008), with a further survey in the field in 2009/10, although the number of respondents has fallen from 26 197 (2004) to 13 699 (2008). Each year, about 3% of respondents have been Asian or Asian British, 2–3% Black or Black British, and 2% Chinese, Mixed or Other ethnic group. The 2004 survey (Healthcare Commission, 2004) elicited an overall response rate of only 42% (27 398/65 899); 44% of White patients responded but far fewer in the minority ethnic groups (30% for the Asian or Asian British group; 33% for the Black or Black British; and 38% for the Mixed, Chinese or Other group). Of those who returned a completed questionnaire, 93% were White, 3% Asian or Asian British, 2% Black or Black British, and 2% either mixed race or from Chinese and other ethnic groups. Ethnic group was missing on 2.8% of responses. The low response rate in the 2004 survey, especially among minority ethnic groups, reduces the utility of the data, although questions are included on medication and talking therapies (Raleigh et al, 2007).

Electroconvulsive therapy

There is one other area that merits investigation: the use of ECT. The central reporting of information on ECT was initiated in the late 1990s and, to date, there have been only two official data collections on the use of ECT by ethnic group for NHS and private patients in England: surveys covering the periods January to March in 1999 and 2002. There are no plans to conduct a further survey as information on the use of ECT will become available from the Mental Health Minimum Data Set. The Healthcare Commission, for example, has indicated that detailed analyses of activity types by ethnic group have been carried out to explore access to different levels of care, including ECT, but these are unpublished.

With respect to the Department of Health surveys, of the 2835 patients reported to have received ECT in 1999, 8.1% (229) were of ethnic group not given/not known (Department of Health, 1999b). In the 2002 survey this proportion had more than doubled, to 18.5% (420/2272) (Department of Health, 2003b). The surveys do not ask about patient experience, but show that the proportion of patients formally detained under the Mental Health Act who consented to ECT treatment was low and showed no increase (29% in 1999; 28% in 2002). No breakdown is available by ethnic group to establish whether numbers of patients who were treated without their consent but with the agreement of a second opinion appointed doctor were higher among Black and minority ethnic groups. An analysis of cases referred to second opinion appointed doctors for consideration of treatment with ECT found no ethnic bias (Middleton, 2002). However, a Mind (2001) survey of the experiences of 418 patients given ECT found that among those from minority ethnic groups 50% found it unhelpful, damaging or severely damaging in the short term and 72% in the long term (v. 27% and 43% respectively of all survey respondents).

Further research is needed on the experience of ECT by patients from minority ethnic groups, including studies of how consent is obtained and side-effects are explained.

Suicide

Suicide was one of the three service areas of particular concern looked at in detail in the 2003 Framework for Action. It highlighted the significantly raised risk of suicide and attempted suicide among young women born in India or East Africa and men born in Ireland, identifying a reduction in this as essential for meeting the key national target of a 20% reduction in the suicide rate by 2010. Despite this focus, Delivering Race Equality is silent on the lack of comprehensive ethnic data on suicide. In Britain, there is currently no collection of information on ethnic group when a death is registered. Moreover, country of birth is now becoming an increasingly unsatisfactory proxy for the size of different ethnic communities: the 2001 national population census (Office for National Statistics, 2003) showed that half of those belonging to minority ethnic groups were born in Britain. Nevertheless, extensive use has been made of official mortality statistics to investigate patterns of suicide by country of birth (Raleigh & Balarajan, 1992; Raleigh, 1996; Harding & Maxwell, 1997). The omission of ethnic group from civil registration procedures has undoubtedly substantially limited our ability to investigate differences revealed by studies of suicide rates among immigrants (Aspinall, 2002) among ethnic group populations.

Alternative data sources are limited. The National Confidential Inquiry into Suicide and Homicide by People with Mental Illness reports information on suicides of people from minority ethnic groups within 12 months of contact with mental health services, including suicide method and the patients' social and clinical characteristics (Hunt et al, 2003). Its second 5-year report was published in 2006, including tables recording ethnic origin and clinical characteristics (Appleby et al, 2006: pp. 50, 51). Several studies have utilised this source (Hunt et al, 2006; Meehan et al, 2006), including one focusing on ethnic group (Bhui & McKenzie, 2008). The Office for National Statistics' longitudinal study (www.ons.gov.uk/about/who-we-are/our-services/longitudinal-study/index.html) is a potential source of information in the longer term, given that ethnically coded data from the 1991 and 2001 national population censuses have been added to the cohort, although there is a significant delay in linking death registrations to the study (Equalities Review Panel, 2007). Information in the Hospital Episode Statistics database is of limited value as it relates only to deaths in hospital (hospital case fatalities), which account for a negligible proportion of suicides, even among those in contact with mental health services in the year before death. The incompleteness of ethnic coding, although now substantially improved, is a further limitation.

A recent study of suicide rates among people of South Asian origin in England and Wales (McKenzie *et al*, 2008) used the South Asian Group Recognition Algorithm (SANGRA) computer program (Nanchahal *et al*, 2001). This technology yielded findings for the whole of the South Asian population, not just immigrants, and the study offers the currently best available evidence. However, such methods are feasible with only a few ethnic groups (notably, South Asians and Chinese) and more information is needed – acquired through processes of systematic review and national testing and accreditation – on how well SANGRA and similar algorithms (such as Nam Pehchan) ascertain individuals of South Asian origin. Inaccuracies are likely to arise with these programs owing to numerator/denominator incompatibility: the numerator uses an operational definition of ethnicity derived from name information, whereas the denominator is usually based on individuals' self-assignment to census categories (Aspinall, 2009).Nevertheless, it is difficult to see how suicide rates in this population could be ascertained or findings replicated by other means in the absence of ethnically coded death registration data.

The recording of ethnicity at birth and death registration

During the past decade, two particular developments offered the possibility of improving the information base. The first was the suggestion in the government's consultation on its White Paper *Civil Registration: Vital Change* (Office for National Statistics, 2002) that ethnic group be recorded at birth and death registration. A robust case for such inclusion was made by the London Health Observatory and London Health Commission (Aspinall *et al*, 2003) and it was also strongly supported in the Civil Registration Review of 2003 (General Register Office, 2003). Further, the proposals, contained in a Draft Regulatory Reform Order that was intended to amend current legislation on civil registration, were propitious: 'It is likely that if the draft Order becomes law, the National Statistician will want to pilot the collection of ethnic group at birth and death registration ... Consultation has provided substantial support for the collection of these additional data items' (Cabinet Office, 2004: p. 63). However, the enabling legislation was rejected by Parliament on the grounds that it was too complex for the regulatory reform process, bringing the process to make this change to an end as there was no other legislative route available.

The Equalities Review Panel (2007: p. 88) has since recommended that 'In England, Wales and Scotland (as appropriate) specific action should be taken to urgently ... introduce ethnicity coding as part of civil registration of birth and death that will enable the variations in infant mortality and life expectancy to be routinely monitored by ethnicity'. However, there are no developments currently underway.

The recording of ethnicity by coroners

A second major development was the Department of Health's working towards the collection of information on ethnicity by coroners (Department of Health, 2003a). The National Institute for Mental Health in England and others have argued that suicide prevention strategies would be better supported and more effective if information on current or latest occupation and ethnic status were available as aggregate data, and have requested that coroners provide this information when reporting cases to the General Register Office. The government's 'fundamental review' of death certification and investigation (Secretary of State for the Home Department, 2003) supported this 'good case in an important area' and recommended that 'from the earliest feasible date, coroners should wherever they can return information on ethnicity and latest occupation status when reporting self-inflicted deaths to the Registrar' (p. 135). The report highlighted the fact that although there are grounds for thinking that suicide rates among young Asian women may be abnormally high, 'without good ethnicity data well founded preventive action is hard to design' (p. 136).

Even though the public would not be able to access this information on any particular person, the suggestion of its recording is not without controversy. The model consent forms for post-mortem examination ask relatives to provide on a voluntary basis information about the religion of the deceased, and the Department of Health (2003c: p. 21) has noted that: 'Home Office experience in piloting the routine capture of data relating to the ethnic origin or faith of persons whose death has been reported to the coroner has engendered a degree of concern and suspicion in some areas', suggesting that additional work is necessary on the acceptable capture of this information.

To date this development has also come to nothing: in response to a written question asking what progress had been made on the recording of ethnicity data by coroners (House of Commons, 2009), the Secretary of State for Justice stated: 'At present coroners do not collect data on the ethnicity of the deceased in deaths which are referred to them. As part of our work to implement the coroner reforms included in the Coroner and Justice Bill we will be reviewing the statistical data currently collected by coroners and considering whether any changes are required'. This was confirmed in a survey sent out by the London Development Centre to London coroners to find out about the level of ethnicity data they record in suicide cases. The survey found that 'record of ethnicity in suicide cases, in the majority of coroner's inquests, was not collected either through coroner's report or through information provided by the police. Protocols or strategies for recording ethnicity data did not exist and there are no plans to develop these' (NHS London Development Centre, 2009). In the event, the Coroners and Justice Act 2009 did not address the issue of ethnicity recording.

Data linkage

This leaves options such as data linkage. The utility of this approach has been demonstrated by the Office for National Statistics in the compilation of data on infant mortality for England and Wales by ethnic group, and by an important initiative in Scotland that has linked individual census records with health and population data (Bhopal *et al*, 2005). The NHS Information Centre's Mental Health Information Review, conducted in 2008, has recommended as a high priority for the Department of Health the establishment of data linkage between the Mental Health Minimum Data Set (MHMDS) records of those who have been receiving specialist mental healthcare and Office for National Statistics mortality records (NHS Information Centre, 2009*b*): as the MHMDS is ethnically coded, this should provide mortality data by ethnic group for a large part of the population.

Workforce data and the adult mental health services mapping exercise

Both the 2003 Framework for Action and Delivering Race Equality's 5-year action plan emphasise the importance of achieving an ethnically diverse mental health workforce representative of the population at all levels and of developing the cultural capability of that workforce. Two data-sets are of utility in monitoring these objectives: the adult mental health service mapping (AMHSM) exercise and the NHS annual staff censuses.

The AMHSM exercise produces an annual inventory of the full range of specialist services provided for adults with mental health problems (University of Durham, 2005). The aim of the mapping was to obtain an accurate statement on the numbers of teams and staff in place each year. The importance of the AMHSM is that it provided data on a wide range of professional disciplines working in mental healthcare that are otherwise concealed in the NHS staff censuses, including the number of crisis resolution, assertive outreach and early intervention teams and the number of staff employed in the new staff roles, including graduate, gateway, support and recovery, Black and minority ethnic community development, and carer support workers.

Some concerns have been raised over data quality, including implausible gaps that probably reflect missing data and the use of head-count rather than whole-time equivalent statistics in a few areas (Association of Public Health Observatories, 2007). Nevertheless, this source has been important in monitoring the employment of community development workers for Black and minority ethnic groups, the establishment of a network of such workers being a key recommendation of *Inside Outside* (Sashidharan, 2003) and an important component of the Delivering Race Equality action plan. The purpose of this development was to address the perceived failure of mental health services to accommodate the needs and help-seeking behaviour of members of minority ethnic communities. The AMHSM publishes the numbers of community development workers reported to have been appointed in each mapping year, from which the Association of Public Health Observatories (2007) has developed indicators on regional rates per million total population and Black and minority ethnic population, for those aged 18–64. Delivering Race Equality had stated that primary care trusts would recruit 500 community development workers by December 2006. Yet, in autumn 2005, 66% of local implementation teams had scored 'weak' on the numbers they had in place, 'reporting that they had less than half the target number, with no plans to remedy this by December 2006' (Commission for Social Care Inspection & Healthcare Commission, 2007: p. 25). In January 2006, the Durham mapping data showed just 160 community development workers in post. The target was therefore revised to 500 whole-time equivalent community development workers in post by December 2007, with at least 50% (250 nationally) in post by March 2007. Even this target has not been met, with reports of 'well over 200 CDWs in post' by August 2007 (Department of Health, 2007c) and 'over 400 new CDWs' by December 2008 (House of Commons, 2008). By December 2009 450 CDWs had been recruited (Wilson, 2009).

The ethnically coded census of medical and dental staff employed at 30 September each year in the Hospital, Public Health Medicine and Community Health Services (HCHS) of the NHS in England collects data on specialty group and organisational type ('community psychiatry' and 'other psychiatry'). This enables some measure of the representativeness of the workforce using 2001 national population census data. The advantage of the HCHS censuses is that they provide accurate data for whole-time equivalent medical staff at the level of medical specialty and subspecialty and information on staff seniority gradation (but are uninformative on other professional disciplines working in mental healthcare).

New collections

The Mental Health Minimum Data Set

Among new routine data sources introduced by the Department of Health is the statistical base for NHS mental healthcare, the Mental Health Minimum Data Set (MHMDS) (Glover, 2000; NHS Information Authority, 2001). This comprises individual records for each period of all types of care received by a patient from specialist mental health services. Established as a standard in 1999 and subsequently rolled out across England, the MHMDS became a mandatory central return on 1 April 2003. Like some other data-sets supporting the National Service Frameworks, the MHMDS uses the ethnic group categorisation of the 2001 national population census. It is a nation-ally defined framework of patient data centrally reported and held locally by mental health trusts, and it shows all periods of in-patient, out-patient, day care patient and community care, thus being much wider than the Hospital Episode Statistics collection. The data-set is providing patient-centred data across the spectrum of specialist mental healthcare, including detailed data on the use of the Mental Health Act and the care programme approach (CPA) in mental health. The MHMDS is seen as central to the development of clinical audit and the assessment of patient outcomes after intervention.

The completeness of ethnicity coding in the MHMDS data was used by the Healthcare Commission for several purposes: existing commitments and national priorities assessment in 2009/10, for mental health service providers (mental health and primary care trusts that provide in-patient services) and primary care trusts (as commissioners); acute in-patient service review; and to contextualise the results of its annual mental health census. Its use by the Healthcare Commission (and now Care Quality Commission) has widened to include a detailed analysis of activity types by ethnic group to explore access to different levels of care, including: hospital admissions and median length of stay, complexity of care, community psychiatric nurse contacts, consultant psychotherapy contacts, day care attendance, social worker contacts, clinical psychology days, out-patient attendances, occupational therapy attendances, detention under the Mental Health Act, supervised discharge, days in medium security, days in psychiatric intensive care units, home-based care days, community bed-days, CPA plans, ECT provision, social services assessment, home visit help, non-NHS residential care, non-NHS sheltered work, social worker involvement, and Health of the Nation Outcome Scales (HoNOS) scores (NHS Information Centre, 2007).

Some services do not complete the MHMDS, including learning (intellectual) disability services, high secure hospitals, child and adolescent mental health services (CAMHS) and independent hospitals. In the first two reports (October 2008 and March 2009) from MHMDS annual returns the results were published as 'experimental statistics' because the design of the analysis is new and there are some data-quality issues: this caveat has been dropped for most of the content of the third report (November 2009). Nevertheless, the MHMDS will undoubtedly transform the information-poor environment described in the Framework for Action. The first report and experimental statistics from the MHMDS annual return for the years 2003–2007, for example, provide information on ethnicity data quality. In 2006–2007, over 80% of people in contact with psychiatric services and 96% of psychiatric in-patients had a valid ethnicity record, showing: the ethnic group of NHS mental health service users in 'admitted', 'only non-admitted' and 'no care' categories; the number of people using NHS adult and elderly secondary mental healthcare by ethnic group; the ethnic group of patients formally detained in hospital; the most restrictive legal status of people who were in-patients by broad ethnic group; and the CPA level for individual service users and for the highest CPA level recorded for each person by ethnic group (NHS Information Centre, 2008b). Of 45 584 MHMDS records for individuals who had had in-patient stays (bed-days) in 2006–2007, none showed ethnicity 'not stated' and 2704 (5.9%) showed 'invalid' ethnic group; of 736 784 records for individuals with no bed-days, no records had ethnic group not stated and 156 385 (21.2%) had 'invalid' ethnic group (Healthcare Commission et al, 2008). In 2008–2009, valid ethnic coding was present for 85.6% of people (14.4% coded 'not stated' or 'invalid' or 'missing') and was 96.6% in the admitted category.

Although the data-set has been designed to allow detailed monitoring of ethnic variations in healthcare provided, concern remains over large variations between regions in the extent of valid ethnic coding, which is unrelated to the size of the minority ethnic populations within the regions (Association of Public Health Observatories, 2007). In addition, the Healthcare Commission et al (2008) have recommended that the submission of MHMDS should be made mandatory for all independent providers of in-patient mental health services.

The Count Me In censuses

The first national mental health and ethnicity census, the National Census of Inpatients in Mental Health Hospitals and Facilities in England and Wales, was undertaken on 31 March 2005 (Healthcare Commission, 2005). Now commonly known as Count Me In, the census covers all mental health in-patients in England and Wales and its main aims are to obtain robust baseline numbers of in-patients (informal/voluntary and detained) from Black and minority ethnic groups using mental health services on a specified date and to encourage all mental health providers to have accurate and comprehensive sustainable ethnic monitoring/record-keeping procedures in place that will yield high-quality data on patient ethnicity in the future. From 2006, the Healthcare Commission has undertaken the census annually, those for 2006, 2007, 2008 and 2009 being extended to include in-patients in NHS and independent mental health and learning (intellectual) disability hospitals and facilities. The final census was carried out in March 2010.

This source has a number of advantages. The census provides comprehensive national coverage of patients in both NHS and independent services (unlike the Hospital Episode Statistics and MHMDS), thus enabling differences between the two types of provider to be analysed (Raleigh et al, 2008). Further, of all the routine sources for mental health data (including the Hospital Episode Statistics and MHMDS), the census has the most complete ethnic coding. In the Count Me In census for 2008, of a total of 31 020 mental health patients (including those in the independent sector), there were just 327 cases of ethnic group not stated (1.1%) and no cases of invalid ethnic group (Healthcare Commission et al, 2008). Finally, rich data are collected on patient characteristics. In addition to 'ethnic category', the census collects such data items as 'assessment of ethnicity' (including codes for self, staff, and relatives), 'language/dialect' (categories and free text), 'religion and faith groups' (categories and free text), and 'sexual orientation' ('patient known to staff as asylum seeker' was also collected in the 2005 census).

The key benefit of the Count Me In censuses lies in the range of data collected, which includes: type of ward (security level and whether single sex or not), CPA level, incidents of seclusion and hands-on restraint, information on self-harm, accidents and physical assaults, length of stay from admission to census day (including patients hospitalised for 1 year or more), whether detained on admission, section of Mental Health Act 1983 under which detained, and referral source.

There are, or course, some limitations to the census. First, it is a one-day snapshot and so does not capture all-year in-patient activity. As Raleigh (2008) has noted, this would skew some of the findings towards long-stay patients (underestimating admissions and detentions of short duration and overestimating median duration of stay from admission to census day). Second, information is lacking on diagnosis, case-mix and socioeconomic factors; nor is the means available to obtain diagnosis and case-mix by linkage to the Hospital Episode Statistics data-set. Thus, the census is not able to throw light on the debate about the high hospital admission rates for psychosis among people of Black Caribbean origin. Also, no adjustment to the detention ratios and other analyses is possible for these variables (Raleigh, 2008). Third, for around a quarter of patients ethnicity is reported by staff or relatives rather than via self-assignment, although the reasons for this are not recorded.

The DRE Dashboard

A further development launched in September 2008 – late in the Delivering Race Equality 5-year action plan – is the 'DRE Dashboard'. This is a tool to help strategic health authorities, primary care trusts and mental health trusts to measure their progress on race equality in mental health at local and regional levels and to identify success, gaps and risks. There are a total of 26 indicators, covering a range of areas to aid understanding about access and outcomes, that are cross-referenced against the 12 characteristics specified in the action plan that Delivering Race Equality hoped would describe mental health services in 2010. The DRE Dashboard has also set out to track six headline indicators as part of a national data collection exercise: access to early intervention; access to crisis resolution/home treatment; use of assertive outreach services; access to psychological therapies; implementation of supervised community treatment under the 2007 Amendments to the Mental Health Act 1983; and recruitment and impact of community development workers. As part of the NHS Information Centre 'Omnibus' returns for the final quarter of 2008/09, specially collected surveys were undertaken asking primary care trusts to report numbers of users of crisis resolution/home treatment, early intervention in psychosis and assertive outreach teams. At the same time, the 13 primary care trusts with first-wave services in the new IAPT programme supplied reports of numbers referred to and entering services and numbers finishing treatment and moving towards recovery. A study by the North East Public Health Observatory has examined how far these four new types of mental healthcare have been used in the care of people from minority ethnic groups (Glover & Evison, 2009). The indicators highlight some of the basic data needed to measure progress on race equality, the aims of the DRE Dashboard initiative being to catalyse the collection of timely information on a regular basis.

Conclusion

Delivering Race Equality and related reports all emphasise that high-quality data on ethnicity are essential for mental health providers and that they should record users' ethnicity and other relevant data such as religion and language. As a 5-year national and local action plan, however, Delivering Race Equality is frequently parsimonious on the 'specifics' of monitoring ethnicity and service use and how routine data collections can be used, despite the Department of Health's pronouncement that 'self-identified ethnicity and preferred spoken language of all service users must be documented routinely and recorded in information systems' (Sashidharan, 2003). Surprisingly, it says nothing about the substantial potential of the Hospital Episode Statistics database – a comprehensive record of every in-patient admission – and the need and means for improving the completeness of data items such as ethnic group and the recording of ECT. Indeed, this physical intervention is not mentioned at all, despite the current lack of routine ethnicity and other data that can be used to assess equity of access and appropriateness of use. Delivering Race Equality sets out no specific actions for primary care, although this is the setting for 90% of treatment of mental ill health, and does not mention how the MHMDS could be exploited. With respect to suicide, the proposed collection of ethnicity data by coroners flagged in earlier reports is not revisited and there is no reference to current proposals to collect ethnic-group data at death registration in the reforms of civil registration.

Since the publication of Delivering Race Equality in 2003, substantial progress has been made in filling some of the gaps identified, but little in remedying others. The Count Me In censuses have been a major success and provide an extremely rich body of evidence on users of NHS and independent in-patient mental health services. They have enabled progress to be assessed with respect to three of the dozen goals of Delivering Race Equality: to reduce admission rates, to reduce detention rates, and to reduce seclusion among Black and minority ethnic groups. On the first two counts there has been no progress, no reduction in these rates. The Count Me In census shows no consistent disparity in the use of seclusion between Black and minority ethnic in-patients and White British in-patients, with the exception of the 'other Black' group (Wilson, 2009). The efforts of the Healthcare Commission to include indicators on Hospital Episode Statistics ethnicity coding levels in its annual performance assessments of NHS organisations since 2003 have undoubtedly significantly contributed to the capturing of ethnicity data that is now of quality (and, consequently, utility) for most mental health trusts. The other major data-collection success has been the Mental Health Minimum Data Set (MHMDS), which is beginning to be exploited to assess equity of access to mental health services. The drawback with respect to both the Hospital Episode Statistics and the MHMDS is that they are not mandatory for independent providers of in-patient mental health services, where 14% of patients were treated in 2008.

The amount of progress made in other areas has been disappointing. The proposed reforms of the civil registration and coroners' service that promised to deliver ethnic coding for deaths have come to nothing, the recording of ethnicity by coroners having been omitted from the Coroners and Justice Act 2009. One recent research study had to use name recognition algorithms to derive suicide rates for people of South Asian ethnic origin and this currently represents the only feasible approach with respect to the full size of the community (immigrants and those born in Britain). The pleas for ethnic coding of death registration data made at the time the modernisation of civil registration was first mooted in 2002 are still being voiced and costly data linkage seems to be the only alternative solution available.

Although some progress has been made in securing ethnic coding on registration of new patients at GP surgeries (through its incentivisation in the Quality and Outcomes Framework), it is likely that the records of a substantial proportion of existing patients on general practice registers lack ethnic coding. Again, various scrutiny bodies have regularly recommended the filling of this information gap through ethnicity data collection, but few tangible developments are in prospect. The Ethnicity and First Language Recording System under the new directed enhanced services (Department of Health, 2009) may help to increase ethnicity coding levels for registered patients. The NHS Care Records Service (www.nhscarerecords.nhs.uk), a secure service that is linking patient information from different parts of the NHS electronically, too, may provide a longer-term solution but these electronic records will still need to be populated with patients' ethnicity from some source or other.

The MHMDS and Hospital Episode Statistics are likely to become the key sources for informing progress towards race equality in mental healthcare. As the Count Me In census – which was set up explicitly to help health services move towards achieving the Government's 5-year plan in Delivering Race Equality – is in its final year, the scope of the MHMDS is likely to be enhanced by the transfer to it of some of the census's data items.

The most notable barrier to the exploitation of Hospital Episode Statistics – the hitherto poor levels of ethnic coding – has now been removed. Whereas the censuses have provided annual cross-sectional 'stock data', a snapshot of the in-patient population at a single point in time, the MHMDS and Hospital Episode Statistics will, between them, provide 'flow data' for patients treated in community and in-patient settings. It is also encouraging that other specific information gaps are being filled by new collections such as the Improving Access to Psychological Therapies (IAPT) Minimum Data Set and the DRE Dashboard indicators.

References

Academy of Medical Sciences (2009) *Research in General Practice: Bringing Innovation into Patient Care. Workshop Report.* Academy of Medical Sciences.

Alexander, Z. (1999) *Study of Black, Asian and Ethnic Minority Issues.* Department of Health.

Appleby, L., Shaw, J., Kapur, N., *et al* (2006) *Avoidable Deaths: Report of the National Confidential Inquiry into Suicide and Homicide by People with Mental Illness.* TSO (The Stationery Office).

Aspinall, P. J. (2002) Suicide amongst Irish migrants in Britain: a review of the identity and integration hypothesis. *International Journal of Social Psychiatry,* **48,** 290–304.

Aspinall, P. J. (2006) Informing progress towards race equality in mental healthcare: is routine data collection adequate? *Advances in Psychiatric Treatment,* **12,** 141–151.

Aspinall, P. J. (2009) Suicide rates in people of South Asian origin in England and Wales. *British Journal of Psychiatry,* **194,** 566–567.

Aspinall, P. J., Jacobson, B. & Polato, G. M. (2003) *Missing Record: The Case for Recording Ethnicity at Birth and Death Registration.* London Health Observatory.

Association of Public Health Observatories (2007) *Indicators of Public Health in the English Regions. 7: Mental Health.* APHO.

Barber, N., Rawlins, M. & Franklin, B. D. (2003) Reducing prescribing error: competence, control, and culture. *Quality and Safety in Health Care,* **12,** 29–32.

Bardsley, M., Hamm, J., Lowdell, C., *et al* (2000) *Developing Health Assessment for Black and Minority Ethnic Groups: Analysing Routine Health Information.* Health of Londoners Project & NHS Executive.

Bhopal, R., Fischbacher, C. M., Steiner, M., *et al* (2005) *Ethnicity and Health in Scotland: Can We Fill the Information Gap?* University of Edinburgh/General Register Office for Scotland (http://www.chs.med.ed.ac.uk/phs/research/Retrocoding%20final%20report.pdf).

Bhugra, D. & Bahl, V. (eds) (1999) *Ethnicity: An Agenda for Mental Health.* Gaskell.

Bhui, K. S. & McKenzie, K. (2008) Rates and risk factors by ethnic group for suicides within a year of contact with mental health services in England and Wales. *Psychiatric Services,* **59,** 414–420.

British Medical Association & NHS Employers (2006) *Revisions to the GMS Contract 2006/7. Delivering Investment in General Practice.* BMA & NHS Employers.

Cabinet Office (2004) *The Draft Regulatory Reform (Registration of Births and Deaths) (England and Wales) Order Explanatory Document.* TSO (The Stationery Office) (http://www.cabinetoffice.gov.uk/regulation/documents/regulatory_reform/pdf/edbirt.pdf).

Cochrane, R. (1977) *Mental illness in immigrants to England and Wales: an analysis of mental hospital admissions, 1971.* Social Psychiatry, 12, 15–35.

Cochrane, R. & Bal, S. S. (1988) Ethnic density is unrelated to incidence of schizophrenia. *British Journal of Psychiatry,* **153,** 363–366.

Commission for Social Care Inspection & Healthcare Commission (2007) *No Voice, No Choice. A Joint Review of Adult Community Mental Health Services in England.* Commission for Healthcare Audit and Inspection.

Connolly, A., Rogers, P. & Taylor, D. (2007) Antipsychotic prescribing quality and ethnicity – a study of hospitalised patients in south east London. *Journal of Psychopharmacology*, **21**, 191–197.

Dawson, I. (2006) *Outpatient Data Quality Report 2003–04 and 2004–05*. The Information Centre.

Dean, G., Walsh, D., Downing, H., *et al* (1981) First admissions of native-born and immigrants to psychiatric hospitals in South-East England 1976. *British Journal of Psychiatry*, **139**, 506–512.

Department of Health (1999a) *National Service Framework for Mental Health*. Department of Health.

Department of Health (1999b) *Electro Convulsive Therapy: Survey Covering the Period from January 1999 to March 1999, England (Statistical Bulletin 1999/22)*. Department of Health.

Department of Health (2000) *The NHS Plan: A Plan for Investment, A Plan for Reform*. Department of Health.

Department of Health (2002) *National Suicide Prevention Strategy for England*. Department of Health.

Department of Health (2003a) *Delivering Race Equality: A Framework for Action*. Department of Health.

Department of Health (2003b) *Electro Convulsive Therapy: Survey Covering the Period from January 2002 to March 2002, England (Statistical Bulletin 2003/08)*. Department of Health.

Department of Health (2003c) *Isaacs Report Response. Response to the Report by Her Majesty's Inspector of Anatomy*. Department of Health.

Department of Health (2004a) *Race Equality Action Plan*. Department of Health.

Department of Health (2004b) *National Standards, Local Action: Health and Social Care Standards and Planning Framework 2005/06–2007/08*. Department of Health.

Department of Health (2005a) *Delivering Race Equality in Mental Health Care, An Action Plan for Reform Inside and Outside Services and The Government's Response to the Independent Inquiry into the Death of David Bennett*. Department of Health.

Department of Health (2005b) *Hospital Episode Statistics (Data Quality Indicators: Component Scores for Data Year 2002/2003)*. Department of Health (not available online: for further information, contact NHS Information Centre).

Department of Health (2007a) *A Practical Guide to Ethnic Monitoring in the NHS and Social Care*. Department of Health.

Department of Health (2007b) *Single Equality Scheme 2007–2010*. Department of Health.

Department of Health (2007c) Delivering Race Equality. Programme Progress. 10 August 2007. Department of Health (http://www.dh.gov.uk/en/Healthcare/Mentalhealth/Policy/BMEmentalhealth/DH_4114939).

Department of Health (2009) *The National Health Service Act 2006: The Primary Medical Services (Directed Enhanced Services) (England) (Amendment) Directions 2009*. Department of Health.

Department of Health & Healthcare Commission (2008) *Report On Self Reported Experience of Patients from Black and Minority Ethnic Groups*. Department of Health & Healthcare Commission.

De Ponte, P. & Jacobson, B. (2007) *Equal Access, Equal Care? Can London Deliver the Race Equality Action Plan for Mental Health?* London Health Observatory, Care Services Improvement Partnership & London Development Centre.

Equalities Review Panel (2007) *Fairness and Freedom: The Final Report of the Equalities Review*. Cabinet Office.

Fitzgerald, C. (2004) *Ethnicity Coding in HES: How Good is HES Ethnicity Coding and Where do the Problems Lie?* Department of Health.

General Register Office (2003) *Civil Registration: Delivering Vital Change*. Office for National Statistics.

Glover, G. R. (1987) 993W: birthplace not stated or born at sea. *Psychological Medicine*, **17**, 1009–1012.

Glover, G. R. (1989*a*) Differences in psychiatric admission patterns between Caribbeans from different islands. *Social Psychiatry and Psychiatric Epidemiology*, **24**, 209–211.

Glover, G. R. (1989*b*) The pattern of psychiatric admissions of Caribbean-born immigrants in London. *Social Psychiatry and Psychiatric Epidemiology*, **24**, 49–56.

Glover, G. R. (2000) A comprehensive clinical database for mental health care in England. *Social Psychiatry and Psychiatric Epidemiology*, **35**, 523–529.

Glover, G. (2003) Use of routinely collected data on psychiatric in-patient care. *Advances in Psychiatric Treatment*, **9**, 300–307.

Glover, G & Evison, F. (2009) *Use of New Mental Health Services by Minority Ethnic Groups in England*. North East Public Health Observatory.

Goldberg, D. & Bridges, K. (1987) Screening for psychiatric illness in general practice: the general practitioner versus the screening questionnaire. *Journal of the Royal College of General Practitioners*, **37**, 15–18.

Goldberg, D. & Huxley, P. (1992) *Common Mental Disorders: A Biosocial Model*. Routledge.

Harding, S. & Maxwell, R. (1997) Differences in mortality of migrants. In *Health Inequalities. Decennial Supplement* (series DS no. 15) (eds F. Drever & M. Whitehead), pp. 108–121. TSO (The Stationery Office).

Health and Social Care Information Centre (2009) *Quality and Outcomes Framework (QOF) for April 2008–March 2009, England: Records and Information about Patients*. The Information Centre (http://www.ic.nhs.uk/webfiles/QOF/2008-09/England%20tables/QOF0809_National_Organisational.xls).

Healthcare Commission (2004) *Patient Survey Report 2004 – Mental Health*. Healthcare Commission.

Healthcare Commission (2005) *Count Me In. Results of a National Census of Inpatients in Mental Health Hospitals and Facilities in England and Wales*. Healthcare Commission.

Healthcare Commission (2008) *The Pathway to Recovery. A Review of NHS Acute Inpatient Mental Health Services*. Healthcare Commission.

Healthcare Commission, Mental Health Act Commission, Care Services Improvement Partnership, *et al* (2008) *Count Me In 2008: Results of the 2008 National Census of Inpatients in Mental Health and Learning Disability Services in England and Wales*. Commission for Healthcare Audit and Inspection.

House of Commons (2008) Hansard, HC, Written Answers for 17 December 2008. Col. 911W. Mental Health Services: Ethnic Groups. TSO (The Stationery Office).

House of Commons (2009) Hansard, HC, Written Answers for 22 January 2009 (pt 0006). Col. 1595W [250400]. Coroners: Ethnic Groups. TSO (The Stationery Office).

House of Lords & House of Commons (2004) *Joint Committee on Human Rights: Third Report of the Session 2004–05*. TSO (The Stationery Office).

Hunt, I. M., Robinson, J., Bickley, H., *et al* (2003) Suicides in ethnic minorities within 12 months of contact with mental health services. National clinical survey. *British Journal of Psychiatry*, **183**, 155–160.

Hunt, I. M., Kapur, N., Robinson, J., *et al* (2006) Suicide within 12 months of mental health service contact in different age and diagnostic groups: national clinical survey. *British Journal of Psychiatry*, **188**, 135–142.

Improving Access to Psychological Therapies Team (2008) *Improving Access to Psychological Therapies (IAPT) Equality Impact Assessment (EqIA)*. Department of Health.

Information Centre (2009) *In-patients Formally Detained in Hospitals under the Mental Health Act 1983 and Patients Subject to Supervised Community Treatment: 1998–99 to 2008–09*. Information Centre.

Information Standards Board for Health and Social Care (2008) *Data Standards: Ethnic Category (DSC Notice: 11/2008)*. Department of Health.

Kumarapeli, R., Stepaniuk, R., de Lusignan, S., *et al* (2006) Ethnicity recording in general practice computer systems. *Journal of Public Health*, **28**, 283–287.

Lakhani, M. (2008) *No Patient Left Behind: How can We Ensure World Class Primary Care for Black and Minority Ethnic People? Report of the Group Chaired by Professor Mayur Lakhani*. Department of Health.

Lawson, R. & Guite, H. (2005) Psychological therapies for common mental illness: how effective and equitable is provision? *Primary Care Mental Health*, **3**, 5–12.

Lelliott, P., Paton, C., Harrington, M., *et al* (2002) The influence of patient variables on polypharmacy and combined high dose of antipsychotic drugs prescribed for in-patients. *Psychiatric Bulletin*, **26**, 411–414.

McKenzie, K., van Os, J., Fahy, T., *et al* (1995) Psychosis with good prognosis in Afro-Caribbean people now living in the United Kingdom. *BMJ*, **311**, 1325–1328.

McKenzie, K., Bhui, K., Nanchahal, K., *et al* (2008) Suicide rates in people of South Asian origin in England and Wales: 1993–2003. *British Journal of Psychiatry*, **193**, 406–409.

Meehan, J., Kapur, N., Hunt, I. M., *et al* (2006) Suicide in mental health in-patients and within 3 months of discharge: national clinical survey. *British Journal of Psychiatry*, **188**, 129–134.

Mental Health Act Commission (2001) *Ninth Biennial Report 1999–2001*. TSO (The Stationery Office).

Mental Health Act Commission (2003) *Minutes of Board Meeting, 20 November*. Mental Health Act Commission.

Mental Health Act Commission (2008) *Risks, Rights, Recovery. Twelfth Biennial Report 2005–2007*. TSO (The Stationery Office).

Mental Health Act Commission (2009) *Coercion and Consent: Monitoring the Mental Health Act 2007–2009. MHAC Thirteenth Biennial Report 2007–2009*. TSO (The Stationery Office).

Middleton, H. (2002) *An Evaluation of Data Collected by the Mental Health Act Commission*. National Institute for Health and Clinical Excellence (http://www.library.nhs.uk/cardiovascular/ViewResource.aspx?resID=117919&tabID=289&catID=744).

Mind (2001) *Shock Treatment*. Mind.

Mind (2002) *Factsheets. Statistics 3: Race, Culture and Mental Health*. Mind (http://www.mind.org.uk/Information/Factsheets/Statistics/Statistics+3.htm).

Ministry of Justice (2007) Collecting Ethnicity Data. *Mental Health Unit Bulletin*, October, p. 3.

Mohammed, M. A., Cheng, K. K., Rouse, A., *et al* (2001) Bristol, Shipman, and clinical governance: Shewart's forgotten lessons. *Lancet*, **357**, 463–467.

Nanchahal, K., Mangtani, P., Alston, M., *et al* (2001) Development and validation of a computerised South Asian Names Recognition Algorithm (SANGRA) for use in British health-related studies. *Journal of Public Health Medicine*, **23**, 278–285.

NHS Information Authority (2001) *Mental Health Minimum Data Set – Data Manual*. NHSIA.

NHS Information Centre (2007) *Mental Health Minimum Dataset (MHMDS): Information Standards Board Submission for Inherited Standard*. The Information Centre (http://www.isb.nhs.uk/docs/MHMDS-ISB.pdf).

NHS Information Centre (2008a) *Mental Health Information. Consultation Feedback Document: Communication Issues*. The Information Centre.

NHS Information Centre (2008b) *Mental Health Bulletin: First Report and Experimental Statistics from Mental Health Minimum Dataset (MHMDS) Annual Returns, 2003–2007*. The Information Centre.

NHS Information Centre (2009a) *Mental Health Bulletin. Third report from Mental Health Minimum Dataset (MHMDS) Annual Returns, 2004–2009*. NHS Information Centre.

NHS Information Centre (2009b) *Mental Health Information Review Recommendations*. The Information Centre.

NHS London Development Centre (2009) *Well Being: Coroners Data Recording Survey*. London Development Centre (http://www.londondevelopmentcentre.org/mental-wellbeing/mental-health-and-well-being/well-being-and-inclusion/well-being.aspx).

Norfolk, Suffolk & Cambridgeshire Strategic Health Authority (2003) *Independent Inquiry into the Death of David Bennett*. NSCSHA.

North Central London Strategic Health Authority (2004) *A Review of Race Relations (Amendment) Act Implementation by NHS Organisations within the North Central London Sector*. NCLSHA.

Office for National Statistics (2002) *Civil Registration: Vital Change. Birth, Marriage and Death Registration in the 21st Century*. TSO (The Stationery Office).

Office for National Statistics (2003) *Census 2001: National Report for England and Wales*. TSO (The Stationery Office).

Patel, K., Winters, M., Bashford, J., *et al* (2003) *Engaging and Changing: Developing Effective Policy for the Care and Treatment of Black and Minority Ethnic Detained Patients*. National Institute for Mental Health in England.

Paton, C. & Lelliott, P. (2004) The use of prescribing indicators to measure the quality of care in psychiatric inpatients. *Quality and Safety in Health Care*, **13**, 40–45.

Raleigh, V. S. (1996) Suicide patterns and trends in people of Indian subcontinent and Caribbean origin in England and Wales. *Ethnicity and Health*, **1**, 55–63.

Raleigh, V. (2008) Collection of data on ethnic origin in England. *BMJ*, **337**, 645–46.

Raleigh, V. S. & Balarajan, R. (1992) Suicide levels and trends among immigrants in England and Wales. *Health Trends*, **24**, 91–94.

Raleigh, V. S., Irons, R., Hawe, E., *et al* (2007) Ethnic variations in the experiences of mental health service users in England. Results of a national patient survey programme. *British Journal of Psychiatry*, **191**, 304–312.

Raleigh, V. S., Polato, G. M., Bremner, S. A., *et al* (2008) Inpatient mental healthcare in England and Wales: patterns in NHS and independent healthcare providers. *Journal of the Royal Society of Medicine*, **101**, 544–551.

Royal College of Psychiatrists (2006) *Consensus Statement on High-Dose Antipsychotic Medication (Council Report CR138)*. Royal College of Psychiatrists.

Sashidharan, S. P. (2003) *Inside Outside: Improving Mental Health Services for Black and Minority Ethnic Communities in England*. National Institute for Mental Health in England.

Scottish Government (2008) *GP Contract Agreement for 2008/09. NHS Circular: PCA(M) (2008)12. Primary and Community Care Directorate (Primary Care Division)*. Scottish Government.

Secretary of State for the Home Department (2003) *Death Certification and Investigation in England, Wales and Northern Ireland. The Report of a Fundamental Review 2003* (Cm 5831). TSO (The Stationery Office).

Shah, R., McNiece, R. & Majeed, A. (2001) Socio-demographic differences in general practice consultation rates for psychiatric disorders among patients aged 16–64. *Health Statistics Quarterly*, **11**, 5–10.

Spiegelhalter, D. J. (2002) Funnel plots for institutional comparison. *Quality and Safety in Health Care*, **11**, 390–391.

Taylor, D. M. (2004) Prescribing of clozapine and olanzapine: dosage, polypharmacy and patient ethnicity. *Psychiatric Bulletin*, **28**, 241–243.

University of Durham (2005) *Adults of Working Age Mental Health Service Mapping Exercise 2005/6*. University of Durham.

Wilson, M. (2009) *Delivering Race Equality in Mental Health Care: A Review*. Department of Health & National Mental Health Development Unit.

CHAPTER 29

Towards social inclusion in mental health?

Justine Schneider and Carole J. Bramley

Summary This chapter explores the uses of the terms social exclusion and social inclusion in a mental health context. We briefly describe the origins of the term social exclusion and analyse its connotations in relation to four key dimensions: the relative, multifactorial, dynamic and transactional. We discuss Levitas's three discourses concerning social exclusion (the redistributionist, moral underclass and social integrationist) and present a case in favour of a fourth perspective, societal oppression. Focusing on social inclusion as a remedy for the ills of social exclusion, we discuss implications for contemporary mental health policy, practice and research. We highlight the potential contribution of social psychology to social inclusion theory. We conclude that a better theoretical understanding of causal mechanisms is needed to enable the development of more socially inclusive mental health services.

Applying the principles of social inclusion to adults with mental health problems is increasingly seen as desirable. In the UK, the National Social Inclusion Programme has been established to take forward the recommendations of the Social Exclusion Unit's influential report and action plan Social Exclusion and Mental Health (Office of the Deputy Prime Minister, 2004a,b).

Much has been written about the history of the concept of social exclusion (Percy-Smith, 2000). It became influential in social policy at national and international levels during the 1990s (Dahrendorf et al, 1995; Rodgers et al, 1995; Room, 1995). The European Union set up an observatory on national policies to combat social exclusion in 1991, and reinforced the theme by requiring national governments to submit annual reports on how they are tackling the issue. This is one factor that keeps the theme live in UK policy circles and it tends to be adopted by interest groups whenever an injustice is perceived or policy priority is sought. In the media, 'social exclusion' seems to have passed into everyday use:

> Of all the disadvantaged groups in society, the disabled are the most socially excluded. Until relatively recently, many were hidden away from the rest of society in institutions. But the problems that Britain's estimated 8.5 m

disabled people face have not gone away – life opportunities remain severely restricted for many. (*The Guardian Society*, 1999, 28 July, p. 7)

The railways must combat the 'social exclusion' that leads to professional people using trains three to four times more than non-professionals, the Rail Passenger Council said yesterday. It also called for increased, focused investment for rural railways. (*The Independent*, 2000, 19 June, p. 8)

Ways need to be found to help pupils with emotional and behavioural difficulties in Northern Ireland to avoid them being socially excluded, it was claimed today. (*Belfast Telegraph Newspapers*, 2003, 16 September).

Used as a term of condemnation, 'social exclusion' makes the accuser's position clear, but it begs the question 'Who is excluding whom from what?' In the examples given above, society appears to be excluding disabled people in general, the railways to be excluding non-professional people from using trains, and schools to be excluding certain children from their peers by suspending them from school. Beneath these answers lies a further layer of assumptions: that social exclusion can be remedied; that it should be addressed as a matter of public concern; and that responsibility for doing so is located in some agency. From the examples given, these may be large and indeterminate (society), private enterprises (the railways) or public bodies (education). Government is invoked to ensure that its own departments and other agencies take seriously their alleged responsibility for preventing social exclusion, and psychiatry has also been called to order with regard to the matter.

In the UK today, there is a strong consensus that the state has a role in reducing social exclusion; this follows directly from much European economic and social policy and it is also the understanding of the United Nations. But these supra-national bodies are predominantly concerned with gross forms of exclusion such as mass unemployment, slavery, disenfranchisement and oppression on ethnic grounds. Subtler forms of exclusion are at work in relation to the situation of people with mental health problems. It may help to understand the significance of social inclusion and its relevance to mental healthcare if we first undertake some conceptual analysis.

Defining social exclusion

Exclusion is a complex concept and many uses of the term fail to do justice to its connotations. Social exclusion tends to be used to describe the position of an individual or group in relation to others, or in relation to benefits that society is supposed to offer, for example physical security, adequate nutrition, shelter, family life, employment, social support, community participation and political involvement. Often, for 'social exclusion' we can substitute the words 'disadvantage', 'poverty' or 'discrimination' without any loss of meaning. Yet it is overly simplistic to condemn everything one dislikes as 'exclusion' and everything one aspires to as 'inclusion'. The analysis presented below identifies four key dimensions of social exclusion:

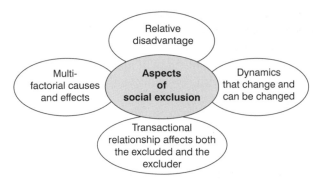

Fig. 29.1   Four key dimensions of social exclusion.

the relative, the multifactorial, the dynamic and the transactional (Fig. 29.1). Each of these implies certain remedies for exclusion or approaches to inclusion, and thereby offers indications for mental healthcare and other agencies tasked with addressing social exclusion.

The relative dimension

First, the concept of inequality underlies most definitions of social exclusion, making it essentially a relative concept, akin to notions of deprivation or disadvantage. This is the most common understanding of social exclusion, and is reflected in the accusations against schools and rail companies cited above.

The multifactorial dimension

Second, social exclusion is inherently multifactorial: in addition to describing the position of an individual or a group in relation to other people or groups, the concept implies that this disadvantage is due to more than one factor (Burchardt *et al*, 2002). These factors may be interrelated, such as poverty, poor housing, poor education and poor health. Such an amalgam of problems has also been described as 'multiple deprivation'. This is why the use of the term social exclusion in relation to rail passengers gives pause for thought. One might think that people who cannot afford to take the train are not disadvantaged in any other way, but describing their situation as social exclusion draws attention to the possibility that without this mode of transport they are also at risk of missing out on other entitlements, perhaps education or employment.

The dynamic dimension

Third, beliefs regarding multiple deprivation are far from new, but the concept of social exclusion adds another dimension, emphasising the processes that operate to create and sustain it. Exclusion is not a fixed

399

state, it may be transient, recurrent or a more long-term experience (Burgess & Propper, 2002). Hence, social exclusion is essentially dynamic: people move in and out of the conditions that lead to exclusion, for example poverty, unemployment or ill health. Giddens (1998) stated that exclusion is concerned with mechanisms that work to disconnect groups of people from social mainstreams. This is sometimes referred to as a cycle of disadvantage or deprivation. The patterns and processes by which these movements into and out of social exclusion come about are therefore of interest to those concerned with social change, in particular if the mechanisms seem to be amenable to intervention. Reflecting this dynamic dimension, in 2004 the Social Exclusion Unit (now the Social Exclusion Task Force) published a series of reports entitled 'Breaking the Cycle' (www.cabinetoffice.gov.uk/social_exclusion_task_force/publications. aspx#published97).

The transactional dimension

Finally, and most distinctively, social exclusion locates individuals or groups in relation to wider structures of society, so it has a transactional dimension. From this perspective, exclusion limits the interactions that are possible between individuals, families, communities, regions and even nations. Since these interactions are reciprocal, not only the excluded are affected: exclusion affects all of society, for better or worse.

Prison is an example of social exclusion that is planned and implemented by a system established to protect society and punish deviants. Slavery is an extreme form of social exclusion that both dehumanises individuals and deprives society of their full participation. Each describes a dyadic relationship (criminal justice system–prisoner, owner–slave) that is understood to have goals beyond the immediate interests of the parties directly involved. These higher goals are formulated in abstract terms: 'law and order' or 'economic prosperity'.

This transactional aspect of social exclusion indicates that remedies cannot be found solely from the perspective of the excluded. Exclusion cannot exist unless someone or something brings it about, be it through inadvertence, the operation of a system (e.g. institutional racism) or active discrimination by individuals. A transactional understanding of social exclusion is of particular importance in the promotion of political engagement and avoidance of conflict.

The higher goal of 'social cohesion' has been introduced as the justification for actions to reduce social exclusion. In the face of the rapid changes brought about through economic integration and migration across the continent of Europe, social cohesion has emerged as a major policy objective in the UK as in other European nations (Levitas, 2005): social exclusion poses a threat of social disintegration and, with it, economic failure.

What do we mean by socially excluded?

In short, when we say that individuals are socially excluded, we mean that they are disadvantaged and that this affects several aspects of their lives. Disadvantage is a necessary but not a sufficient condition of social exclusion. We also mean that they were not born disadvantaged and need not remain that way. Finally, exclusion is a two-way street: it affects people's status as members of a community and their political influence as members of a state; consequently, the wider society is also affected to the extent that it creates or tolerates social exclusion.

Social exclusion and the state

As outlined above, to proceed from the identification of social exclusion as an ill to the adoption of a remedy, one moves through an understanding, explicit or implicit, of how the state and society interact. It may be helpful to consider these responses in relation to alternative 'discourses' of social exclusion. Levitas (1998) describes a discourse as a set of interrelated concepts acting as a 'matrix' through which to understand the world. Noting that the term discourse has to some extent replaced 'ideology' within social science, she points out that use of the word draws attention to the importance of language 'not simply as a way of expressing the substance of political positions and policies, but as that substance' (1998: p. 3). In relation to social exclusion, Levitas identifies three discourses (Box 29.1, items 1–3).

The redistributionist discourse

The redistributionist discourse is mainly about poverty: it sees income inequality as the cause of exclusion, and economic mechanisms such as taxation and welfare benefits as means to reduce it. The redistributionist

---

Box 29.1 Discourses of social exclusion

1 The redistributionist discourse: exclusion results from poverty and can be prevented by redistribution of wealth
2 The moral underclass discourse: individuals are responsible for their own exclusion, through their behaviour or cultural choices
3 The social integrationist discourse: 'exclusion' = 'unemployment', so paid employment eliminates exclusion
4 The societal oppression discourse: exclusion is the fault of the excluders, not the excluded

(Items 1–3 after Levitas, 1998)

discourse on social exclusion does not account for non-material causes of exclusion such as discrimination experienced by minority ethnic groups or disabled people.

The moral underclass discourse

The moral underclass discourse is concerned with the behaviour or the culture of individuals, for example young people, ex-offenders, single mothers or adults lacking basic skills, whose apparent failures and inadequacies are seen as the cause of their own exclusion. Remedies might include programmes targeted at specific social groups, for instance work-related training and parenting classes. With its focus on individuals and families, this discourse gives little attention to the structural or institutional factors that contribute to exclusion, such as inadequate housing, lack of amenities and labour market forces.

The social integrationist discourse

The social integrationist discourse sees inclusion mainly in terms of paid employment, to the extent that 'inclusion' and 'employment' are virtually synonymous. This is the understanding of social exclusion that dominates European social policy. It is also the nearest discourse to contemporary policy on social inclusion in England, illustrated by the emphasis on economic integration in the work of the Social Exclusion Task Force (2007): 'Britain has enjoyed a strong economy and growing prosperity in recent years, but we would be more prosperous still if the talents of each and every member of the community could flourish. Social exclusion and wasted human potential are harmful to the country as well as to those individuals suffering from them'.

For the most part, the social integrationist perspective fails to address exclusion in the workplace and gives little importance to unpaid work within society, which includes voluntary work, caring for dependants, neighbourhood and political involvement, and other activities associated with the strengthening of communities and the welfare of individuals.

A fourth discourse: societal oppression

These three discourses identify respectively poverty, culture and unemployment as the prime causes of social exclusion. We would like to put forward for consideration a fourth perspective, the societal oppression discourse (for its origins see, e.g., Adams et al, 2002). Societal oppression is mediated through interpersonal relationships, inter-group dynamics or institutional systems, and it appears to operate independently of the other three discourses. Social inclusion requires the more powerful actors to recognise the part that they play in oppressing the excluded. To some extent, this discourse is the inverse of the moral underclass discourse. In both perspectives, sectors of society are identified in terms of their personal attributes and are disadvantaged as a consequence. In the moral underclass discourse this unfavourable treatment is judged to be the fault of the victim, but in the societal oppression discourse, it is blamed on an unjust, powerful overclass. Like the other three discourses, the societal oppression discourse can be used to enhance our understanding of how to promote social inclusion. It may, for example, be applicable to the coercive role that psychiatrists have as agents of the state when implementing parts of the Mental Health Act.

A meta-discourse

The richness and utility of the concept of social exclusion is that it can be used to condemn a wide range of social ills and to justify any policy response that promises to remedy them. Groups whose political beliefs or discourses do not coincide can all decry it with a single voice, although they will differ over what to do about it. We may therefore call social exclusion and inclusion a meta-discourse; with these terms people from different political perspectives find a common language of condemnation and praise.

Social exclusion and mental health

'Social exclusion' began to appear in the mental health literature around the turn of the century (Sayce, 1998; 2001; Morris, 2001). The Social Exclusion Unit's report on mental health and social exclusion (Office of the Deputy Prime Minister, 2004a) showed just how far people with mental health problems fit the definition of the 'socially excluded'. Responses are identified in the UK National Action Plan on Social Inclusion 2003–2005, which states that 'The fight against poverty is central to the UK Government's entire social and economic programme. Tackling the roots of social exclusion – in particular, discrimination, inequality and lack of opportunity – is an essential part of the vision of a successful and prosperous society. And breaking down barriers to employment goes hand in hand with promoting social inclusion' (Department of Work and Pensions, 2003: p. 3)

The report was followed by an action plan on mental health and social exclusion (Office of the Deputy Prime Minister, 2004b), which evolved into the National Social Inclusion Programme, about which more is said below.

From exclusion to inclusion

Relativity

Prescriptions for alleviating social exclusion in mental healthcare may be derived from each of the dimensions and discourses identified here. For example, one remedy implied by the relativity of social exclusion is to reduce the differences between people with mental health problems and

403

> **Box 29.2** Direct payments
>
> 'The Community Care (Direct Payments) Act, introduced in 1996, gave local au-
> thorities the power to offer people a cash payment instead of direct services ...
> The payments can be used to pay an agency to provide the support the individual
> wants, as well as to directly employ personal assistants to enable the person to
> live the way they want'
>
> (Ridley & Jones, 2002: pp. 643–644)

others. One major difference lies in the purchasing power of each group, with a high proportion of people with mental health problems reliant on social security benefits for their income. In this respect, the promotion of 'direct payments' is a step towards greater social inclusion (Box 29.2). Holding the budget for their own care has potential to place individuals with mental health problems on a par with people who have the financial resources to buy what they need. In practice, the opportunity is rarely realised, owing to low take-up of direct payments (Ridley & Jones, 2002; Newbiggin & Lowe, 2005). Nevertheless, financial strategies like these fit well within the redistributionist discourse, and their shortcomings reflect its blind spots: inequality is inevitably part of exclusion, but exclusion has other, additional causes. In terms of our dimensions, it is compounded from multiple sources. For a person seeking direct payments, poor education, low levels of social support or living in an area where there is a poor supply of care alternatives pose additional obstacles to social inclusion.

Multiple deprivation

Responses to multiple disadvantages need to be multifaceted. In mental healthcare, this implies a need for concerted action from a range of public sector agencies, including health, social care, education and housing. An example in mental health is the development of care planning to incorporate assessment of diverse needs, mainly through the care programme approach (CPA). Not only is this more inclusive, it may also be more effective (Schneider *et al*, 2002; Carpenter *et al*, 2004).

The discourse surrounding oppression is particularly relevant to the analysis of the multiple sources of exclusion. There is an imbalance of power between service providers and service users or carers. Knowledge about mental illness and decision-making power are unequally held. Para-doxically, therefore, being the focus of attention of mental health services can contribute to exclusion. Noble & Douglas (2004) reported that service users want more involvement in decision-making about their own care, whereas carers want good information and communication with services. Services that work to increase participation and user (or carer) autonomy are essential components of a strategy to reduce social exclusion.

Dynamic theories about the origins and outcomes of mental health problems are familiar: one such is the vulnerability–stress–coping (or restitution) model of mental illness. Moreover, given the cyclical nature of some mental health problems and the therapeutic orientation of services, a dynamic understanding of social exclusion translates easily to mental health. From a dynamic perspective, the process whereby a person becomes socially excluded can be intercepted and countered. The discourses indicate possible tactics for doing so, but we have also seen that each discourse may be criticised for not considering some aspect of social inclusion. In particular, an intervention that helps one aspect of inclusion may harm another. Direct payments may reduce the relative disadvantage but might also entrench the individuals' dependence on benefits, preventing increasing social inclusion when their illness improves or remits. A dimensional approach to social exclusion helps us to examine the unintended effects of strategies to promote inclusion.

Social transactions

The relational nature of mental healthcare offers numerous opportunities for social inclusion to be increased or decreased. One burgeoning field of research and development concerns stigma, a barrier to social inclusion that operates at the level of public attitudes and can affect the self-confidence of people with mental health problems (Rusch *et al*, 2005; Thornicroft, 2006).

Demos and ethnos

Huxley & Thornicroft (2003) differentiate between two types of social inclusion: that which corresponds to the Greek idea of *demos* – the political community – which grants (or withholds) rights; and that which corresponds to *ethnos* – the cultural community – which relates to belonging. A person's membership of the demos means that he or she has the legal status of citizen and may participate in political life, but this does not necessarily involve acceptance as a member of the cultural community (the ethnos). The involuntary nature of some mental healthcare means that people may be detained against their wishes. The nature of this interaction is inherently exclusionary for the individuals affected, as it separates them from their usual social environment and also deprives them of fundamental rights. In doing so, it contravenes both ethnos and demos.

Implications for psychiatrists

To return to the questions implied at the outset, can social exclusion be remedied, should it be addressed and, if so, what responsibility does the psychiatrist have in this? The development of the National Social Inclusion Programme to oversee the implementation of the Social Exclusion Unit's

---

Box 29.3 The seven areas addressed in the National Social Inclusion Programme

- Employment
- Income and benefits
- Education
- Housing
- Social networks
- Community participation
- Direct payments

---

report Mental Health and Social Exclusion (Office of the Deputy Prime Minister, 2004a) demonstrates the government's response in England to the moral question: it should be addressed. This programme is designed to coordinate government departments and is divided into seven areas, listed in Box 29.3. Therefore, the responsibility for fostering social inclusion is seen to lie with government departments.

Psychiatrists are clearly expected to play their part: in April 2007 social inclusion was named as a policy priority for mental health services over the next few years (Appleby 2007a). Step-by-step guides to socially inclusive mental health services are available (Department of Health, 2006a,b). However, the emphasis placed on breaking down traditional barriers could pose a threat to psychiatrists' professional identities: 'Employment, housing and a strong social network are as important to a person's mental health as the treatment they receive' (Appleby, 2007b: p. 1). A socially inclusive approach may also demand skills, such as community development and conflict resolution, that are not normally acquired though psychiatric training. This is reflected in their inclusion in the list of 'essential shared capabilities' for the mental healthcare workforce (Hope, 2004).

There remains the question of whether social exclusion can be remedied. The National Social Inclusion Programme's Inclusion Database (www. socialinclusion.org.uk/good_practice/?subid=78) contains information on over 500 projects that 'enable people with mental health issues to engage with their local communities'. It is organised into nine 'life domains' (Box 29.4). The database gives examples of what is being done in the name of social inclusion in mental health, but the rationale behind these activities is not explained and, as we have already been pointed out, there is danger in using the term 'social inclusion' simplistically to convey general approval.

Repper & Perkins (2003) provide a descriptive account of strategies to promote social inclusion from a mental healthcare perspective, with plenty of advice underpinned by practical experience. They report evidence that social inclusion can in certain circumstances be promoted by mental

---

Box 29.4 The life domains of the Social Inclusion Database

- Employment and training for work
- Education
- Housing
- Arts and cultural activities
- Physical exercise and sports activities
- Volunteering
- Faith-based groups
- Finance
- Neighbourhoods

---

health services. However, if sustainable and replicable strategies for social inclusion are to be put in place, a clearer understanding of effective mechanisms to bring it about is required. In the next section we highlight theoretical frameworks from social psychology that might explain why certain types of organisational structure and interpersonal activity may be more conducive to social inclusion than others. Such frameworks enable the formulation of strategies to promote inclusion or diminish exclusion.

Social psychology

Social identity theory

Social identity theory is an attempt to understand inter-group discrimination. Its authors, Tajfel & Turner (1979), posit that membership of social groups forms part of a person's self-concept and predict that people are positively biased towards their own group (the 'in' group). The theory brings together two fundamental cognitive concepts: mechanisms of classification, by which people, events and objects are placed into categories; and mechanisms of comparison, by which people compare their group with other groups. The product of the classification and comparison processes is 'social identification', which has an impact on a person's self-esteem. If membership of a group has a positive effect on self-esteem, then the individual's social identification with that group (the 'in' group) increases, leading the person to incorporate the group membership as part of their self-image. At the same time, a negative bias is predicted towards other groups (the 'out' groups). This bias can result in discrimination, leading to low self-esteem among 'out'-group members and a negative self-image (self-stigma). This theoretical framework of social identity has been expanded in relation to people with mental health problems to explain stigma and to indicate how the impact of discrimination may be countered (e.g. Link & Phelan, 2001; Corrigan & Matthews, 2003).

Allport's contact hypothesis

Allport (1954) offers an alternative theoretical framework that might guide interventions to promote social inclusion in mental health. His theory, which has been developed mainly in relation to race and ethnicity, is known as Allport's contact hypothesis. Identifying 'in' and 'out' groups, the theory states that equalising the status between the two groups, for example through the pursuit of a common goal, will promote direct contact and that the familiarity that ensues offers an opportunity to disconfirm stereotypes. This in turn increases perceived similarity between the two groups and promotes greater liking. It is principally the positive contact (prolonged, meaningful, pleasant interaction) that has the desired effect, and this is generalisable to many types of group (Pettigrew & Tropp, 2006).

Conclusions

There is strong commitment to social inclusion in UK mental health policy and, more broadly, in European social policy. Social inclusion is a worthy goal of mental health services, but its attainment requires extensive social change. Within services, structures, systems and the balance of power between clinician and patient will have to be re-examined. Beyond services, social exclusion is perpetuated by public prejudice, by far-reaching discrimination and by the association between mental illness and other indicators of deprivation. The dimensions and discourses described here indicate many areas for intervention and various approaches that could be adopted.

Social psychology offers theoretical frameworks that may be used to identify promising interventions and predict their effects on social inclusion, but a more developed account of the mechanisms and causes of social inclusion in mental healthcare is needed. Social inclusion in mental health may be described as 'a discourse in search of a theory'. A coherent theory of social inclusion in mental health could act as a fulcrum, turning policy commitment into systemic change. Without such a theory, the title of this chapter must remain a question.

References

Adams, R., Dominelli, L. & Payne, M. (2002) *Anti-Oppressive Practice*. Palgrave Macmillan.

Allport, G. W. (1954) *The Nature of Prejudice*. Addison-Wesley.

Appleby, L. (2007a) *Mental Health Ten Years On: Progress on Mental Health Care Reform*. Department of Health (http://www.dh.gov.uk/en/Publicationsandstatistics/Publications/PublicationsPolicyAndGuidance/DH_074241).

Appleby, L. (2007b) *Breaking Down Barriers: The Clinical Case for Change* (Gateway Ref. 8187). Department of Health (http://www.dh.gov.uk/en/Publicationsandstatistics/Publications/PublicationsPolicyAndGuidance/DH_074579).

Burchardt, T., Le Grand, J. & Piachaud, D. (2002) Degrees of exclusion: developing a dynamic, multidimensional measure. In *Understanding Social Exclusion* (eds J. Hills, J. Le Grand & D. Piachaud), pp. 30–43. Oxford University Press.

Burgess, S. & Propper, C. (2002) The dynamics of poverty in Great Britain. In *Understanding Social Exclusion* (eds J. Hills, J. Le Grand & D. Piachaud), pp. 44–61. Oxford University Press.

Carpenter, J., Schneider, J., McNiven, F., *et al* (2004) Integration and targeting of community care for people with severe and enduring mental health problems: users' experiences of the Care Programme Approach and Care Management. *British Journal of Social Work*, **34**, 313–333.

Corrigan, P. W. & Matthews, A. K. (2003) Stigma and disclosure: implications for coming out of the closet. *Journal of Mental Health*, **12**, 235–248.

Dahrendorf, R., Frank, F. & Hayman, C. (1995) *Report on Wealth Creation and Social Cohesion in a Free Society*. Commission on Wealth Creation and Social Cohesion.

Department of Health (2006a) *Vocational Services for People with Severe Mental Health Problems: Commissioning Guidance* (Gateway Ref. 5659). Department of Health (http://www.dh.gov.uk/en/Publicationsandstatistics/Publications/PublicationsPolicyAndGuidance/DH_4131059).

Department of Health (2006b) *From Segregation to Inclusion: Commissioning Guidance on Day Services for People with Mental Health Problems* (Gateway Ref. 5658). Department of Health (http://www.rcpsych.ac.uk/pdf/Segregationinclusion.pdf).

Department of Work and Pensions (2003) *UK National Action Plan on Social Inclusion 2003–2005*. Department of Work and Pensions (http://www.dwp.gov.uk/docs/nap-2003-2005.pdf).

Giddens, A. (1998) *The Third Way: The Renewal of Social Democracy*. Polity Press.

Hope, R. (2004) *The Ten Essential Shared Capabilities for Mental Health Care: A Framework for the Whole of the Mental Health Workforce* (Gateway Ref. 3453). Department of Health (http://www.dh.gov.uk/en/Publicationsandstatistics/Publications/Publications PolicyAndGuidance/DH_4087169).

Huxley, P. & Thornicroft, G. (2003) Social inclusion, social quality and mental illness. *British Journal of Psychiatry*, **182**, 289–290.

Levitas, R. (1998) *The Inclusive Society? Social Exclusion and New Labour*. Macmillan Press.

Levitas, R. (2005) *The Inclusive Society? Social Exclusion and New Labour* (2nd edn). Macmillan Press.

Link, B. G. & Phelan, J. C. (2001) Conceptualizing stigma. *Annual Review of Sociology*, **27**, 363–385.

Morris, D. (2001) Citizenship and Community in Mental Health: a joint national programme for social inclusion and community partnership. *Mental Health Review*, **6**, 21–24.

Newbiggin, K. & Lowe, J. (2005) *Direct Payments and Mental Health: New Directions*. Pavilion/JRF.

Noble, L. M. & Douglas, B. C. (2004) What users and relatives want from mental health services. Service research and outcomes. *Current Opinion in Psychiatry*, **17**, 289–296.

Office of the Deputy Prime Minister (2004a) *Mental Health and Social Exclusion: Social Exclusion Unit Report*. ODPM.

Office of the Deputy Prime Minister (2004b) *Action on Mental Health: A Guide to Promoting Social Inclusion*. ODPM.

Percy-Smith, J. (2000) Introduction: the contours of social exclusion. In *Policy Responses to Social Exclusion: Towards Inclusion?* (ed. J. Percy-Smith), pp. 1–21. Open University Press.

Pettigrew, T. F. & Tropp, L. R. (2006) A meta-analytic test of intergroup contact theory. *Journal of Personality and Social Psychology*, **90**, 751–783.

Repper, J. & Perkins, R. (2003) *Social Inclusion and Recovery: A Model for Mental Health Practice*. Baillière Tindall.

Ridley, J. & Jones, L. (2002) Direct what? The untapped potential of direct payments to mental health service users. *Disability and Society*, **18**, 643–658.

Rodgers, G., Gore, C. & Figueiredo, J. (eds) (1995) *Social Exclusion: Rhetoric, Reality, Responses*. International Institute for Labour Studies.

Room, G. (ed.) (1995) *Beyond the Threshold. The Measurement and Analysis of Social Exclusion*. Policy Press.

Rusch, N., Angermeyer, M. C. & Corrigan, P. W. (2005) Mental illness stigma: concepts, consequences, and initiatives to reduce stigma. *European Psychiatry*, **20**, 529–539.

Sayce, L. (1998) Stigma, discrimination and social exclusion: what's in a word? *Journal of Mental Health*, **7**, 331–343.

Sayce, L. (2001) Social inclusion and mental health. *Psychiatric Bulletin*, **25**, 121–123.

Schneider, J., Carpenter, J., Wooff, D., *et al* (2002) Community mental health care in England: associations between service organisation and quality of life. *Health and Social Care in the Community*, **10**, 423–434.

Social Exclusion Task Force (2007) *Context for Social Exclusion: What Do We Mean by Social Exclusion?* TSO (The Stationery Office) (*http://www.cabinetoffice.gov.uk/social_exclusion_task_force/context.aspx*).

Tajfel, H. & Turner, J. (1979) An integrative theory of intergroup conflict. In *The Social Psychology of Intergroup Relations* (eds G. W. Austin & S. Worchel). Brooks Cole.

Thornicroft, G. (2006) *Shunned: Discrimination against People with Mental Illness*. Oxford University Press.

Index

Compiled by Linda English